Ultrasound for Medical Education and Primary Care

Edited by

JING GAO
Montana College of Osteopathic Medicine
Rocky Vista University
Montana, USA

WEN HE
Department of Ultrasound
Beijing Tiantan Hospital
Beijing, China

J. BRIAN FOWLKES
Department of Radiology
University of Michigan
Michigan, USA

WILEY

Published by John Wiley & Sons, Inc., Hoboken, New Jersey.

For general information on our other products and services or for technical support, please contact our Customer Care Department within the United States at (800) 762-2974, outside the United States at (317) 572–3993 or fax (317) 572–4002.

Wiley also publishes its books in a variety of electronic formats. Some content that appears in print may not be available in electronic formats. For more information about Wiley products, visit our web site at www.wiley.com.

Library of Congress Cataloging-in-Publication Data Applied for:

Paperback ISBN: 9781394381050

Cover Design: Wiley
Cover Images: © therads/stock.adobe.com, © PIJITRA PHOMKHAM/Shutterstock, © Chaikom/Shutterstock

Set in 10/12pt STIXTwoText by Straive, Pondicherry, India

Printed in Singapore
M137350020626

Contents

List of Contributors

Ryan Brauman
Rocky Vista University, College of Osteopathic Medicine, Ivins, Utah, USA

Camille Z. Bentley
Rocky Vista University, College of Osteopathic Medicine, Parker, Colorado, USA

Valentina Bonnefil
Rocky Vista University, College of Osteopathic Medicine, Ivins, Utah, USA

Kevin Brighton
Rocky Vista University, College of Osteopathic Medicine, Parker, Colorado, Ivins, Utah, USA

Ethan Burke
Rocky Vista University, College of Osteopathic Medicine, Ivins, Utah, USA

Tyler Burke
Rocky Vista University, College of Osteopathic Medicine, Parker, Colorado, USA

Stella Chan
Rocky Vista University, College of Osteopathic Medicine, Ivins, Utah, USA

Thomas Chandy
Rocky Vista University, College of Osteopathic Medicine, Parker, Colorado, Ivins, Utah, USA

Johnson Chen
Department of Radiology, Weill Cornell Medicine, Cornell University, New York, USA

Daniel Daskalakis
Rocky Vista University, College of Osteopathic Medicine, Ivins, Utah, USA

Edwin Seldon Davis
Rocky Vista University, College of Osteopathic Medicine, Ivins, Utah, USA

Li-Juan Du
Department of Ultrasound, Beijing Tiantan Hospital, Capital Medical University, Beijing, China

Lindsay Ellison
Rocky Vista University, College of Osteopathic Medicine, Ivins, Utah, USA

Xiang Fei
Department of Ultrasound, The First Medical Center, General Hospital of PLA, Beijing, China

Andrew Fisher
Rocky Vista University, College of Osteopathic Medicine, Ivins, Utah, USA

Jacquelyn Flor
Rocky Vista University, College of Osteopathic Medicine, Ivins, Utah, USA

Kathryn Forneris
Rocky Vista University, College of Osteopathic Medicine, Ivins, Utah, USA

J. Brian Fowlkes
Department of Radiology, University of Michigan, Ann Arbor, Michigan, USA

Jennifer Frazee
Rocky Vista University, College of Osteopathic Medicine, Parker, Colorado, Ivins, Utah, USA

Jing Gao
Rocky Vista University, Montana College of Osteopathic Medicine, Billings, Montana, USA

Ryan Geist
Rocky Vista University, College of Osteopathic Medicine, Ivins, Utah, USA

Ning Guo
Department of Ultrasound, Shanghai Sixth People's Hospital, Shanghai Jiaotong University School of Medicine, Shanghai, China

Jonathan Hansen
Rocky Vista University, College of Osteopathic Medicine, Ivins, Utah, USA

Ashna Haque
Rocky Vista University, College of Osteopathic Medicine, Ivins, Utah, USA

Wen He
Department of Ultrasound, Beijing Tiantan Hospital, Capital Medical University, Beijing, China

Pintong Huang
Department of Ultrasound in Medicine, the Second Affiliated Hospital, Zhejiang University School of Medicine, Hangzhou, China

Grace Isaacson
Rocky Vista University, College of Osteopathic Medicine, Ivins, Utah, USA

Boris Joutovsky
Rocky Vista University, College of Osteopathic Medicine, Ivins, Utah, USA

Christine Kai
Rocky Vista University, College of Osteopathic Medicine, Ivins, Utah, USA

Shane Kaysen
Rocky Vista University, College of Osteopathic Medicine, Ivins, Utah, USA

Oliver Kripfgans
Department of Radiology, University of Michigan, Ann Arbor, Michigan, USA

Raymond Kwong
Rocky Vista University, College of Osteopathic Medicine, Ivins, Utah, USA

Jason Lee
Rocky Vista University, College of Osteopathic Medicine, Ivins, Utah, USA

Rebecca Lee
Rocky Vista University, College of Osteopathic Medicine, Ivins, Utah, USA

Abigail Limov
Rocky Vista University, College of Osteopathic Medicine, Ivins, Utah, USA

Megan Maar
Rocky Vista University, College of Osteopathic Medicine, Ivins, Utah, USA

Nena L. Mason
Geisel School of Medicine at Dartmouth, Hanover, New Hampshire, USA

Rachel McCann
Rocky Vista University, College of Osteopathic Medicine, Ivins, Utah, USA

Giovanni Montesano
Rocky Vista University, College of Osteopathic Medicine, Ivins, Utah, USA

Andy Nigh
Rocky Vista University, College of Osteopathic Medicine, Ivins, Utah, USA

Austin Page
Rocky Vista University, College of Osteopathic Medicine, Ivins, Utah, USA

Telyn Peterson
Rocky Vista University, College of Osteopathic Medicine, Ivins, Utah, USA

Anton Pham
Rocky Vista University, College of Osteopathic Medicine, Ivins, Utah, USA

Jill Pitcher
Rocky Vista University, College of Osteopathic Medicine, Parker, Colorado, Ivins, Utah, USA

Mateen Razaan
Rocky Vista University, College of Osteopathic Medicine, Ivins, Utah, USA

Yun-Yun Ren
Department of Ultrasound, Obstetrics & Gynecology Hospital, Fudan University, Shanghai, China

Richard Rodriguez-Brizuela
Rocky Vista University, College of Osteopathic Medicine, Parker, Colorado, USA

Courtney Shill Russell
Rocky Vista University, College of Osteopathic Medicine, Ivins, Utah, USA

Mikala Russell
Rocky Vista University, College of Osteopathic Medicine, Ivins, Utah, USA

Robert Russell
Rocky Vista University, College of Osteopathic Medicine, Ivins, Utah, USA

Zoya Sandhu
Rocky Vista University, College of Osteopathic Medicine, Ivins, Utah, USA

Michael Stephens
Rocky Vista University, College of Osteopathic Medicine, Parker, Colorado, Ivins, Utah, USA

Andy Thai
Rocky Vista University, College of Osteopathic Medicine, Ivins, Utah, USA

Kelli Tichy
Rocky Vista University, College of Osteopathic Medicine, Ivins, Utah, USA

Anthony Tran
Rocky Vista University, College of Osteopathic Medicine, Ivins, Utah, USA

Andrew Wojtanowski
Rocky Vista University, College of Osteopathic Medicine, Parker, Colorado, USA

Dale Woodbury
Rocky Vista University, College of Osteopathic Medicine, Ivins, Utah, USA

Chun-Xia Xia
Department of Ultrasound, Beijing Tongren Hospital, Capital Medical University, Beijing, China

Kalvin Zee
Rocky Vista University, College of Osteopathic Medicine, Ivins, Utah, USA

Man Zhang
Department of Radiology, University of Michigan, Ann Arbor, Michigan, USA

Ming-Bo Zhang
Department of Ultrasound, the First Medical Center, General Hospital of PLA, Beijing, China

Wei Zhang
Department of Ultrasound, Beijing Tiantan Hospital, Capital Medical University, Beijing, China

Han-Xue Zhao
Department of Ultrasound, Beijing Tongren Hospital, Capital Medical University, Beijing, China

Yuan-Yi Zheng
Department of Ultrasound, Shanghai Sixth People's Hospital, Shanghai Jiaotong University School of Medicine, Shanghai, China

Qing Zhong
Rocky Vista University, College of Osteopathic Medicine, Ivins, Utah, USA

Jia-an Zhu
Department of Ultrasound, Peking University People's Hospital, Beijing, China

List of Illustrators

Chapter No.	Chapter Title	Name of Illustrators
Chapter 1	Introduction to Diagnostic Ultrasound	Lucas Vijay Srivastava Chandra
Chapter 2	Head and Neck Soft Tissue	Ryan Braumann
Chapter 3	Chest and Lung	Alexandra Moody and Andy Thai
Chapter 4	The Heart	Alexandra Moody and Lucas Vijay Srivastava Chandra
Chapter 5	Gastroenterology	Lucas Vijay Srivastava Chandra
Chapter 6	Obstetrics and Gynecology	Ria Sandhu
Chapter 7	Genitourinary System	Andy Thai
Chapter 8	Peripheral Vascular Ultrasound	Andy Thai
Chapter 9	Musculoskeletal Ultrasound	Ria Sandhu and Lucas Vijay Srivastava Chandra
Chapter 10	Extracranial Arteries	Andy Thai
Chapter 11	The Endocrine System	Daniel Daskalakis and Lucas Vijay Srivastava Chandra
Chapter 12	FAST/EFAST and Emergency Medicine	Alexandra Moody
Chapter 13	Ultrasound-Guided Procedures	Andy Thai
Chapter 14	Ultrasound in Resuscitation	Tyler Knight Burkhart
Chapter 15	Ultrasound of the Breast	Ria Sandhu

All illustrators: Rocky Vista University, College of Osteopathic Medicine, Ivins, Utah, USA

Preface

Ultrasound has become a very favorable imaging tool in medical education and clinical patient care due to its high safety, accuracy, portability, and low cost. Many medical schools in the United States have added ultrasound to their preclinical and clinical curricula. Ultrasound is also an important course in postgraduate training and continuing medical education.

This book is for medical students, residents, primary care physicians, and sonographers who are beginning their study of medical ultrasound. Therefore, the authors worked to deliver a textbook in a learner-friendly manner by using easy-to-understand text, images, tables, and review questions. The design of this book is based on the ultrasound education curriculum at Rocky Vista University and references in the literature. Readers can use the brief introduction of anatomy, clinical indications for ultrasound, normal appearance, and common pathologies of ultrasound images in each chapter as references to guide their ultrasound image acquisition and interpretation.

The author team of this book consists of senior radiologists, ultrasound scientists, clinical physicians, experienced medical educators, and medical students. We hope this textbook can provide readers with a reference and serve as a practical guide in their initial study and continuing clinical practice. Many of our colleagues have helped in the creation of this book. We thank all the authors for their dedicated efforts and the support from the institutions, medical associations, and ultrasound manufacturers, as well as academic collaborations among domestic and international medical institutions.

Jing Gao, MD, Wen He, MD, J. Brian Fowlkes, PhD

Acknowledgments

The editors would like to thank the following persons for their contributions to the creation of this book. Our sincere thanks to all of the authors of the chapters for their dedication to this effort. We greatly appreciate the editing assistance of Anthony Tran, DO, Julian Ortiz, DO, Juhyun Lee, DO, Andrew Phan, DO, Connor Haskins, DO, Austin Meyer, DO, Jacob King, DO, Candance Wong, DO, Joshua Mongillo, MPH, and Lynne Stephenson, MS. Special thanks to members of the AIUM staff for coordinating reviews and contributing and organizing comments that helped improve the content including Therese Cooper, MS, RDMS, Peter Magnuson, BA and Emily Mullen, BS. We also appreciate the helpful comments on various portions of the materials we received from Richard Barr, MD, PhD, Janice Boughton, MD, Bryann Bromley, MD, Therese Cooper, MS, RDMS, Charlotte Henningsen, MS, RDMS, Richard Hoppman, MD, Thomas Marini, MD, Irene Ma, MD, PhD, and Kathy Minton, MA.

CHAPTER 1

Introduction to Diagnostic Ultrasound

Grace Isaacson[1], Boris Joutovsky[1], Oliver Kripfgans[2], and J. Brian Fowlkes[2]

[1] Rocky Vista University, College of Osteopathic Medicine, Ivins, Utah, USA

[2] Department of Radiology, University of Michigan, Ann Arbor, Michigan, USA

A Brief History on the Invention of Clinical Ultrasound

In the year 1790, an Italian physiologist named Lazarro Spallanzani was fascinated with bats and their ability to navigate effortlessly through complete darkness. He marveled at the accuracy with which they could catch their prey without light. Among his numerous experiments with blindfolded bats, he had discovered that they could still maneuver their surroundings without difficulty. He then plugged their ears. Upon observing that their flight became severely erratic, he hypothesized that it was the bat's sense of sound, and not their sight, which provided their primary mode of navigation. In his own words, he stated, "The ear of the bat serves more efficiently, or at least for measuring distances" [1]. He determined from his experiments that bats must emit ultrasonic waves that are inaudible to human ears, and that it was the echoes from these waves bouncing off objects that allowed bats to sense distance, direction, and ultimately their own location in space. Today, we credit Spallanzani as the first to study anything related to ultrasound physics [1]. Echolocation at the time was considered an anomaly and was met with great skepticism by his fellow scientists. Two Harvard students, Robert Galambos and Donald Griffin, would prove his theory over a century later [1].

In 1877, 86 years after Spallanzani's experiments with bats, Jacque and Pierre Curie observed that putting pressure on various crystals created electricity and thus are credited with the discovery of piezoelectricity [2]. It was this discovery that allowed ultrasound transducers to become a reality. In 1915, a physicist by the name of Paul Langevin would use this technology to create the "first transducer," which could detect objects, including submarines, at the bottom of the ocean that was used during World War I, and further developed for use during World War II [3]. These developments laid significant groundwork for the use of ultrasound in medicine. In 1942, Karl Dussik transmitted an ultrasound beam through the human skull with the hope that he could detect brain tumors [4]. He was credited with being the first to use sonography to make a medical diagnosis. After 1951, developments in breast ultrasound imaging and broad field view B-mode sonography demonstrated the feasibility of the application of handheld device and compounding technique in real-time B-mode sonography [5, 6].

In 1958, Ian Donald and colleagues were the first to incorporate this technology into the medical field of obstetrics and gynecology [7]. From there, ultrasound technology made great strides in the field of science, especially in screening for fetal anomalies.

Ultrasound technology has permanently taken a sophisticated and invaluable role in medical diagnostics and treatment. It has utility in clinical and diagnostic settings, such as physical examinations, procedural guidance, and the monitoring of treatment efficacy [8]. The clinical application of ultrasound provides imagery and mechanisms for detecting movement and flow in vascular, organ, and musculoskeletal systems in the human body. Because ultrasound does not emit harmful ionizing radiation, it is ideal for frequent follow-up examinations [8].

Ultrasound is operator dependent. Knowledge of anatomy, pathology, ultrasound principles, ultrasound artifacts and bioeffects, and patient clinical information are all important for operators to perform and interpret ultrasound examinations adequately in clinical patient care [8, 9].

The Basic Physics and Instrumentations of Ultrasound

Sound, Waves, and the Range of Human Hearing

Sound is a form of mechanical energy that travels through matter and is created by a vibrating source. This mechanical energy produces a phasic pattern of oscillations, which is characteristic of waveforms. Unlike light waves, sound waves require a medium to propagate [8]. Individual particles of the medium exhibit particle motion parallel to the direction of traveling longitudinal sound waves. This allows for acoustic propagation of mechanical energy in a domino-like fashion [10].

Acoustic Parameters

Sound waves, like all waves, are defined by the following parameters: frequency (MHz), wavelength, amplitude, power, and intensity [8]. While frequency and amplitude are determined by the source, the propagation speed of a sound wave is determined by the medium, and frequency and wavelength are related through the propagation speed [8, 10].

The spectrum of sound may be described in relation to the frequency range of human hearing. In most humans, the range of hearing lies between 20 and 20,000 Hz [10]. Sound frequencies below 20 Hz are referred to as infrasound, while sound frequencies above 20,000 Hz are referred to as ultrasound. Medical ultrasound typically ranges from 1 to 50 MHz (much higher than that of human hearing). Frequency (f) is the number of oscillations of a wave or particle per second and is independent of the medium. It is expressed in Hertz (Hz). These oscillations may be pictured as the cyclic compressions and rarefactions on a spring. As you push one end of the spring, the energy is propagated longitudinally along the coils, similar to that of molecules of a medium propagating a sound wave. The amplitude of the wave at a given moment of time is the distance from the mean position of the particle to the actual position of the particle. The peak amplitude is the distance between the mean and the maximal displacement. The period (T) of the wave is the time it takes for each oscillation to occur, expressed in seconds (s), and is the inverse of the frequency [8, 9].

Wavelength (λ) is the distance traveled in one oscillation and may be represented as one complete cycle or the distance from compression to the next compression or rarefaction to the next rarefaction on a longitudinal wave. For a sound speed of 1600 m/sec, the wavelengths in ultrasound application vary from 0.8 mm at 2 MHz to 0.08 mm at 20 MHz. Frequency and wavelength are inversely related; as frequency increases, wavelength decreases [8–10].

The Interactions Between Ultrasound and Tissues

When ultrasound waves are sent into the body, they interact with various media (e.g. air, bone, and tissue). Some of these waves are scattered, and some are absorbed and dissipated mostly as heat [10]. The echoes that are reflected or scattered back to the transducer are translated from electrical information to a sonographic image by the ultrasound machine. The amplitude of echoes returned (backscatter) is determined by a property of tissue called the acoustic impedance along with any effects associated with directional scattering and losses along the returning path [8]. This intrinsic property of a medium is determined by the density of the medium multiplied by the propagation speed of the sound wave [11].

Acoustic impedance is a measure of an individual particle's resistance to the mechanical energy contained in the acoustic field (Table 1.1) [11]. This resistance is proportional to both the density and propagation speed of the wave. The importance of this concept comes into play when determining the amplitude of the echoes returned to the transducer by two media with different acoustic impedances.

TABLE 1.1 **Acoustic impedance values of various media.**

ACOUSTIC IMPEDANCE OF VARIOUS MEDIA	
MEDIUM	**ACOUSTIC IMPEDANCE (MRayl)**
Air	0.0004
Fat	1.38
Water	1.48
Kidney	1.62
Liver	1.65
Bone	7.8

Source: Data from [11].

tWhen ultrasound pulses hit a large smooth surface of two media of different acoustic impedances, mechanical energy is reflected back to the transducer. This is called specular reflection, and the intensity of the echoes reflected is related to the difference in the acoustic impedances of the media [8, 11].

Reflection specifically occurs at tissue interfaces, which are junctions of tissues with different acoustic impedances [8, 9]. Therefore, if the sound waves pass through tissues of similar impedances (homogeneous tissues or fluid), few or no echoes will be produced, and the area being imaged will look dark or anechoic. Sound waves passing through tissues with large differences in acoustic impedances produce larger amplitude echoes and, therefore, produce bright or hyperechoic appearance in the image. It is the amplitude of the reflected sound that determines the relative brightness of the image. Air has a much lower acoustic impedance compared to soft tissues or bone. Therefore, when an ultrasound beam hits an interface between air and tissue, there is a large reflection of the ultrasound, and very little ultrasound is transmitted to the tissue distal to the air [8, 9].

Snell's law, which is often used to describe light waves, can also be used to describe the reflection and refraction interactions of ultrasound waves at an interface (Fig. 1.1). As ultrasound hits a linear interface at 90°, the echo from that interface will travel back to the transducer. In contrast, if it hits a linear interface at any angle less than 90°, the echo may miss the transducer and escape detection [10]. It will instead reflect at an angle equal to the angle of incidence, similar to light reflecting off a mirror. Refraction refers to a change in the direction of sound transmission after hitting an interface of two tissues with different speeds of sound transmission [11]. For example, when a beam hits an interface at an angle other than 90°, the portion that continues forward changes direction (bends). Refraction is an important cause of incorrect localization of a structure on an ultrasound image, which will be discussed in greater detail under artifacts.

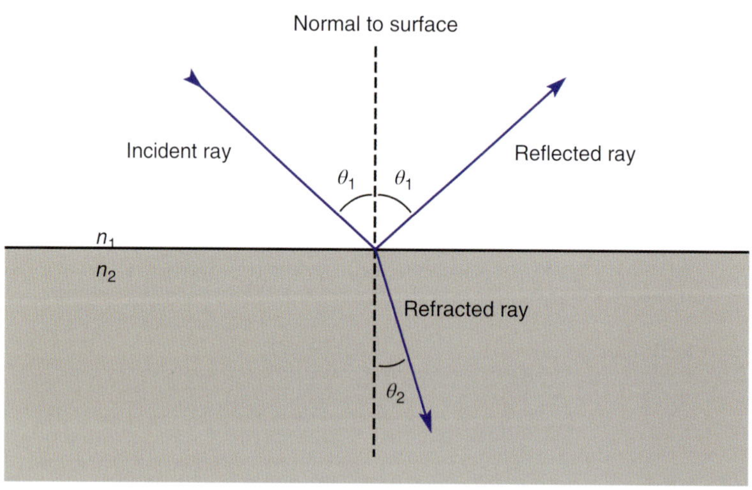

FIGURE 1.1 This illustration explains ultrasound wave propagation at an interface (Snell's law). Waves traveling in the medium n_1 and hitting the interface of n_1 and n_2 at 90° produce echoes that travel back toward the transducer. Waves hitting at <90° (θ_1) produce waves that are reflected at the same angle and may escape detection. The portion of these waves that then travel into n_2 will be refracted to travel along a new direction (θ_2) that depends on the relative values of n_1 and n_2.

Scattering occurs when ultrasound pulses encounter rough and irregular tissue structures [11]. The echoes are reflected in a wide range of angles, which reduces their intensity. When this scattering is caused by structures in the tissue that are smaller than the wavelength of sound, we get a pattern in the ultrasound image termed speckle, resulting from interference among these scattered signals. Speckle gives a textured or grainy appearance to most biological tissues and organs on imaging. The use of multiple beams coming from different directions helps to address this issue by averaging out speckle in the image, which in turn yields reduced noise and improved image contrast and subsequently better delineation of anatomical features, such as a focal lesion in the liver.

Any time an ultrasound wave is sent through a tissue, there is some reduction of intensity due to attenuation. There are two significant factors that contribute to attenuation. One is the scattering by the mechanisms described above. The other is absorption, which is mechanical energy dissipated typically as heat. This conversion of energy into heat is the most important contributor to attenuation in ultrasound [8, 10].

Higher frequencies have shorter wavelengths and thus give the operator higher axial (and lateral) resolution images, allowing for better discrimination between tissues. This is why higher-frequency waves are more helpful for imaging superficial structures. However, one must consider depth when selecting a given frequency for ultrasound, as higher-frequency waves are also attenuated more for a given distance compared to lower-frequency waves [11, 12]. Lower-frequency ultrasound waves have longer wavelengths that penetrate deeper into tissue due to a decreased cumulative attenuation but provide the operator poorer discrimination between tissues. Optimizing the choice of transmitted frequency for a variety of clinical scenarios is one of the fundamental challenges faced in ultrasound. Adjusting the amplitude of the transmission could obtain a deeper penetration of tissues, but regulations and safety issues limit the maximum pressure amplitudes that can be transmitted into tissue. This is where coded excitation can come into play. Coded excitation is a technology in ultrasound that allows the user to increase the signal-to-noise ratio for a given frequency and thus increase imaging depth without increasing the amplitude. Coded excitation methods use transmitted pulses that are much longer than typical imaging transmission pulses. The increased temporal energy in the pulse improves signal-to-noise ratios, but additional signal processing is needed to prevent loss of axial resolution. Axial resolution can be recovered by a matched filter process (circuit or algorithm), specific to the code embedded into the transmitted pulse [13].

The relationship between frequency and wavelength is connected through the sound speed of the medium, that is, the product of frequency and wavelength is equal to the propagation speed of the wave (m/s). As stated previously, the frequency of a wave is determined by the transmitting source and therefore must remain constant in the equation. While frequency is constant, the propagation speed will change depending on the density and stiffness of the tissue through which the ultrasound waves travel. As a property of the medium, the sound speed then sets the wavelength for the given frequency. Based on the relative compressibility of the medium, the speed of ultrasound through gases is low, liquids high, and solids the highest [8, 10, 11]. Similarly, the propagation speed is much faster in bone and fluid-filled organs than in air (Table 1.2) [8]. A balance of all these factors (propagation velocity and associated wavelength, imaging depth, etc.) plays a role in obtaining a high-quality image.

$$v = f\lambda$$

Velocity (v) is equal to the frequency (f) multiplied by the wavelength (λ).

TABLE 1.2 Propagation speeds of ultrasound through various media.

DENSITY AND PROPAGATION SPEED OF VARIOUS MATERIALS		
MEDIUM	**DENSITY (kg/m^3)**	**SPEED (m/s)**
Air	1.2	331
Fat	925	1450
Water	1000	1540
Muscle	1050	1547
Bone	1400–1900	4080

Source: Data from [8].

Another factor that affects the amount of attenuation is the distance traveled by the wave. The longer the ultrasound waves must travel and the higher their frequency, the greater the cumulative attenuation. The type of medium (e.g. tissue) also affects the amount of attenuation. Water and blood attenuate ultrasound by a barely appreciable degree, while cortical bone presents a virtually impermeable barrier due to its impedance mismatch to tissue and its attenuation (Table 1.3). Ultrasound equipment typically compensates for nominal tissue attenuation and automatically increases the amplitude (and thus overall brightness) of the signal in deeper areas of the image, commonly referred to as time-gain compensation (TGC). The attenuation experienced by waves in various media is quantified using the attenuation coefficient (α), having typical units of dB/cm-MHz, showing the increasing amount of attenuation with distance traveled and with increasing ultrasound frequency. This coefficient helps in assessing the amount of attenuation that ultrasound waves experience in certain media. The ratio of the two echo

TABLE 1.3 Attenuation coefficients of various media at a frequency of 1 MHz.

ATTENUATION COEFFICIENTS OF VARIOUS MEDIA ($f = 1$ MHz)	
MEDIUM	**(α = dB/cm)**
Blood	0.2
Fat	0.48
Liver	0.5
Muscle	1.09
Air	1.64 (20°C)
Bone (cortical-trabecular)	6.9–9.94

Source: Culjat et al. [14] and Christensen et al. [15].

amplitudes (intensities) is often expressed on a logarithmic scale, decibels (dB) [14, 15]. For example, if the ratio of two echo amplitudes is two, then expressed in dB, this would be $20 \log(2) = 6\,\text{dB}$. In terms of intensities, a ratio of 2 would be $10 \log(2) = 3\,\text{dB}$.

Transducers and Sound Beams

Ultrasound (US) technology generates imaging through the conversion of energy between its different forms. The change of mechanical to electrical energy is referred to as the piezoelectric phenomenon, while the inverse conversion of electrical to mechanical energy is known as the reverse piezoelectric phenomenon [10].

To produce waves, an external electric voltage stimulates crystalline material within transducers to undergo vibrational and compressive kinetic movements capable of emitting US waves [16]. Therefore, the production of a US beam is accomplished using the reverse piezoelectric phenomenon. Contrarily, incoming beams that are reflected from tissues hit the crystalline material, causing a kinetic change that generates an electric signal, demonstrating the piezoelectric phenomenon in the detection of incoming acoustic signals.

Structural components of transducers optimize the piezoelectric effect to produce clear ultrasonographic images. Transducers typically consist of the piezoelectric plate, a matching layer, and a backing layer. A lens may also be present in transducers. Each transducer may have a varying number, size, shape, and arrangement of transducer elements used for different applications [10].

The piezoelectric element of US transducers may consist of a synthetic ceramic material, such as lead zirconate titanate (PZT). The thickness of the plate determines the frequency of vibration. Appropriate thickness allows waves to resonate under the constructive interference wave theory, thus reinforcing each other. Resonance is seen when the plate thickness is one-half the wavelength of the desired frequency [13]. Electrical activation of thinner plates produces higher frequencies [16].

The backing layer dampens the oscillation of the piezoelectric plate to reduce the duration of the ultrasound pulse. The acoustic insulator of transducers localizes plate vibrations and prevents energy from flowing into the transducer housing. An acoustic matching layer is seen anterior to the piezoelectric plate and functions to match the high impedance of the plate to the relatively lower impedance of the tissue and to place outgoing waves in phase so that resonance occurs [10]. This improves transmission into soft tissues as well as reception from tissues. Generally, improved reception is more crucial since there is an upper limit of power transmitted into soft tissue. The more acoustic signal the matching layer lets through to the piezoelectric plate, the better the resulting image [16].

The transducer description given here is a classic construction scenario. There are many new technologies that have been applied in transducer construction such as composite materials for the piezoelectric layer and even replacing the piezoelectric with alternative ways of producing and receiving ultrasound such as the capacitive micromachined ultrasound transducer (CMUT). These are beyond the level of discussion presented here, and readers interested in further details are referred elsewhere [17, 18].

Ultrasound Beam Shape

Once the ultrasound leaves the transducer, the beam that is produced has multiple characteristics that can be viewed and studied. These are discussed below.

Non-focused Source

A planar disc transducer, sometimes referred to as a single-element (planar) transducer, is a non-focusing source from which an ultrasound beam is emitted. When emitting a (near) continuous wave (CW) at a given frequency, the pathway of the beam can be divided into the near field (Fresnel zone) and the far field (Fraunhofer zone) (Fig. 1.2). The beam width in the near field is approximately the transducer width, or aperture [13]. At the end of the near field comes a point where the beam reaches its last maximum intensity of constructive interference along its axial route (Fig. 1.2). This marks the position at which the beam begins to spread laterally at an angle known as the angle of divergence [13]. Larger transducers and lower wavelengths minimize the angle of divergence, while smaller transducers and higher wavelengths increase the angle at which the beam spreads. The near field is influenced by the same properties, such that a longer near field will result in a smaller angle.

Focused Source

Transducers with focusing capability are commonly used in medical imaging and produce beams that exhibit different wave properties than the unfocused transducers discussed above. As the beam leaves the transducer, it gradually decreases in width until it

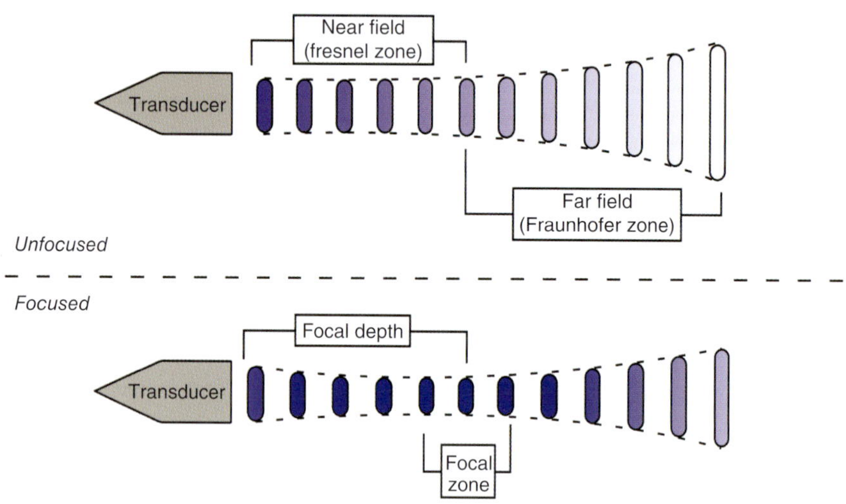

FIGURE 1.2 General shape of US beam (top) unfocused transducer: the near field is of equal width as the transducer and begins diverging after the natural focal point, becoming the far field. The angle of divergence represents the lateral spread of the beam once it passes the focal point. (Bottom) Focused transducer: beam width gradually decreases as the beam leaves the transducer, reaching its minimal width at the focal point. After the focal point, the beam diverges similarly to the unfocused US beam.

reaches the focus, or its narrowest point. The focus also has the highest intensity of the entire beam and produces the highest spatial resolution. The focal length is the distance from the transducer to the focal point. Once the ultrasound beam reaches its focal point, it begins to diverge in a similar pattern seen in unfocused beams (Fig. 1.2).

Alternative Beamforming

It must be noted that the descriptions above are for the traditional approaches to transmitting ultrasound. There have been several advances made that include the use of planar transmitters, similar to non-focused source described above, that are combined with beam steering from multiple angles. Receiving echoes from these different transmits can be combined with receive beamforming for high frame rate ultrasound imaging. For further information, the reader is referred elsewhere [19].

Image Formatting

A variety of transducer types have been developed to optimize imaging requirements based on the examination performed. The clinical application of transducer formats will be discussed thoroughly in the following chapters.

As the application for which the ultrasound imaging varies, so does the format (Fig. 1.3). Linear array transducers (Fig. 1.3a) are composed of an array of elements oriented in a straight line, typically producing a rectangular image as the beam is transmitted into tissues perpendicular to the array. Linear array transducers are commonly used in vascular, musculoskeletal, and superficial structure ultrasound examinations. Curvilinear transducers (Fig. 1.3b) are similar to linear designs, but the elements are on a slightly curved surface. While both transducers offer a wide field of view, the curvilinear transducer's field of view expands with increasing tissue depth [13]. These transducers are useful when a broad image is required that is not obstructed by bones or gas. This may include evaluations of the abdomen, pelvis,

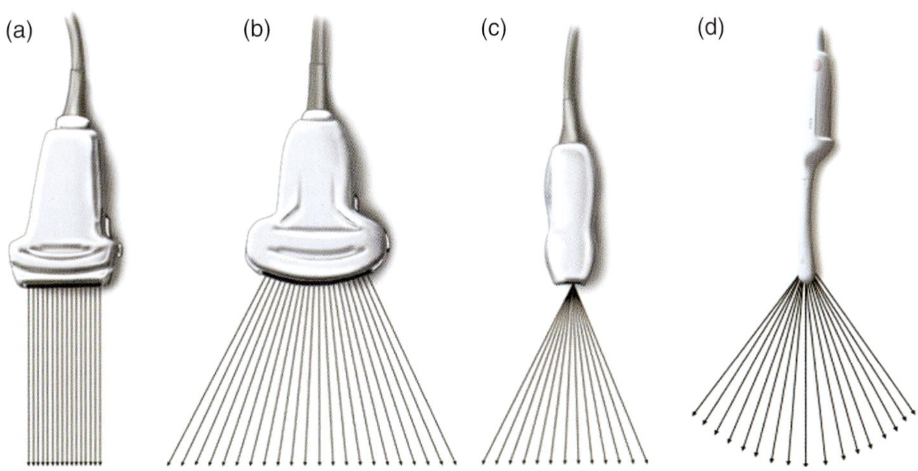

FIGURE 1.3 Transducers. Transducer formats for linear array (a), curvilinear array (b), phased array (c), and endocavity array (d).

obstetrics, and gynecological organs [16]. Phased array transducers (Fig. 1.3c) with smaller transducer footprints are useful in performing transthoracic imaging of the heart. Endocavitary transducers (Fig. 1.3d) are inserted into body cavities or surgical openings to allow transducers to be placed closer to target tissues. This allows operators to scan these structures with higher frequencies, improving spatial resolution and diminishing image distortions and artifacts [13]. Note that combinations of these imaging approaches can be made, such as using some beam steering with linear arrays to create trapezoidal image formats.

Use of 3D/4D imaging has expanded the use of ultrasound imaging by allowing manipulation of images into an alternate imaging plane, the coronal plane, and for displaying a three-dimensional image. Both of these imaging methods can provide additional diagnostic information for clinical use. 3D imaging can be conducted with a curvilinear array and endocavity transducers that are rotated slowly along multiple 2D image planes to compose a 3D image [16]. An alternative method of providing a 3D image includes the use of a 2D transducer that is steered along the traditional lateral and elevational directions [16].

Resolution and Image Characteristics

Spatial resolution allows operators to distinguish between two objects located at two different positions in space. Axial resolution is the ability to identify such objects at different positions along the axis of the ultrasound beam, one behind the other [20]. Axial resolution is improved with higher frequencies due to shortened wavelengths and when using shorter pulse lengths [10]. It does vary to some degree with tissue depth as the bandwidth of the pulse changes with depth due to frequency-dependent attenuation.

Lateral resolution differentiates reflectors that are located side-by-side, perpendicular to the US beam [20]. Lateral resolution is improved with narrower beam width, proximity to focal plane, higher frequency, and higher scan line density [10].

As spatial resolution improves at higher frequencies, it is subject to greater attenuation [16]. Lower frequencies must, therefore, be used to reach deeper tissues, with the associated reduction in spatial resolution. Ultrasound technology incorporates broad-bandwidth technology to optimize image quality and balance the benefits seen in high and low frequency beams.

Bandwidth is defined as the range of frequencies that a transducer can produce and detect. Pulsed wave ultrasound can produce a wider range of frequencies, and short pulses have larger bandwidths. By producing beams with a larger bandwidth, a greater spectrum of reflected echoes can be detected from tissues insonated, ultimately improving spatial resolution [21]. In simple terms, larger bandwidth allows the production of shorter pulses, which allows for better separation of echoes from closely spaced targets.

The capability of differentiating the time over which events occur is known as temporal resolution [10]. The rate at which images are produced influences temporal resolution, with higher frame rates being more capable of distinguishing moving objects in time. Increasing the number of scan lines in an image can improve lateral resolution but will decrease frame rates. Decreasing frame rates will worsen temporal resolution [16]. This is also true in deeper structures, where increased depth requires lower frame rates due to longer beam travel time and worsening temporal resolution.

The distinction of echo amplitudes, seen by grayscale differences in displayed pixels, is referred to as contrast resolution [16]. These differences in contrast are used to identify objects in an image, and the combination of spatial and contrast resolutions limits the size of objects that can be seen [13]. Background noise may sometimes be seen from electrical sources and/or speckle, sometimes resulting in difficulty distinguishing true echoes and diminishing contrast resolution. Noise can be reduced by averaging several images over time or with spatial compounding [16].

Display Modes

Amplitude Mode (A-Mode)

One of the earliest forms of medical ultrasound was the amplitude mode, or A-mode. As echoes return from tissues, the amplitude of the received signal on the transducer was portrayed on a cathode ray oscilloscope (CRO). On a CRO, the vertical axis corresponds to the amplitude of the returning echoes while the horizontal axis corresponds to the time scale for the echo return (Fig. 1.4a). As the strength of echoes increases, amplitude rises as well. Increased time along the horizontal axis implies

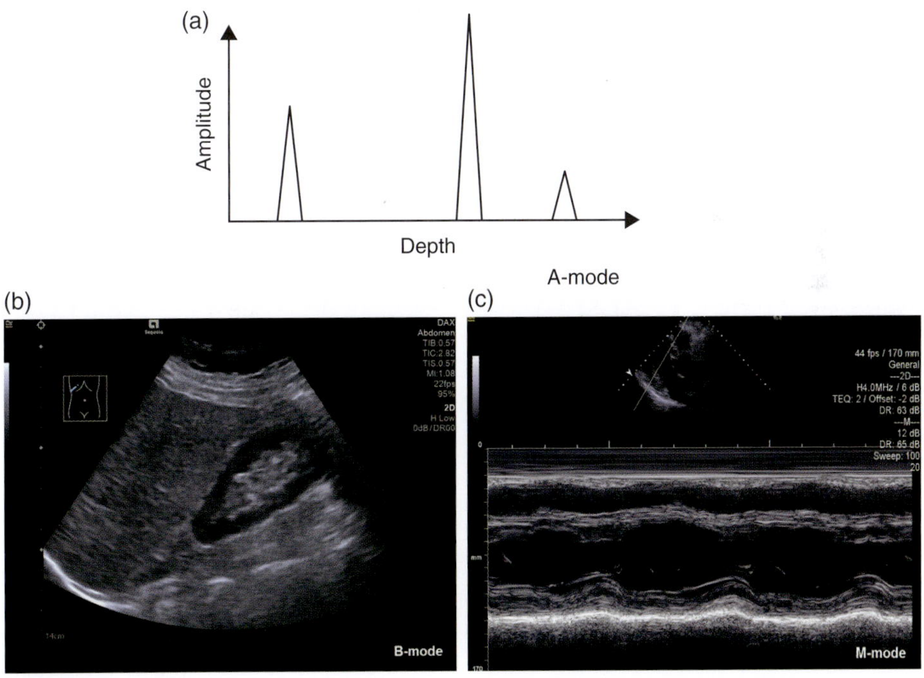

FIGURE 1.4 Ultrasound display modes: (a) Amplitude mode (A-mode) represents the amplitude of returning echoes projected along the *x*-axis at varying times along the *y*-axis corresponding to tissue depths. (b) Brightness mode (B-mode) is a common 2D image display for anatomic structures based on the intensity of gray pixels (related to echo strength) and depth of the tissue imaged. (c) Motion mode (M-mode) uses a user-selected line through the B-mode image (top half) and portrays the movement of structures along that line over time (bottom half).

that the echoes travel further distances and are located deeper within the body and further from the transducer. A-mode produces a one-dimensional image of returning echoes. The image produced when using A-mode ultrasonography is a simple time trace of this signal [10, 20].

Brightness Mode (B-Mode)

Returning echoes are portrayed as gray dots of varying brightness corresponding to echo amplitude (Fig. 1.4b). Strong echoes produce increased brightness. Weak echoes produce dark regions in the image as they are returning from nonreflective tissue. Vertical direction within the image corresponds to the distance between the reflector and the transducer. The use of multiple scan lines produced from the transducer's surface is properly positioned horizontally to generate a 2D image of the structures through which the beams pass. Most ultrasound machines display images with up to 256 shades of gray. This is now a common mode used for diagnostic imaging [20].

Motion Mode (M-Mode)

M-mode generates an electronic trace of a moving object lying along the path of a single ultrasound beam. The transducer is placed in one fixed position in relation to the moving structure. If the distance between the transducer and the reflector changes due to movement, the corresponding image will display that change as a function of time (Fig. 1.4c). Stationary structures will remain in place, while moving structures will move along the vertical axis of the screen as a function of time (horizontal axis). Among many of its uses, M-mode is often displayed simultaneously with B-mode to study cardiac valves, calculate fetal heart rate, and evaluate lung motion [20].

Other Imaging Modes

There are other ultrasound imaging modes that have been developed over time such as elastography that have not been covered here. The reader is referred elsewhere for additional information [22].

Real Time and Freeze

US machines can image dynamic movement of tissues with their capacity to produce high frame rates for real-time imaging. This is useful in observing moving organs and serves as a major advantage of US imaging when compared to diagnostic tools such as CT or MRI.

The freeze function allows the operator to interrupt the real-time acquisition at a given moment and analyze the features of the image and store it for further investigation. When frozen, the transducer usually stops transmitting US pulses [10]. When the image is frozen, the most recently collected images are temporarily stored in a series known as a cine loop. The entire cine loop or portions of it can then be archived.

Doppler Ultrasound

Doppler ultrasound can be used to detect motion, such as blood flow [13]. Moving components within the body function serve as reflectors for sound emitted by the transducer. Their change in velocity alters the frequency that returns to the transducer. This change in frequency is used in continuous wave (CW) ultrasound systems to determine the Doppler shift [16].

Wave fronts from targets moving toward the transducer are more tightly packed, resulting in a higher-frequency wave than the one emitted. In contrast, lower frequencies are seen when targets are traveling away from the transducer [16]. The magnitude of the Doppler shift frequency is proportional to the relative velocity between the source and the observer [13]. Therefore, as the velocity of moving structures such as red blood cells increases, the Doppler shift also increases.

The angle of approach by the transducer impacts the Doppler shift [16]. The angle between the direction of sound emission and the direction of blood flow should be less than 60° (Fig. 1.5) to reliably measure Doppler shift. Flow velocity (Doppler frequency) is reduced in relation to the increase in cosine of the Doppler angle, and the cosine of angles greater than 60° varies rapidly [13].

$$\text{Doppler shift} = \frac{2 \times \text{reflector speed} \times \text{incident frequency} \times \cos(\text{angle})}{\text{Propagation speed}}$$

According to the above equation, Doppler shift is directly related to the reflector speed (tissue velocity), the incident frequency (frequency of the transmitted ultrasound), and the cosine of the angle of incidence. Propagation speed is the speed of sound in the medium and is inversely related to the Doppler shift [23].

Doppler signals are mostly applied when studying blood flow but can also be used when analyzing tissue motion [16]. Blood signals are most commonly of low amplitude and high frequency shift. Tissue signals appear as high amplitude and low-frequency shifts due to the relatively slower velocities when compared to blood flow in vessels of appreciable size, for example, capillary velocities are too small for most Doppler systems to detect separately from tissue motion. The use of a wall filter

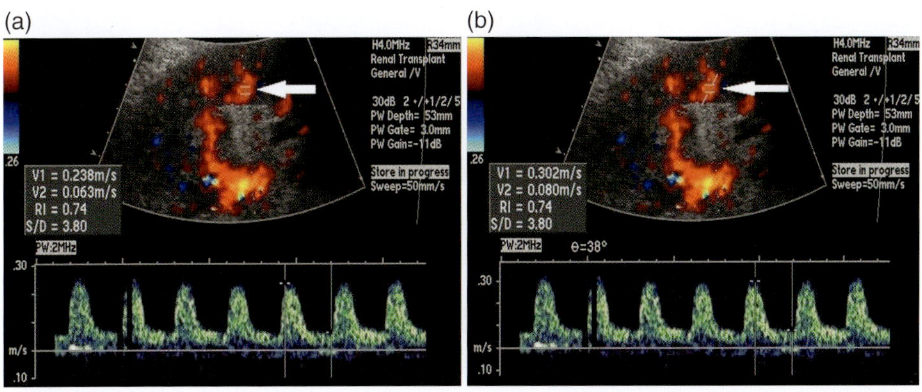

FIGURE 1.5 The operator should use Doppler angle correction when measuring flow velocity using spectral Doppler. There is a difference in flow velocity measured without (a, white arrow) and with (b, white arrow) using Doppler angle correction (0.238 versus 0.302 m/s).

allows the ultrasound machine to distinguish Doppler produced by blood flow compared to the surrounding tissues [10].

Important Note: While the Doppler effect described above is the origin of the Doppler modes seen on ultrasound machines, the actual measurement methods used to detect motion may not detect the actual frequency shift. In fact, the actual Doppler effect as measured by CW ultrasound is rarely used. Other "Doppler" modes use phase shift. This can be easily seen by the fact that there can be aliasing as will be described below. The Doppler effect itself does not alias. However, we commonly retain the terms color Doppler and pulsed Doppler even though the methods rely on phase shift methods. Perhaps more properly, these should be, and sometimes now are, termed color flow and pulsed wave [24].

Spectral Doppler (Pulsed Wave) and 2D Color Flow Images

Velocity changes within a specific area can be analyzed using spectral Doppler, also called pulsed wave [23]. Velocity information that is read from a single location is represented as a frequency shift (vertical axis) as a function of time (horizontal axis) [13]. Positive or negative on the vertical axis corresponds to the direction of the Doppler shift, while the grayscale (sometimes colorized) shows the strength of the Doppler signal (Fig. 1.6).

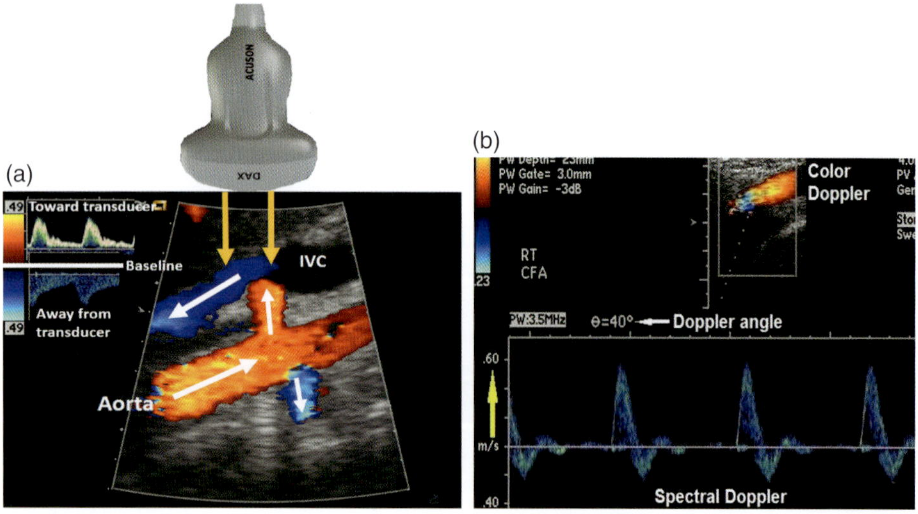

FIGURE 1.6 (a) Color flow imaging representing the mean Doppler frequency and flow direction is superimposed on the B-mode image. Doppler displays positive (red color and spectrum above the baseline) representing flow toward the transducer and negative Doppler frequency shifts (blue and spectrum below the baseline) representing flow away from the transducer at a specific location over time. White arrows show the direction of blood flow, and yellow arrows indicate the nominal direction of transmitted sound beams. IVC, inferior vena cava. (b) Vertical distance in the spectral trace corresponds to the Doppler shift (flow velocity) scale (yellow arrow). A Doppler angle (white arrow) less than 60° is recommended to keep the direction of the transmitted sound beam as parallel to the direction of blood flow as possible, which can better measure the flow velocity. RT, right; CFA, common femoral artery.

The Doppler signal can be portrayed as a 2D color image superimposed on a B-mode image (Fig. 1.6). Color flow Doppler corresponds to the Doppler shift (actually phase shift) and depicts direction of flow and mean velocities (not corrected for angle) [13]. By convention, blood flow toward the transducer is seen as red and blood flow away from the transducer is seen in blue (although the user can typically reverse this color scale if desired). A complication in color flow Doppler is the potential for aliasing, in which color flow direction information in vessels may be distorted, making accurate determination of blood flow direction difficult [21, 23]. Spectral Doppler can alias as well if the pulse repetition frequency (PRF), also referred to by other names such as Scale, is not set properly. Power Doppler is similar to color flow Doppler but displays the power of the Doppler signal rather than its velocity [25]. Therefore, it does not have the same aliasing issue while having the advantages of being less dependent on Doppler angle and providing increased sensitivity.

Continuous Versus Pulsed Wave Doppler

A continuous wave (CW) Doppler uses two transducer elements, with one transmitting a CW ultrasound signal and the other receiving the Doppler shifts. The CW ultrasound allows for highly accurate Doppler measurements in high-velocity flow such as aortic valve stenosis. A disadvantage of CW Doppler is the range ambiguity since there is no arrival time information as with pulsed ultrasound [23]. Pulsed wave (PW) Doppler is characterized by a single transducer that serves in both sending and receiving Doppler signals. Compared to CW Doppler, pulsed wave Doppler has improved control over the specific area being interrogated but is limited in Doppler accuracy and in high-velocity measurements due to aliasing [23].

Artifacts

Artifacts can cause visual misrepresentations and may distort the representation of anatomical structures. Operators must identify artifacts to interpret diagnostic ultrasound images correctly.

A major artifact is acoustic shadowing that can also be used for certain diagnoses. Shadows are formed when beams are unable to pass through a strongly attenuating or reflecting structure [13]. Shadows normally project directly posterior to the structure along the beam axis, typically vertically for linear arrays and radially in phased or curvilinear arrays (Fig. 1.7). Shadowing is formed by large stones, calcifications, and bones, which are caused mainly by sound absorption, refraction, and reflection. Acoustic shadowing can also interfere with lung images due to US scattering at the interface between tissue and air, while the presence or absence of shadowing may also be diagnostic for some conditions.

Reverberations are reflections of multiple repeated pulses and echoes formed by strongly reflecting interfaces [16]. Strong reflective tissues that are relatively shallow are the most common sources of reverberations. As a strong echo returns to the transducer, it may be reflected from the transducer toward the tissue. It then returns to the transducer as a second, weaker echo (Fig. 1.7). This subsequent echo is known as the reverberation. As reverberations are produced from the ultrasound wave traveling to the transducer twice or more, the ultrasound machine registers them as traveling

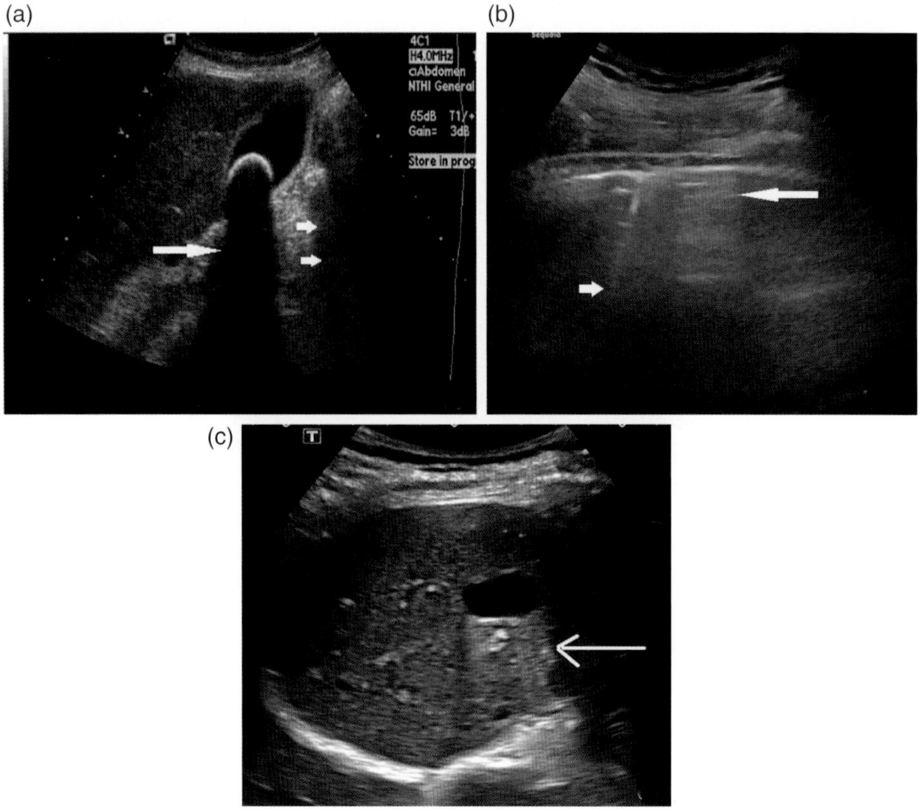

FIGURE 1.7 Common ultrasound artifacts. (a) Shadows posterior to highly reflective gallstones (long white arrow) and bowel gas (short white arrows). (b) Reverberations appear as multiple echoes produced by strong reflecting interfaces (A-line, long white arrow). Comet tails (B-lines, white short arrow) are formed by hyperechoic reflections perpendicular to what is being imaged in the lung ultrasound. (c) Posterior acoustic enhancement (white arrow) is shown as the ultrasound beam travels through an anechoic and low attenuation structure to produce an image artifact observed posterior to a liver cyst.

a further distance and portrays them as objects located deeper than the reflecting surface from which they originate [26].

Reverberations can be identified from authentic echoes by their response to gentle pressure on the skin. A genuine echo will move closer to the transducer at the same rate by which the transducer is pressed deeper against the skin, while the separation of reverberation bands will decrease at twice the rate due to their multiple pathways.

Reverberations are common in images of liquid-filled areas or in dental implants [27]. For example, the anterior bladder wall may demonstrate reverberations due to multiple reflections between it and the transducer, which are readily seen in the anechoic, urine-filled bladder. Two types of reverberations are ring-down and comet-tail artifacts (Fig. 1.7). Ring-down reverberations display a bright vertical line from objects such as an air bubble that travels down the image, while comet tails are hyperechoic trails that are seen in structures such as lung surface irregularities, foreign bodies, and cholesterol deposits in the gallbladder wall. Comet-tail artifacts result from echoes bouncing back and forth within two reflective surfaces of

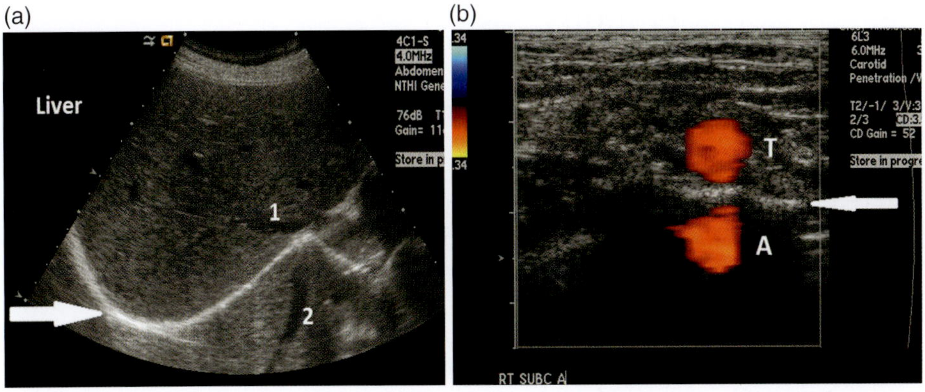

FIGURE 1.8 Images containing true structures and artificial ones appearing as a mirror image adjacent to an echogenic-curved reflector such as the diagram (a, white arrow) and subclavicle bone (b, white arrow). (a) In B-mode ultrasound image, the artifactual liver parenchyma and hepatic vein (2) appear similar to true liver and hepatic vein (1). (b) In color flow imaging, artifactual vessel (A, artifactual vessel) is a mirror to the true subclavian artery (T, true vessel). RT, right; SUBC A, subclavian artery.

an object, but with some energy of each interaction returning to the transducer. As echoes return to the transducer, each new echo produces a weaker signal resembling a comet tail on the US machine when viewed together [26].

Acoustic enhancement (Fig. 1.7c) is also known as posterior acoustic enhancement due to locally increased transmission to the tissue posterior to a structure that contains liquid [26]. As the US beam travels from tissues through weakly attenuating structures such as a cyst or blood vessel, it returns to the transducer with greater intensity than adjacent areas that travel through uniform tissue. This is displayed as structures seen immediately posterior to these structures as having increased echogenicity. The enhancement artifact assists in making the diagnosis of a cystic structure.

Mirror images appear when echoes go through multiple reflections, causing an altered image formation [26]. A beam that hits a bright reflector may hit an object on its return to the transducer. The echo thus takes a longer path to reach the transducer and registers on the machine as a second object that is deeper than the bright reflector. A mirror image is thus created in B-mode (Fig. 1.8a) and color flow imaging (Fig. 1.8b) [28]. In addition, scattering from the object may be sufficiently strong to again reflect from the mirroring surface and return an echo to the transducer along the original beam path. The mirror image can disappear with transducer adjustments, whereas a real object will remain on the screen after transducer adjustments [26, 28].

Safety of Diagnostic Ultrasound

Acoustic energy from US beams has direct interactions with the scanned tissues [20]. The physical effects on tissues can be both thermal and nonthermal. Although no direct causal relationship has been shown between the use of diagnostic ultrasound and adverse bioeffects in humans, the output of diagnostic ultrasound is regulated in the United States by the Food and Drug Administration (FDA) to minimize any potential bioeffects [21].

General Considerations

Minimizing the time that an ultrasound field is on is crucial in limiting patient exposure. By using periodic pulses, pulsed wave (PW) Doppler reduces the time under which a subject is irradiated when compared to continuous wave (CW) Doppler [21]. Spectral Doppler and M-mode imaging are stationary modes such that the exposure is along a single beam path. Imaging modes such as color flow imaging, power Doppler, and B-mode are scanned modes, and beams are primarily fired to different locations to increase the field of view such that the ultrasound power is more widely distributed.

Reduction of beam intensity, peak negative pressure, and exposure time are of prime importance in preventing unnecessary bioeffects [21]. Therefore, the as low as reasonably achievable (ALARA) principle is recommended when performing ultrasound examinations [29, 30]. Intensity can be measured as the temporal peak intensity, the greatest intensity at any point in time, or the spatial peak intensity, the largest intensity anywhere in the ultrasound field, for example, the focal point. The average intensity value during the ultrasound pulse is defined as the pulsed average intensity [20]. Another quantification of intensity is the temporal average intensity, which is the average value within the entire pulsed repetition period. For pulsed wave ultrasound, the temporal average intensity is related to the duty factor, or the fraction of time that the ultrasound beam is being transmitted through tissues [21]. A small duty factor signifies longer periods between pulses, decreasing the temporal average intensity. These intensity parameters serve as important factors when studying the possibility of bioeffects in tissues. Considering these values along with the overall exposure time, or dwell time, can increase operator awareness of the possibility of causing bioeffects [16–21]. The operators should follow the ALARA principle to guide how to perform ultrasound exams by using system controls to reduce ultrasound intensity and pressure, limit dwell time and examination time while maintaining image quality and efficient and effective diagnostic scanning and performing ultrasound exams only when medically indicated.

Thermal Effects

Acoustic energy is converted into heat within tissues. The risk of bioeffects, therefore, rises with increasing temperature and duration of exposure. The duration of exposure, type of tissue imaged, spatial focusing, rate of temperature increase, and ultrasound frequency can all influence the risk of bioeffects.

The thermal index (TI) can be used to assess potential heating from a transducer in specific equipment settings. It is displayed on ultrasound machines as a ratio of acoustic power currently being produced and the maximal acoustic power required to raise the tissue temperature 1°C in adults [16].

The American Institute of Ultrasound in Medicine (AIUM) provides a recommendation of the maximum scanning time at each TI where one can be reasonably assured against adverse bioeffects caused by thermal changes in patient tissue [30]. The TI may be displayed on US screens for operators to assess possible adverse effects based on the TI value and the duration of their imaging time. Monitoring the TI and reducing exposure time allows for risk reduction and minimization of temperature increases in keeping with the ALARA principle.

Greater temperature increases are possible in spectral Doppler, with less seen in color Doppler, and the least seen in B-mode imaging. But the TI is designed to help the operator minimize output regardless of the mode, while needing to keep in mind dwell time.

Acoustic Cavitation

Ultrasound interacts with gas bodies in a process known as cavitation, which may result in physical tissue changes [21]. Generated microbubbles can interact with the ultrasound to produce fluid motion, including jetting. Bubble collapse may lead to shearing forces within tissues and high temperatures in and around the bubbles. Cavitation can produce heat and free radicals, scatter acoustic energy, and microstreaming of fluid, all potential sources for mechanical changes [21].

Beam properties, such as frequency and pulse duration, have been shown to impact cavitation. Tissue fluid parameters, including density, viscosity, compressibility, heat conductivity, and surface tension, impact cavitation as well.

Ultrasound contrast agents contain microbubbles that have the potential for cavitation. Adverse effects of microbubbles have been demonstrated when operating with a mechanical index (MI) >0.4 in mammalian tissues when contrast agents are present. The mechanical index is defined in the following section. AIUM recommendations for limiting gas body bioeffects when operating at MI >0.4 include minimizing contrast dose, MI, and total exposure time [31].

Mechanical Index

As the TI serves to monitor the potential for thermal energy increases in tissues, the mechanical index (MI) is used to gauge the likelihood of mechanical effects due to cavitation [21]. MI is proportional to the acoustic pressure and inversely proportional to the square root of the ultrasound frequency. This means that higher acoustic pressures are needed for higher-frequency ultrasound to have the same potential for cavitation. The display of the MI allows the operator to more easily monitor this potential for effects. Studies have shown an MI of 0.4 as the threshold for pulmonary capillary hemorrhage and an MI of 1.4 for intestinal capillary hemorrhage. These values were reported for laboratory animals, and further research must be done to better understand possible bioeffects in humans [30, 32]. Again, the objective is to minimize the MI while maintaining diagnostic image quality.

Tissue Type

As mentioned earlier in this chapter, ultrasound beam absorption and attenuation vary with tissue type. Fluids such as amniotic fluid, blood, or urine have low ultrasound attenuation, while bone absorbs acoustic energy quite well. Reducing output power while increasing gain becomes important when imaging bony structures to minimize exposure, which is the reason the TI has three forms that are selectable on the ultrasound machines depending on the imaging situation. TIS is for soft tissue, TIB for bone distal to the transducer, and TIC for bone near the transducer, for example, transcranial ultrasound. More perfused tissues will better dissipate thermal energy and will be cooled down more effectively.

Current AIUM guidelines for obstetric ultrasound discuss that although no causal relationships have been shown between obstetric screening and harmful bioeffects, fetal imaging should only be done when medically indicated. Other non-medical, or nonpurposeful, viewing of the fetus is contraindicated and inappropriate. When performing fetal imaging, the AIUM recommends that dwell times should be minimized, output indices such as the thermal and mechanical index monitored, and that Doppler and elasticity measurements are done appropriately and only when indicated [29, 33].

Soft tissues can shift acoustic energy to higher frequencies, causing amplitude distortion, which results in a shockwave that may expose tissues to disproportionally higher levels of energy [21]. For example, full bladder scanning can result in shockwave formation because fluid has a low attenuation coefficient and thus places higher ultrasound frequencies at posterior structures. Additionally, enhanced attenuation, caused by increasing the ultrasound frequency, can expose these structures to larger energy absorption.

Endocavitary uses of diagnostic ultrasound bring the transducer in closer proximity to sensitive tissue, and surface heating of the transducer itself may serve as a heat source. This increases the general concern for endocavitary scans. However, ultrasound, when used properly, is a safe and effective medical device whose benefits outweigh the potential risks.

Reduction of Ultrasound Output

Organizations, including the FDA and AIUM, helped develop the "Standard for Real-Time Display of Thermal and Mechanical Acoustical Output Indices on Diagnostic Ultrasound Equipment." This serves the purpose of displaying both the TI and MI on the US machine so operators are more aware of the acoustic beam interaction with tissues and will allow operators to perform risk-versus-benefit analyses when conducting ultrasound exams.

It is suggested that machines should be set to examination presets according to the type of examination performed, for example, an OB preset should be used for an OB examination to avoid unnecessary exposure. Direct controls, such as correct diagnostic settings, output power, and focusing, should be taken into consideration by operators to reduce US output. For example, the lowest output power that produces a clear image should be used as well as proper optimization of the beam focus at target tissues to avoid unnecessary exposure [21]. Indirect controls should also be considered. These affect the temporal and spatial distribution of the acoustic beam. Ultrasound imaging modes (B-mode, color Doppler) distribute ultrasound over a larger portion of tissue, while unscanned modes (continuous wave Doppler, spectral or pulsed Doppler, M-mode) apply the ultrasound along a single beam thus increasing the potential for heating. Pulsed repetition frequency (PRF) decreases can result in lower temporal average intensity and thus decrease potential heating. Reduction of burst length in pulses can also reduce patient exposure. Other factors include appropriate transducer selection and appropriate use of receiver gain controls. Image quality can be enhanced without increasing output intensity by using receiver gain and TGC [21].

Scanning time for training and research purposes should be kept to a minimum, and informed consent should be given after explaining the possibility of bioeffects and how the scan relates to what is commonly performed in a clinical examination.

For study purposes, ultrasound should be used conservatively to reduce repetitive and lengthy examinations [29]. Although ultrasound is safer compared to other diagnostic imaging such as CT, operators are responsible for informing patients of the overall safety, maximizing efficiency, and minimizing patient exposure to unnecessary ultrasound when performing any studies.

Knobology

There is considerable variation in the design of user controls between ultrasound vendors (Fig. 1.9). The operator needs to be familiar with the "knobology" (knobs, buttons, functions) on the machine being used to perform ultrasound examinations [34] and understand what these knobs control on the system. This is critical for obtaining high-quality clinical images in a safe and effective manner. For example, increasing the receive gain control or the power control can increase the echo brightness in a B-mode image. But the gain control does not increase the ultrasound exposure to the patient. Similarly, adjusting the TCG can improve image quality without increasing exposure. Thus, understanding how these controls can be used to make images more clinically useful, and which are changing the ultrasound exposure, is important knowledge and should be part of proper training. Most commercial ultrasound machines have functions to preset parameters of ultrasound image processing (image depth, total gain, dynamic range, harmonic imaging, speckle reduction) for specific ultrasound examination (e.g. cardiac, abdomen, OB, arterial, and venous) after selecting a transducer (e.g. linear array and phased array). Preset

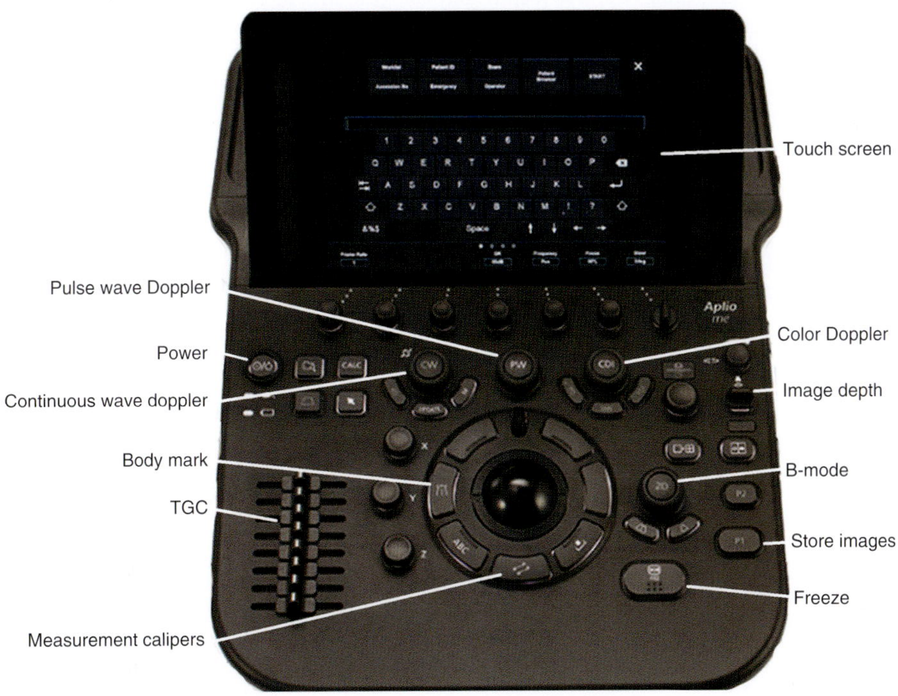

FIGURE 1.9 Knobology of ultrasound machine.

functions potentially improve the performance of ultrasound examinations by using standardized, proper, and consistent image processing and quality.

Commonly used knobology is as follows [34]:

B (or 2D): B-mode (grayscale) ultrasound image
C (or CD): color flow imaging
CW: continue wave Doppler mode
D (P or PW): pulse wave Doppler mode
Depth: change image depth
G: total image gain
Freeze: freeze a frame of image
M: M-mode ultrasound
P (or store): save static image or real-time cine loop
TGC: time-gain compensation
Zoom: zoom in/out of image (or a region of interest)

Summary

Ultrasound principles and instrumentation have been refined for centuries and developed into a mainstay of medical diagnostic imaging. Choosing the correct type of transducer as well as using the appropriate imaging mode will create the optimal images necessary for any medical evaluation. Ultrasound operators must be able to identify physiological structures as well as artifacts for detecting pathologic changes while also minimizing the risks of ultrasound to the patients being scanned.

Review Questions

1. The propagation speed of a wave is determined by which of the following?
   a. Wavelength
   b. Amplitude
   c. Period
   d. Medium
   e. Frequency
2. Which of the following answer choices places media in order of increasing sound propagation speed?
   a. Gas, solid, liquid
   b. Gas, liquid, solid
   c. Solid, liquid, gas

   d. Liquid, solid, gas
   e. Solid, bone, liquid

3. If the wavelength of a medium at a given frequency is 4 mm and the frequency is doubled, what is the wavelength?
   a. 1 mm
   b. 2 mm
   c. 4 mm
   d. 16 mm
   e. 32 mm
4. Using given values of propagation speed and frequency, which of the following can be calculated?
   a. Period
   b. Wavelength
   c. Amplitude
   d. a and b
   e. a and c
5. If the frequency of sound is decreased by ½, how will it affect the wavelength and why?
   a. Stay the same
   b. Decrease, because frequency and wavelength are directly related
   c. Decrease, because frequency and wavelength are inversely related
   d. Increase, because frequency and wavelength are directly related
   e. Increase, because frequency and wavelength are inversely related
6. What transducer properties minimize the loss of lateral resolution of the far field?
   a. A larger transducer width
   b. Lower wavelength
   c. Higher frequencies
   d. Decreased scan line thickness
   e. All of the above
7. What is true for scanning deep tissues?
   a. High transmit frequency is used
   b. It is more difficult to maintain high frame rates
   c. Spatial resolution is maintained
   d. Low scan line densities are preferred
   e. Low attenuation in deep tissue
8. A sound beam traveling perpendicular to blood flow will demonstrate what kind of Doppler effect?
   a. Large Doppler shift
   b. Normal Doppler shift
   c. Small Doppler shift
   d. No Doppler shift
   e. The same Doppler shift as parallel to blood flow

9. Which two factors are located on the ultrasound device screen and should be monitored regularly by the operator to reduce chances of bioeffects?
   - **a.** Beam intensity, dwell time
   - **b.** Duty factor, thermal index
   - **c.** Thermal index, mechanical index
   - **d.** Pulsed average intensity, temporal average intensity
   - **e.** None of the above
10. Which strategy can be used to reduce ultrasound exposure and minimize bioeffects?
   - **a.** Selecting appropriate machine settings prior to starting subject screens
   - **b.** Avoiding repetitive and lengthy examinations
   - **c.** Using the lowest output intensity to produce a clear image
   - **d.** Move or lift the transducer when imaging of a stationary structure is not necessary
   - **e.** All the above

Correct answers: 1. d; 2. b; 3. b; 4. d; 5. e; 6. e; 7. b; 8. d; 9. c; 10. e.

References

1. Kane D, Grassi W, Sturrock R, Balint PV. A brief history of musculoskeletal ultrasound: from bats and ships to babies and hips. *Rheumatology* 2004; 43: 931–933.
2. Curie J, Curie P. Development, via compression, of electric polarization in hemihedral crystals with inclined faces. *Bull Soc Minéral Fr* 1880; 3: 90–93.
3. Langevin P. French Patent No. 505,703. Filed September 17, 1917. Issued August 5, 1920.
4. Dussik KT. On the possibility of using ultrasound waves as a diagnostic aid. *Z Neurol Psychiatry* 1942; 174: 153–168.
5. Wild JJ, Reid JM. Application of echo-ranging techniques to the determination of structure of biological tissues. *Science* 1952; 115(2983): 226–230.
6. Holmes JH, Howry DH, Posakony GJ, Cushman CR. The ultrasonic visualization of soft tissue structures in the human body. *Trans Am Clin Climatol Assoc* 1954; 66: 208–223.
7. Donald I, MacVicar J, Brown TG. Investigation of abdominal masses by pulsed ultrasound. *Lancet* 1958; 1: 1188–1195.
8. Kremkau FW. Sonography principles and instruments. 10th ed. Elsevier, 2022.
9. Abu-Zidan F, Hefny AF, Corr P. Clinical ultrasound physics. *J Emerg Trauma Shock* 2011; 40(4): 501–503.
10. Tole NM. Basic physics of ultrasonographic imaging. Geneva, Switzerland: WHO, 2015.
11. Chan V, Perlas A. Basics of ultrasound imaging. Toronto, ON: Springer, 2011.
12. Barootchi S, Chan HL, Namazi SS, et al. Ultrasonographic characterization of lingual structures pertinent to oral, periodontal, and implant surgery. *Clin Oral Implants Res* 2020; 31(4): 352–359. http://doi.org/10.1111/clr.13573.
13. Hoskins P, Martin K, Thrush A. Diagnostic ultrasound: physics and equipment. 2nd ed. Cambridge, UK: Cambridge University Press, 2010.
14. Culjat M, Goldenberg D, Tewari P, Singh R. A review of tissue substitutes for ultrasound imaging. *Ultrasound Med Biol* 2010; 36: 861–873.
15. Christensen EE, Curry TS, Dowdey JE. Introduction to the physics of diagnostic radiology. 2nd ed. Philadelphia, PA: Lea & Febeger, 1978.
16. Abu-Zidan FM. Basic ultrasound physics, instrumentation, and knobology. In: Zago M (ed.). Essential US for trauma: E-FAST. Ultrasound for acute care surgeons. Milano: Springer, 2014. http://doi.org/10.1007/978-88-470-5274-1_1.

17. Li J, Ma Y, Zhang T, et al. Recent advancements in ultrasound transducer: from material strategies to biomedical applications. *BME Front* 2022; 2022: 9764501. http://doi.org/10.34133/2022/9764501.
18. Brenner K, Ergun AS, Firouzi K, et al. Advances in capacitive micromachined ultrasonic transducers. *Micromachines* 2019; 10(2): 152. http://doi.org/10.3390/mi10020152.
19. Demi L. Practical guide to ultrasound beam forming: beam pattern and image reconstruction analysis. *Appl Sci (Switz)* 2018; 8(9): 1544–1558.
20. Noble V, Nelson B, Sutingco N. Manual of emergency and critical care ultrasound. New York, NY, USA: Cambridge University Press, 2007.
21. Rumack CM, Levine D. Diagnostic ultrasound. [Electronic resource]. Philadelphia, PA, USA: Elsevier, 2018.
22. Bridal SL. Innovative ultrasound imaging techniques: biomedical applications. London, UK and Hoboken, NJ: ISTE Ltd. and John Wiley & Sons, Inc., 2024.
23. Edelman S. Ultrasound physics. Chapter 1. ESP Ultrasound, 2016 http://www.esp-inc.com.
24. Foley WD, Erickson SJ. Color Doppler flow imaging. *AJR* 1991; 156: 1–13.
25. Rubin JM, Bude RO, Carson PL, et al. Power Doppler US: a potentially useful alternative to mean frequency-based color Doppler US. *Radiology* 1994; 190(3): 853–856.
26. Lumb P, Karakitsos D. Critical care ultrasound. Philadelphia, PA: Elsevier Saunders, 2014.
27. Chan HL, Kripfgans OD. Dental ultrasound in periodontology and implantology. Springer Nature Switzerland AG, 2020.
28. Rubin JM, Gao J, Hentel K, Min R. Duplication image in vascular sonography. *J Ultrasound Med* 2010; 29: 1385–1392.
29. American Institute of Ultrasound in Medicine (AIUM). As low as reasonably achievable (ALARA) principle. AIUM 05/19/2020. https://www.aium.org/resources/official-statements/view/as-low-as-reasonably-achievable-(alara)-principle.
30. American Institute of Ultrasound in Medicine (AIUM). Recommended maximum scanning times for displayed thermal index (TI) values. AIUM 09/26/2022 https://www.aium.org/resources/official-statements/view/recommended-maximum-scanning-times-for-displayed-thermal-index-(ti)-values.
31. American Institute of Ultrasound in Medicine (AIUM). Statement on biological effects in tissues with ultrasound contrast agents. AIUM 08/19/2021 https://www.aium.org/resources/official-statements/view/statement-on-biological-effects-in-tissues-with-ultrasound-contrast-agents.
32. American Institute of Ultrasound in Medicine (AIUM). Statement on biological effects of ultrasound in vivo. AIUM 08/19/2021 https://www.aium.org/resources/official-statements/view/statement-on-biological-effects-of-ultrasound-in-vivo.
33. American Institute of Ultrasound in Medicine (AIUM). Prudent use and safety of diagnostic ultrasound in pregnancy. AIUM 05/19/2020 https://www.aium.org/resources/official-statements/view/prudent-use-and-safety-of-diagnostic-ultrasound-in-pregnancy.
34. Zander D, Huske S, Hoffman B, et al. Ultrasound image optimization ("Knobology"): B-mode. *Ultrasound Int Open* 2020; 6: E14–E24. http://doi.org/10.1055/a-1223-1134.

CHAPTER 2

Head and Neck Soft Tissue

Ethan Burke[1], Kelli Tichy[1], Megan Maar[1], and Chun-Xia Xia[2]

[1] Rocky Vista University, College of Osteopathic Medicine, Ivins, Utah, USA

[2] Department of Ultrasound, Beijing Tongren Hospital, Capital Medical University, Beijing, China

Introduction

The complexity of the head and neck region in anatomical structure and content makes this area highly susceptible to a myriad of pathologies, ranging from inflammatory disorders to malignancy. Common practice today includes the use of high-frequency ultrasound for assessment of malignancy, guidance for fine needle aspiration or biopsy, and the diagnosis of lymphatic anomalies [1]. Analysis of ultrasound characteristics for lymph nodes, thyroid glands, and salivary glands is key to the diagnosis of pathologies due to the variety and number of these structures. More than one-third of the total lymph nodes in human body locate in the head and neck region [2, 3].

Alongside other diagnostic methods, clinicians can utilize ultrasound for an office-based real-time assessment to investigate suspicions or confirm a diagnosis for soft tissue pathologies in the neck [1]. Additionally, there are several pathologies associated with the thyroid and parathyroid glands, carotid arteries, and jugular veins that can be found via ultrasound imaging of the neck. These subjects will not be covered here and can be found in the endocrine (Chapter 11) and vascular (Chapter 10) chapters, respectively. This chapter will cover ultrasound assessment of the head and neck, including the normal ultrasound appearances and common pathologies in lymphadenopathy and salivary inflammation.

General Anatomy

The anatomy to follow gives a detailed explanation of the salivary glands and cervical lymph nodes to provide a basis for ultrasound exploration of the head and neck.

Anatomy of the Salivary Glands

Submandibular Gland The submandibular gland lies under the mandible within the posterior region of the submandibular triangle (Fig. 2.1). Due to its posterolateral location, it is partially covered by the mylohyoid muscle, with the superficial and deep divisions identifiable on ultrasound images [4, 5]. The deeper structures of the submandibular gland can, however, be obscured in obese patients [6]. The submandibular duct runs anteromedially from the gland to open at the sublingual caruncle just lateral to the frenulum of the tongue in the oral cavity [5, 6]. The duct runs superior to the mylohyoid muscle and is usually too narrow to be visible by conventional B-mode ultrasound [6, 7]. The facial artery and vein may cross the submandibular gland in their path to and from the face, providing branches to the gland along their respective courses [5].

Sublingual Gland The sublingual glands are the deepest of salivary glands that are located superior to the geniohyoid muscle, just below the intrinsic muscles of the tongue [5]. The almond-shaped structures are lateral to midline and situated within the sublingual space that communicates with the submandibular space at the posterior aspect of the mylohyoid muscle [5, 7]. This communication allows for lesions of the sublingual gland to easily pass into the submandibular space [7]. The submandibular duct also traverses through this space as it courses along its medial portion to open at the sublingual caruncle [8].

Parotid Gland The parotid gland locates on the lateral side of the angle of the mandible and contains the parotid plexus of the facial nerve (CN VII), the retromandibular vein, and the external carotid artery (Fig. 2.1) [5]. While the embedded branches of the facial nerve serve as the divide between superficial and deep lobes of the parotid gland, nearly all branches are too small to be visualized on conventional B-mode ultrasound [6]. The retromandibular vein, therefore, is the landmark used to

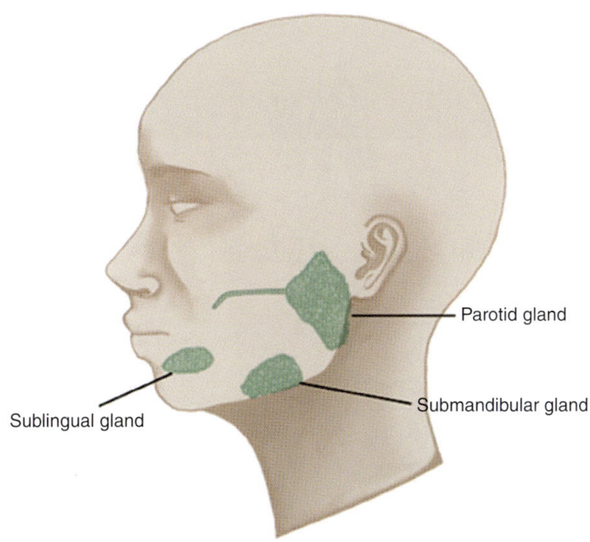

FIGURE 2.1 Illustration of the salivary glands.

detect the lobular separation between superficial and deep partitions on ultrasound images [6]. The parotid duct courses from the gland along the external aspect of the masseter muscle to pierce the buccinator muscle and enter the posterolateral aspect of the oral cavity opposite the 2nd maxillary molar [5, 8].

Anatomy of Cervical Lymph Nodes

Comprehensive sonographic examinations of cervical lymph nodes follow the levels established by the American Head and Neck Society and American Academy of Otolaryngology-Head and Neck Surgery, which include levels I–VII based on anatomical location (Fig. 2.2) [3, 9]. Cervical lymph nodes appear as oval, homogeneous, hypoechoic structures with a hyperechoic hilum on high-resolution ultrasound images [10]. Due to many lymph nodes in the head and neck, a knowledge of the relevant anatomic relations between lymph nodes and their landmarks plays an important role in identifying, documenting, and classifying locations of neck lymph nodes in patients with inflammation or malignancy properly [11].

Level I: Level I is subdivided into **level Ia,** which includes submental lymph nodes, and **level Ib,** which includes submandibular lymph nodes [3, 9]. These lymph nodes are just inferior to the mylohyoid muscle and superior to the lower margin of the hyoid bone [9]. The submental lymph nodes are lateral to midline and medial to the anterior digastric muscle bellies, while the submandibular lymph nodes are anterior to the posterior border of the submandibular glands [9]. Lymph nodes at level Ia have high suspicion of metastases from the malignancy in the anterior oral cavity and lower lip. Level Ib cervical lymph nodes are commonly at risk for metastases from the malignancy in the oral, anterior nasal cavities, and the submandibular gland [12].

Level II: Level II nodes include the upper internal jugular nodes. These lymph nodes form part of the deep cervical chain that extends inferiorly along the internal jugular vein from the base of the skull to the level of the hyoid bone [9].

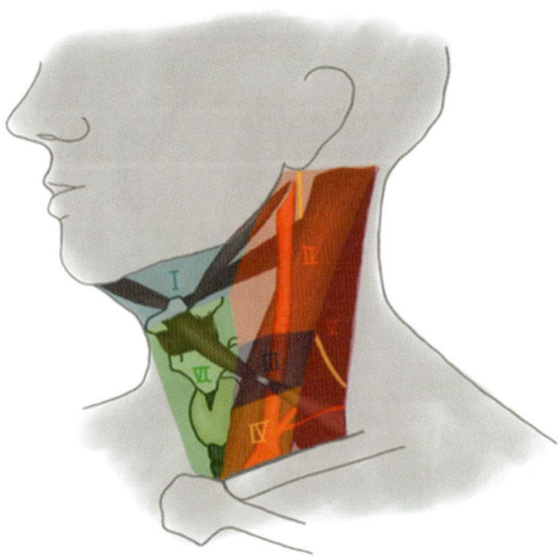

FIGURE 2.2 Illustration of levels of cervical lymph nodes.

They are bordered posteriorly by the posterior border of the sternocleidomastoid muscle [3]. Level II nodes are further divided by the internal jugular vein into level IIa and IIb [12]. **Level IIa** lymph nodes surround the superior portion of the internal jugular vein and contain the jugulodigastric lymph nodes [9]. **Level IIb** lymph nodes are separated posteriorly from the superior portion of the internal jugular vein by a small fat pad. While level IIa lymph nodes are associated with oral or laryngeal cancers, level IIb lymph nodal metastasis is commonly from oropharyngeal or nasopharyngeal cancers directly [12].

Level III: Level III lymph nodes include the middle internal jugular lymph nodes that locate inferior to the hyoid bone and above the inferior margin of the cricoid cartilage along the sternocleidomastoid muscles [3, 9]. The region of their location from the posterior border of the sternocleidomastoid muscle extends to the medial border of the common carotid artery or internal carotid artery [9]. As a continuation of the caudal-most portion of level II lymph nodes, level III lymph nodes receive efferent lymphatics from level II, retropharyngeal, pretracheal, and recurrent laryngeal lymph nodes, creating routes of metastasis from the oral cavity, nasopharynx, oropharynx, and larynx [12].

Level IV: Level IV lymph nodes locate along the lower segment of the internal jugular vein from the inferior border of the cricoid cartilage to the level of the clavicle [9]. They range from the posterior border of the sternocleidomastoid muscle and posterior border of the anterior scalene muscle to the medial border of the common carotid artery [9]. While the cricoid cartilage serves as the only definite border between level III and level IV lymph nodes that are difficult to visualize on conventional B-mode ultrasound, therefore approximating the zone between the hyoid and superior manubrium is used to differentiate these levels [3]. Level IV lymph node metastases are commonly from a malignancy in the esophagus, larynx, thyroid, and trachea [12].

Level V: Level V lymph nodes locate in the posterior triangle that traverse from the posterior edge of the sternocleidomastoid muscle to the anterior border of the trapezius muscle [9]. These are further divided into two divisions using the cricoid cartilage as an anatomical landmark [12]. **Level Va** lymph nodes are the superior half of the level V lymph nodes that locate posterior to levels II and III. **Level Vb** is the inferior half of the level V nodes and directly locates posterior to the level IV region [9]. Level V efferent lymphatics include the drainage from the occipital and retroauricular lymph nodes, occipital scalp, nasopharynx, and thyroid gland [12].

Level VI: Level VI lymph nodes include the pre-laryngeal and pretracheal lymph nodes locate from the inferior margin of the hyoid bone to the superior border of the manubrium and are anterior to both levels III and IV [9]. Level VI lymph nodes are responsible for draining the lower face and anterior neck, floor of the oral cavity, thyroid, and esophagus [12].

Level VII: Level VII lymph nodes include the anterior superior mediastinal lymph nodes and span from suprasternal notch to brachiocephalic artery [9]. They are inferior to level VI [13]. Level VII lymph nodes play an important role in staging thyroid cancer due to their communication with superior levels [14]. These lymph nodes are also associated with metastases from nasopharyngeal and oropharyngeal malignancy due to communication with level II lymph nodes [12].

Indications

Indications for Salivary Glands Ultrasound

Conventional B-mode ultrasound can be used to assess the structure of the salivary glands, including submandibular, sublingual, and parotid glands. Indications for ultrasound include diffuse or recurring salivary gland enlargement and tenderness, abscess, salivary duct obstruction, neoplasm, and cysts [4, 6]. When assessing suspected lesions of the salivary glands, it is important to evaluate these glands in both longitudinal and transverse planes and lymph nodes in the neck to distinguish malignancy from benign conditions in salivary glands and their associated lymph nodes [6].

Indications for Other Soft Tissue Mass

With palpable soft tissue masses in the neck, ultrasound is used in initial diagnostic assessment. An understanding of the varying appearance of lesions on ultrasound can help to determine whether masses are cystic or solid with characteristics of benign or malignant [15]. Ultrasound characteristics of masses include the size, shape, contour, and echotexture of the mass [15]. Ultrasound can also be used to guide fine needle aspiration to provide tissue samples for further histologic confirmation. Additionally, other neck lesions and conditions include parapharyngeal space tumor, thyroglossal duct cyst, parathyroid or thymic cysts, ectopic thyroid, temporomandibular joint effusion, branchial cleft cyst, lipomas, and Zenker's diverticulum [15].

Indications for Cervical Lymph Nodes Ultrasound

Ultrasound scanning of the cervical lymph nodes is indicated to assess enlarged nodes for malignancy, differentiating lymph nodes from other neck masses, performing fine needle aspiration for cytology, and defining primary sources of metastatic disease [4]. While there are criteria to help to differentiate malignancy from benign lesions based on characteristics on B-mode ultrasound and color flow images, such as the location, shape, contour, echotexture, vascularity of the lesion, and changes after a specific treatment (such as radiation therapy for metastasis) [4, 15]. In addition, ultrasound-guided fine needle aspiration provides tissue samples for further histopathology examinations to determine malignant or benign lesions.

Ultrasound Techniques

Imaging Salivary Glands and Neck Soft Tissue

A high-frequency linear array transducer (10–15 MHz) is recommended to assess the salivary glands and cervical lymph nodes that are superficially located [6]. A high-frequency transducer provides good image resolution that allows identifying small lesions and analyzing echotexture and vascularity in the lesion. A 5–10 MHz

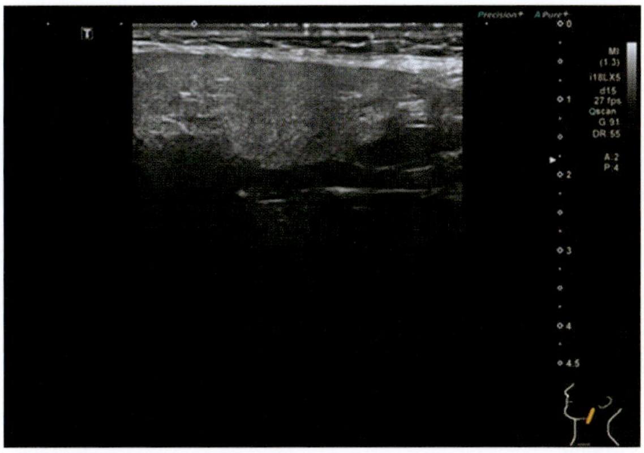

FIGURE 2.3 Longitudinal plane of a normal left parotid gland (B-mode grayscale image).

transducer may be required to image deeper structures in the neck [15]. The normal echogenicity of all major salivary glands is hyperechoic and homogeneous (Fig. 2.3). The increase in echogenicity in glands due to the deposition of fat and/or fibrotic tissue in the glands [6]. Commonly used ultrasound imaging techniques for the neck include B-mode grayscale image, color flow imaging, power, and spectral Doppler.

Techniques for Imaging Lymph Nodes

B-mode: In determining benign versus malignant lymph nodes, B-mode can be used to assess the size, shape (the ratio of shortest diameter to longest diameter), margins, and internal echotexture of the lymph node for differentiating a malignant from benign lymph node [6, 16]. Benign lymph nodes are more likely to be oval and homogenous with echogenic central hilum (Fig. 2.4a), while malignant nodes are rounder and heterogeneous with the pattern of abnormal or absent an echogenic hilum [15, 17]. Scanning in longitudinal and transverse planes should be performed to encompass ultrasound characteristics to identify pathologies [10].

Color flow imaging: Color flow imaging can be helpful in distinguishing malignant from benign lymph nodes based on the vascularity within the node [15]. Generally, a malignant lymph node (primary or metastatic) has hypervascularity.

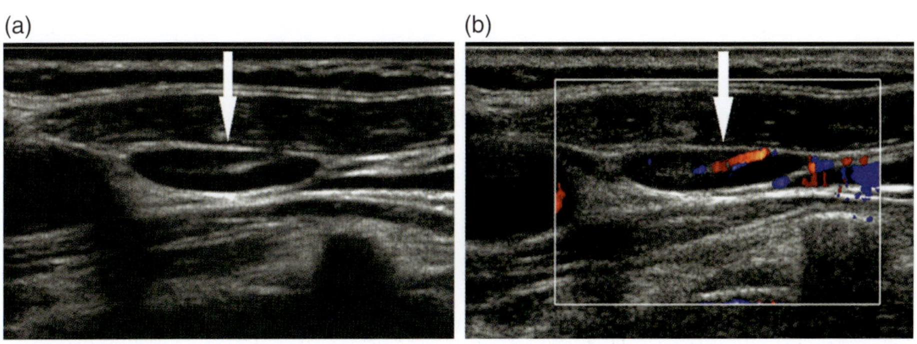

FIGURE 2.4 A normal lymph node (white arrow) in B-mode (a) and color flow (b) images.

Conversely, a benign lymph node has minimal central blood flow (Fig. 2.4b). However, a lymph node with inflammation can also appear with hypervascularity on color flow imaging [18]. Clinical information, other imaging modalities such as PET-CT or magnetic resonance imaging, and biopsy can be used for further assessment to determine benign or malignant lymph nodes when the nature of the lymph node is undetermined by using ultrasound alone.

Pathological Findings

Salivary Glands

Acute Inflammation Acute inflammation of salivary glands can present as enlarged glands with inhomogeneous hypoechoic areas on grayscale image and with increased vascularity on color flow image (Fig. 2.5) [6]. One of the most common causes of inflammation to the salivary glands is due to dental infection, inflammatory responses caused by trauma, ductal obstruction, and some autoimmune diseases [7].

Chronic Inflammation In contrast to acute inflammation, chronic inflammation in salivary gland does not cause gland enlargement or increased blood flow. The gland with chronic inflammation is generally represented by hypoechoic and inhomogeneous echotexture in the gland [6].

Abscess An abscess usually appears hypoechoic or anechoic, with ill-defined borders (Fig. 2.6) and some posterior acoustic enhancement [6]. Hyperechoic areas from microbubbles of gas within the abscess may be seen, but otherwise the abscess is hypoechoic without internal vascularity [6]. Clinically, abscesses are associated with pain and fever and can be drained under ultrasound guidance if the abscess is liquified.

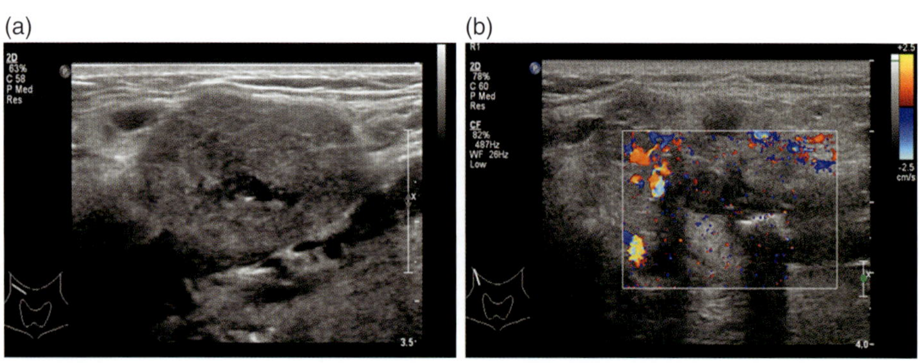

FIGURE 2.5 A submandibular gland with acute inflammation. The gland appears inhomogeneous and hypoechoic on B-mode ultrasound (a) and increased vascularity in color flow imaging (b).

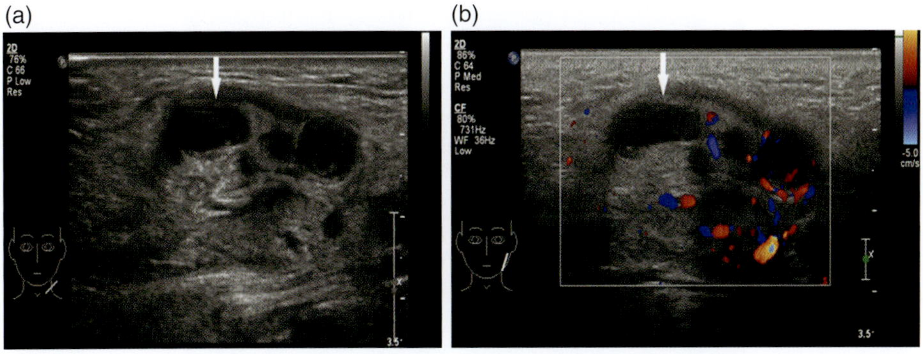

FIGURE 2.6 Abscess in submental gland. The gland shows an anechoic area (white arrow) on B-mode image (a) and no internal blood flow on color flow imaging (b).

Sialolithiasis Sialolithiasis, or salivary calculi, can locate in the parenchyma or duct and appear as hyperechoic spots (lines) with posterior acoustic shadowing (Fig. 2.7) on B-mode ultrasound [6]. These are most often found in the submandibular duct due to the glandular secretions [10]. Depending on the location of the calculi, whether within the duct or the glandular body, dilated salivary ducts can also present due to the obstruction [10]. If a salivary duct is obstructed, the gland becomes swollen due to acute inflammation. The location (parenchyma or a duct) of the obstructive calculi needs to be determined before beginning a treatment [6].

Sialosis Sialosis is painless bilateral swelling of the salivary glands, usually the parotid, without inflammation or neoplastic cause [19]. In ultrasound images, the gland will appear diffusely enlarged, hyperechoic, and homogeneous on a gray-scale image (Fig. 2.8) [6]. As sialosis is a chronic disease process usually associated with alcoholism, diabetes, or bulimia, the vascularity of the gland is not increased on color flow imaging [6, 19]. Ultrasound is helpful in distinguishing sialosis from more sinister masses when devising a method of treatment [20].

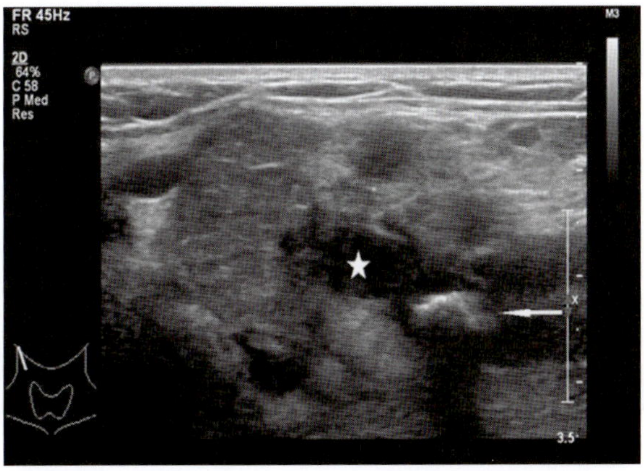

FIGURE 2.7 Hyperechoic calcification-sialothiasis (white arrow) with acoustic shadowing in the dilated submandibular duct (*) on B-mode ultrasound.

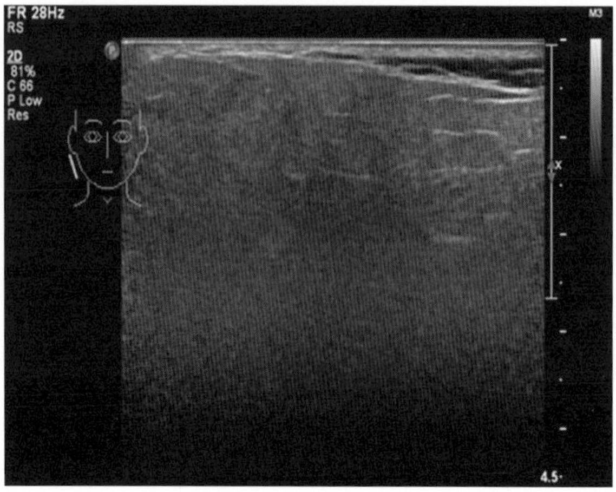

FIGURE 2.8 Visualization of parotid gland sialosis in B-mode ultrasound image.

Sjögren Syndrome Sjögren's syndrome is an autoimmune disorder caused by mononuclear cell invasion of lacrimal and salivary glands and is one of the most notable salivary gland pathologies that can be diagnosed using ultrasound [21]. A gland with Sjogren's appears inhomogeneous with hypoechoic islands due to lymphocytic infiltration and duct dilation, often presenting with increased vascularity in the affected gland (Fig. 2.9) [6, 15]. Findings are usually present in the parotid glands but may be found in all salivary glands in some cases [15]. Because the disease is associated with lymphoproliferative neoplasm, the assessment of cervical lymph nodes is required in the diagnosis and monitoring of regression and progression of the disease [6].

Benign Neoplasm **Pleomorphic adenomas** account for the majority of salivary neoplasms with a predominance in parotid and submandibular glands, appearing as hypoechoic and lobulated lesions [20]. Ultrasound imaging of pleomorphic adenomas reveals well-defined borders with posterior acoustic enhancement that can contain calcifications (Fig. 2.10). These are usually unilateral, benign, and

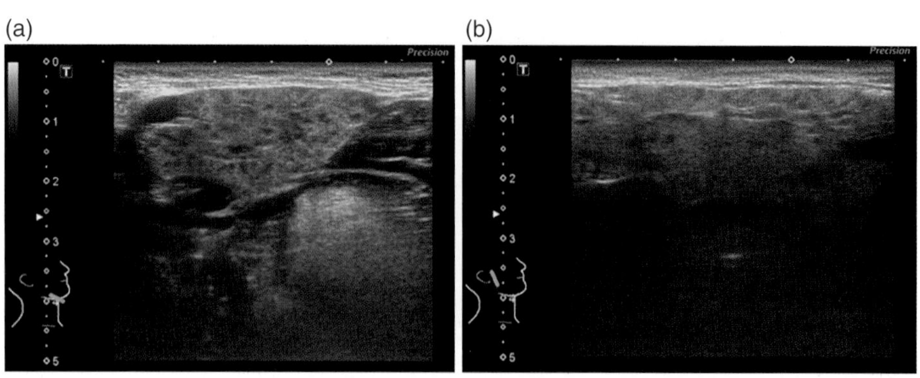

FIGURE 2.9 B-mode ultrasound image recorded from a patient with Sjogren's syndrome of the parotid gland. The affected parotid (a) and submandibular (b) glands appear inhomogeneous in echotexture.

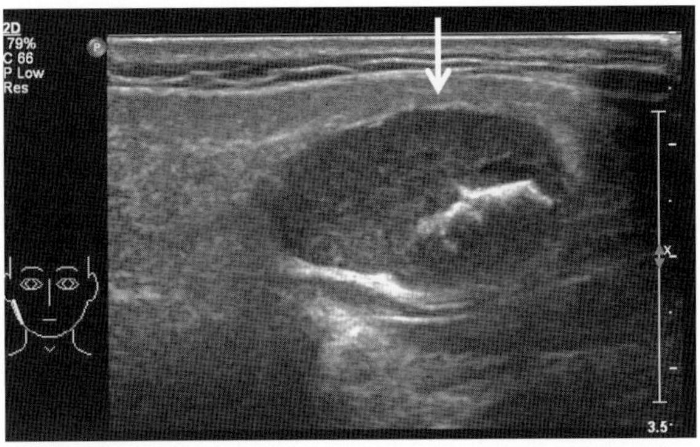

FIGURE 2.10 A pleomorphic adenoma appears well-defined lobulated borders (arrow) on B-mode ultrasound image.

painless. However, biopsy is recommended to rule out malignancy. It is important to note that some caseous mycobacterial diseases may present as hypoechoic salivary gland without central vascularity [6].

Warthin tumors appear different in homogeneity from pleomorphic adenomas on ultrasound. Pleomorphic adenomas appear more homogeneous, while Warthin tumors are heterogeneous [22]. These tumors are hypoechoic with well-defined borders but can contain more anechoic areas and show increased vascularity with an oval-shaped lesion and some characteristics of a cystic structure [6, 15, 22]. The development of these benign and painless neoplasms is associated with smoking. Biopsy is recommended to rule out malignancy or pleomorphic adenomas for managing timely treatment [22].

Malignant Neoplasms Although cytopathology is the gold standard in the diagnosis of malignant salivary gland masses, there are ultrasound imaging characteristics helpful in determining whether biopsy is necessary [15]. Unlike benign neoplasms, malignant neoplasms tend to appear as a hypoechoic mass with irregular shape and ill-defined margins [6]. Lesions may also be less mobile and tender. Submandibular glands should be assessed with a high index of suspicion as nearly 50% of lesions are malignant but may possess benign imaging features [6]. Mucoepidermoid carcinoma, acinic cell carcinoma, and adenoid cystic carcinoma are the most common malignancies of the parotid gland [15].

Other Soft Tissue Masses of the Neck In general, cysts appear as encapsulated anechoic fluid-filled masses. Sebaceous cysts may appear similar, but with less homogeneity in the fluid space. Encapsulated hypoechoic to anechoic masses with ill-defined borders and posterior acoustic enhancement are considered abscesses with hyperechoic microbubbles sometimes able to be visualized on ultrasound [6]. Diffuse inflammation that is unencapsulated indicates cellulitis [15]. Lipomas appear as a solid encapsulated mass that arises from surrounding tissue with hyperechoic horizontal lines due to their connective tissue content [15]. Fine needle aspiration is not considered diagnostic for lipomas, and therefore, diagnosis is generally made on ultrasound. Fistulas and diverticula commonly consist of hypoechoic tracts [15].

Cervical Lymph Nodes

Benign lymph nodes can be differentiated from malignant nodes using size and shape based on the long-to-short axis ratio, and internal structures and volume [23]. Malignant nodes are generally round without an echogenic hilum, while benign nodes are typically elliptical with an echogenic hilum and a central vascular flow pattern [4]. Intranodal hyperechoic calcifications can indicate metastases of a carcinoma to the lymph node [24].

Lymphoma Lymphomas (Hodgkin's or non-Hodgkin's) tend to be difficult to distinguish from other lymphadenopathies using ultrasound [25]. The affected lymph nodes can appear enlarged, hypoechoic, with defined margins, round in shape, and are often found in the upper cervical chain, submandibular region, and the posterior triangle [25]. They can also present as homogeneous or inhomogeneous and can sometimes contain echoic stripes [15]. A lymph node with lymphoma commonly appears greater than 4 cm in diameter, hypoechoic with loss of the echogenic hilum, showing some peripheral vascularity, and affecting multiple or groups of lymph nodes (Fig. 2.11) [15, 26]. A lymph node with an increase in vascularity on color flow imaging suggests a malignant lymph node [15].

Metastatic Lymphadenopathy Ultrasound permits detection of suspicious lymph nodes in early stage of the disease [27]. Ultrasound characteristics of metastatic lymphadenopathy are sometimes similar to that in lymphomas, such as vascularity, size, shape, margins, and echogenicity (Fig. 2.12). Anechoic areas are especially suspicious as they may suggest necrosis [15]. Metastatic lymph nodes may also have borders that appear sharp due to tumor infiltration within the node or ill-defined, indicating tumor invasion [25]. In addition, cervical lymphadenopathy is not uncommon in patients with thyroid carcinoma, lung cancer, and other malignancies in the chest, head, and neck [11].

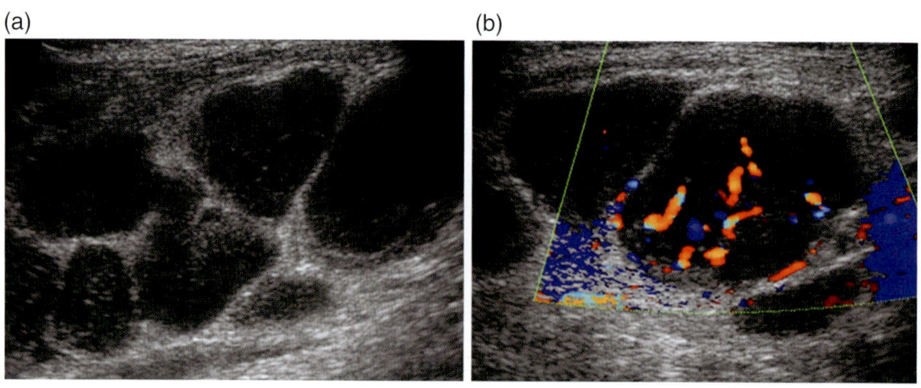

FIGURE 2.11 B-mode (a) and color flow (b) images of cervical lymph nodes from a patient with diffuse large B-cell lymphoma. Multiple cervical lymph nodes appear round-shaped, hypoechoic, hypervascular, and absence of an echogenic central hilum.

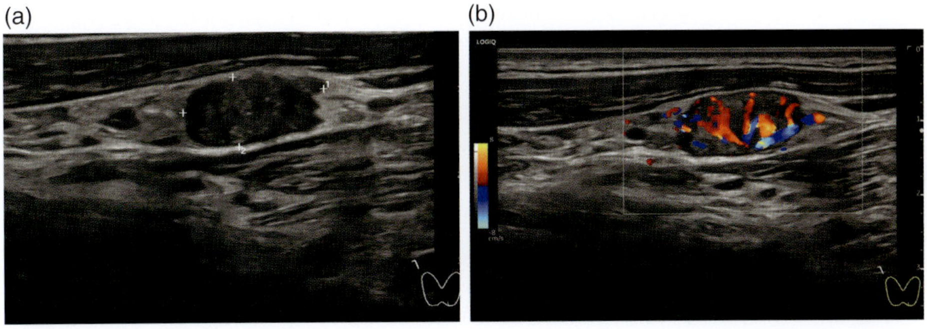

FIGURE 2.12 B-mode (a) and color flow (b) images of metastatic cervical lymphadenopathy from a patient with papillary thyroid carcinoma. The cervical lymph node metastasis presents an irregular shape, unclear margins, the absence of the normal hilum, hypoechogenicity, microcalcifications, and abnormal mixed vascularity.

Summary

With the proper technique and an understanding of the anatomy of the head and neck, ultrasound is a useful tool to readily diagnose pathology and monitor the treatment effects. Ultrasound can be utilized in the emergency department or in a clinical setting when assessing salivary glands, cervical lymph nodes, and soft tissue lesions in the neck, therefore helping to prevent unnecessary invasive procedures and ultimately minimizing patient discomfort. Ultrasound as a point-of-care tool is continuing to expand its application for assisting physicians in the standard of patient care worldwide.

Review Questions

1. Which vascular structures may run across the submandibular gland?
   - **a.** Lingual artery and vein
   - **b.** Facial artery and vein
   - **c.** Maxillary artery and vein
   - **d.** External carotid artery
2. Upon feeling a patient's neck for lymph nodes, you feel a swollen node along the internal jugular vein just inferior to the base of the skull. Which level of lymph nodes is this included in?
   - **a.** Level I
   - **b.** Level II
   - **c.** Level III
   - **d.** Level V
3. A patient comes in with a tender submandibular mass. Upon ultrasound scanning, you find a solid hypoechoic mass with an irregular shape, ill-defined margins, and hypervascularity. Is this lesion more likely to be benign or malignant?
   - **a.** Malignant tumor
   - **b.** Benign tumor
   - **c.** Hemagioma
   - **d.** Lipoma

4. The submandibular gland appears normal in size with minimal vascularity. The gland is hypoechoic and inhomogeneous. Does this presentation more likely represent acute or chronic inflammation?
   a. Acute
   b. Chronic
   c. No inflammation
   d. Cannot be determined
5. A patient presents with the complaint of reduction in facial expression after surgery to the cheek. The patient cannot remember the name of the surgery performed. What structure was the surgery most likely performed on, and what other anatomic structure was concurrently damaged?
   a. Submandibular gland, Mandibular branch of Trigeminal n. (CN V_3)
   b. Submandibular gland, Facial n. (CN VII)
   c. Parotid gland, Mandibular branch of Trigeminal n. (CN V_3)
   d. Parotid gland, Facial nerve (CN VII)
6. A patient, who has been a heavy smoker for 40 years, presents with a mass at the angle of the mandible. The mass is hypoechoic and well defined with anechoic areas and channels on ultrasound. What is the likely pathology?
   a. Pleomorphic Adenoma, benign
   b. Warthin tumor, benign
   c. Mucoepidermoid carcinoma, malignant
   d. Abscess, benign
7. How do you distinguish cellulitis from an abscess on ultrasound?
   a. Cellulitis is an encapsulated, noncompressible mass, while abscesses appear as diffuse, unencapsulated inflammation
   b. Cellulitis is hypoechoic with well-defined borders, while abscesses are hyperechoic with greater homogeneity
   c. Cellulitis appears hyperechoic with horizontal lines throughout due to connective tissue, while abscesses are diffuse loculations with well-defined borders
   d. Cellulitis appears as diffuse loculations distributed throughout tissue, that is not localized, while an abscess is localized and tends to be liquefied

Correct answers: 1. b; 2. b; 3. a; 4. b; 5. d; 6. b; 7. d.

References

1. Sniezek J. Head and neck ultrasound: why now? *Otolaryngol Clin N Am* 2010; 43: 1143–1147.
2. Prativadi R, Dahiya N, Kamaya A, Bhatt S. Chapter 5 ultrasound characteristics of benign vs malignant cervical lymph nodes. *Semin Ultrasound CT MRI* 2020; 38: 506–515.
3. Wagner J, Alleman A. Ultrasonography of cervical lymph nodes. *Radiol Clin North Am* 2019; 57: 485–500.
4. American Institute of Ultrasound in Medicine. AIUM practice guideline for the performance of ultrasound examinations of the head and neck. *J Ultrasound Med* 2014; 33: 366–382.
5. Moore KL, Dalley AF, Agur AMR. Clinically oriented anatomy. 7th ed. Philadelphia, PA: Lippincott Williams & Wilkins, 2014.

6. Bialek EJ, Jakubowski W, Zajkowski P, et al. US of the major salivary glands: anatomy and spatial relationships, pathologic conditions, and pitfalls. *Radiographics* 2006; 26(3): 745–763.
7. Agarwal AK, Kanekar SG. Submandibular and sublingual spaces: diagnostic imaging and evaluation. *Otolaryngol Clin N Am* 2012; 45: 1311–1323.
8. Netter FH. Atlas of human anatomy. 5th ed. Philadelphia, PA: Saunders/Elsevier, 2011.
9. Ahuja AT and Ying M. Pictorial Essay: Sonographic evaluation of cervical lymph nodes. AJR 2005; 184 (5): 1691–1699. doi.org/10.2214/ajr.184.5.01841691.
10. Frank SJ, Koenigsberg T, Gutman D, Koenigsberg M. Applications of 3-dimensional ultrasonography in the neck, excluding the thyroid. *J Ultrasound Med* 2018; 37: 1791–1806.
11. American Institute of Ultrasound in Medicine. AIUM-ACR-SPR-SRU practice parameter for the performance and interpretation of a diagnostic ultrasound examination of the extracranial head and neck. *J Ultrasound Med* 2018; 37: E6–E12.
12. Gregoire V, Ang K, Budach W, et al. Delineation of the neck node levels for head and neck tumors: a 2013 update. DAHANCA, EORTC, HKNPCSG, NCIC CTG, NCRI, RTOG, TROG consensus guidelines. *Radiother Oncol* 2014; 110: 172–181.
13. Hartl D, Breuskin I, Mirghani H, et al. Anatomic variability of the upper mediastinal lymph node level VII. *World J Surg* 2016; 40: 1899–1903.
14. Choi JY, Choi YS, Park YH, at al. Experience and analysis of level VII cervical lymph node metastases in patients with papillary thyroid carcinoma. *J Korean Surg Soc* 2011; 80(5): 307–312.
15. Sofferman RA. Interpretation of ultrasound. *Ultrasound Clinics* 2012; 7(2): 167–190.
16. Jayapal N, Ram SM, Murthy V, et al. Differentiation between benign and metastatic cervical lymph nodes using ultrasound. *J Pharm Bioallied Sci* 2019; 11(6): 338–346.
17. Acu L, Ozhan Oktar S, Acu R, et al. Value of ultrasound elastography in the differential diagnosis of cervical lymph nodes. *J Ultrasound Med* 2016; 35: 2491–2499.
18. Misra D, Panjwani S, Rai S, et al. Diagnostic efficacy of color Doppler ultrasound in evaluation of cervical lymphadenopathy. *Dent Res J* 2016; 13(3): 217–224.
19. Badarinza M, Serban O, Maghear L, et al. Multimodal ultrasound investigation (grey scale, Doppler, and 2D-SWE) of salivary and lacrimal glands in healthy people and patients with diabetes mellitus and/or obesity, with or without sialosis. *Med Ultrasound* 2019; 21(3): 257–264.
20. Kato H, Kawaguchi M, Ando T, et al. Pleomorphic adenoma of salivary glands: common and uncommon CT and MR imaging features. *Jpn J Radiol* 2018; 36: 463–471.
21. Jonsson R, Brokstad KA, Jonsson MV, et al. Current concepts on Sjogren's syndrome – classification criteria and biomarkers. *Eur J Oral Sci* 2018; 126: 37–48.
22. Matsuda E, Fukuhara T, Donishi R, et al. Usefulness of a novel ultrasonographic classification based on anechoic area patterns for differentiating Warthin tumors from pleomorphic adenomas of the parotid gland. *Yonago Acta Med* 2017; 60(4): 220–226.
23. Nishio N, Fujimoto Y, Hiramatsu M, et al. Diagnosis of cervical lymph node metastases in head and neck cancer with ultrasonic measurement of lymph node volume. *Auris Nasus Larynx* 2019; 46: 889–895.
24. Ying M, Bhatia KS, Lee YP, et al. Review of ultrasonography of malignant neck nodes: greyscale, Doppler, contrast enhancement and elastography. *Cancer Imaging* 2014; 13(4): 658–669.
25. Ahuja AT, Ying M, Antonio G, et al. Ultrasound of malignant cervical lymph nodes. *Cancer Imaging* 2008; 8(1): 48–56.
26. Young Chae S, Jung HN, Inseon R, Suh S. Differentiating cervical metastatic lymphadenopathy and lymphoma by shear wave elastography. *Sci Rep* 2019; 9: 12396.
27. Mcqueen AS, Bhatia KS. Head and neck ultrasound: technical advances, novel applications and the role of elastography. *Clin Radiol* 2018; 73: 81–93.

CHAPTER 3

Chest and Lung

Courtney Shill Russell[1], Telyn Peterson[1], and Ming-Bo Zhang[2]
[1] Rocky Vista University, College of Osteopathic Medicine, Ivins, Utah, USA
[2] Department of Ultrasound, the First Medical Center, General Hospital of PLA, Beijing, China

Lung Ultrasound

Introduction

As an imaging modality, ultrasonography can provide robust information to assist in the diagnosis and treatment of several clinically relevant diseases of the chest and lung. The successful use of point-of-care ultrasound (POCUS) to aid in the diagnosis of pleural effusion, peripheral lung masses, pneumonia, and pulmonary edema has been well established [1–4].

Due to the limitation of ultrasound to image tissues/organs through air, the assessment of the deep lung was considered neglected as an imaging modality for evaluation of pulmonary parenchyma compared to X-ray and CT. Although ultrasound cannot directly visualize structures that are not abutting the pleural line, the value of ultrasound for the evaluation of pulmonary pathologies using patterns of ultrasound artifact has been recognized in recent years. POCUS as a time-effective imaging strategy has been developed to image lung and pleural pathologies in clinical patient care [1–4].

Ultrasound Techniques

Lung ultrasound can be used to diagnose various conditions as well as guide procedures to prevent complications, such as pneumothorax. Ultrasonography is more sensitive than radiography at differentiating between fluid and consolidation [5]. Benefits also include radiation-free, portability, repeatability, and low costs [5, 6].

Scanning Protocol

A linear probe or a phased array probe with 3.5–5.0 MHz is ideal for chest and pleural ultrasonography. The penetration is sufficient to scan the thoracic wall and pleural cavity [5]. An intercostal approach is ideal to image the heart, lung, and pleural

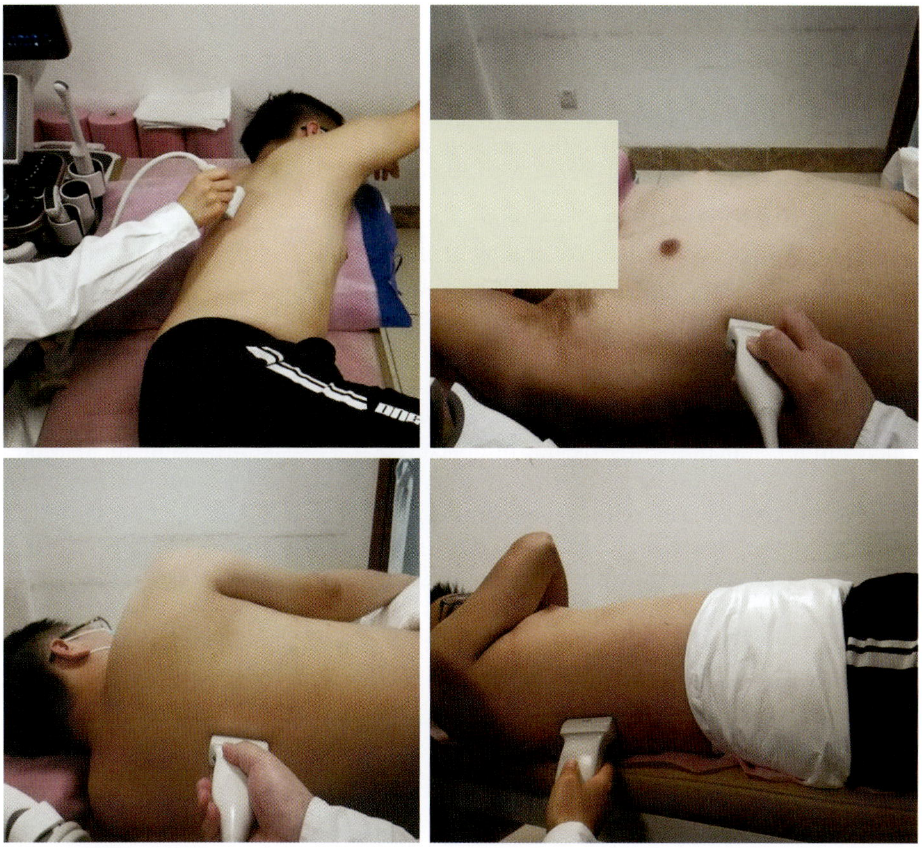

FIGURE 3.1 Images show alternative positions for scanning the chest wall and lungs in unstable patients.

cavity. A higher frequency linear probe (7.5–10 MHz) can be used for visualizing the pleura and chest wall in pediatrics and imaging superficial structures (subcutaneous tissue and chest wall muscle) [7].

Patient Position

The position of the patient is determined by the clinical condition of the patient. For imaging the thoracic cavity in stable patients, the patient can be seated in the upright position with elbows in front resting on a table or countertop. This allows free fluid to rest at the bottom of the thoracic cavity and access to scan the anterior, lateral, and posterior chest wall [5, 7]. There are variations for patients who cannot sit in the upright position. Scanning can be done in the supine or semi-supine position. While scanning in the supine or semi-supine position, the patient's ipsilateral arm should be adducted across the chest toward the contralateral shoulder [5]. This position will give access to the ipsilateral anterior and lateral chest wall. Another position is moving the patient in the full lateral decubitus position with the desired hemithorax to be scanned in the upright position (Fig. 3.1) [5].

Important Ultrasound Artifacts in Lung Scan

Ultrasound artifacts play an important role in the diagnosis of lung and pleura pathology in the developed protocols. The spatial compounding setting on the scanner should be turned off to preserve the artifacts when performing lung ultrasound [8].

Pleural Line in B-mode A smooth, well-defined, straight hyperechoic line is associated with the interfacing of the pleurae. The pleural line has the appearance of marching ants – this is known as lung sliding following inspiration and expiration in real-time B-mode ultrasound. The absence of these lines may be indicative of pathology, such as pneumothorax [9].

Pleural Line in M-Mode With respiration, the lung will create a grainy image under subcutaneous tissue, often called the "seashore" sign in M-Mode (Fig. 3.2). The motion of the pleura creates artifact from the pleural line sliding and appears like a beach with waves coming to the shore. When the lungs' motion and pleural sliding are undetectable with M-mode ultrasound, the sandy beach is replaced with hyperechoic, horizontal, and straight lines known as the "Barcode" sign (Fig. 3.2). The "Barcode" sign suggests a pneumothorax as there is no lung sliding between the visceral and parietal pleura, which can be imaged with ultrasound due to air [9, 10].

A-Lines A reverberation artifact of smooth, equidistant hyperechoic lines that occur when the probe is perpendicular to the pleura (Fig. 3.3). These lines are separated by the thickness of the subcutaneous tissue, which may vary depending on

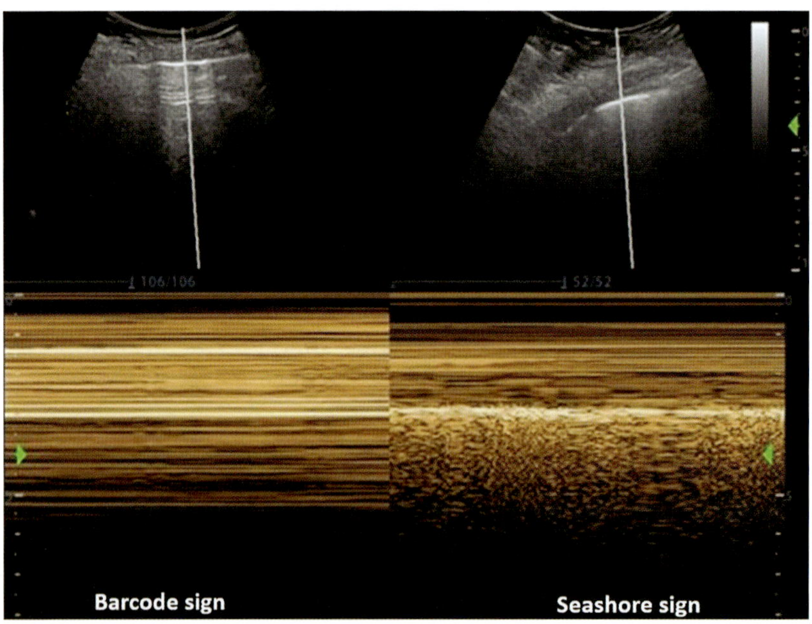

FIGURE 3.2 M-mode ultrasound displays "Seashore" sign in normal pleura or "Barcode" sign in the patient with pneumothorax.

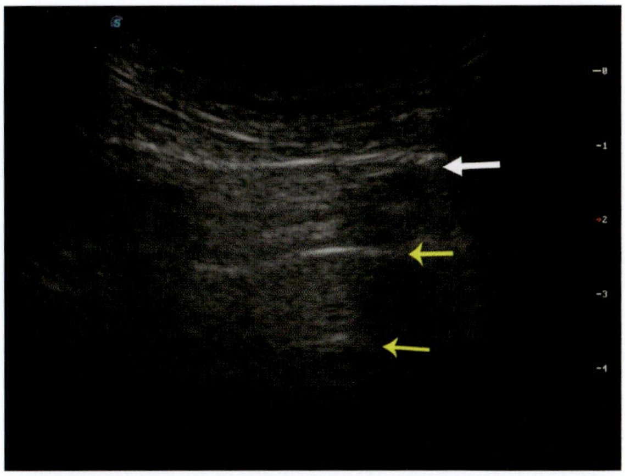

FIGURE 3.3 B-mode lung image shows the pleural line (white arrow) and A-lines (yellow arrows).

ultrasound machine settings. A-lines are present in healthy individuals and may also appear in pneumothorax [9, 10].

B-Lines Normal lung sliding has comet tail artifacts that arise from the pleural line and become extinguishable as they enter a normal air-filled lung. Extension of these comet tail artifacts appears as the lung becomes more fluid-filled in a variety of disease processes that replace the normal air/fluid ratios in a normal lung. These pathologic B-lines appear as laser-like vertical hyperechoic reverberation artifacts that arise from the pleural line, extend to the bottom of the screen without fading, and move synchronously with lung sliding following breathing (Fig. 3.4). B-lines may be present in healthy individuals, but they will be limited to less than three in a visualized area. The presence of B-lines will erase A-lines and is indicative of pathological processes, especially interstitial edema. B-lines will be absent in pneumothorax [1, 4].

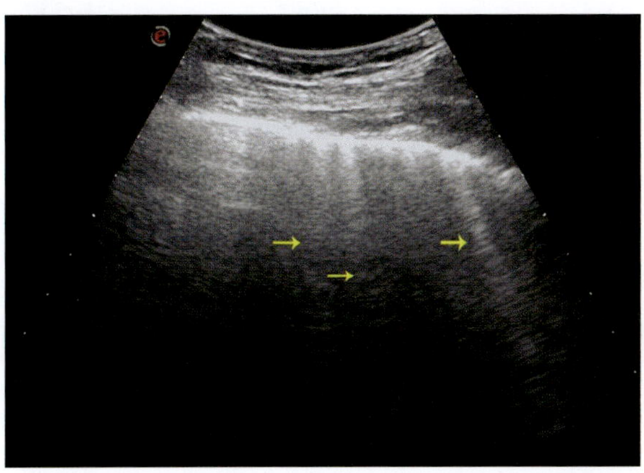

FIGURE 3.4 B-mode image shows B-lines (yellow arrows).

Z-Lines Short, broad, ill-defined vertical comet tail artifacts arising from the pleural line but do not extend to the bottom of the screen and fade by 2–4 cm. They differ from B-lines because they do not erase A-lines or move with respiration.

Ultrasound-Related Anatomy

Ultrasound can provide 2D images of human tissues/organs. Its optimal imaging depth depends on the scanning frequency. The higher the frequency, the higher the resolution and the higher tissue attenuation to the ultrasound waves, the shallower the depth of the image [11]. The top of the ultrasound image (near field) correlates with the most superficial interface, which is close to the transducer. Understanding the relation between ultrasound and anatomy above the pleural space and thoracic cavity is crucial in performing chest and lung ultrasound.

The following sections outline common chest and lung pathologies based on the location from superficial to deep tissues/structures on ultrasound images.

Epidermis, Dermis, and Subcutaneous Tissue

A higher frequency transducer is necessary to examine these superficial structures in the body. Epidermis and dermis are the most superficial hyperechoic structures displayed at the top of the ultrasound image; this layer extends 1–3 mm depending on the body habitus of the person undergoing ultrasound examination (Fig. 3.5) [12]. Subcutaneous adipose is considerably more hypoechoic than surrounding muscles, fascia, and dermal layers, and its layers are easily identifiable when compressed by the transducer. Adipose tissue, as mentioned in other chapters, is slightly more hyperechoic than liquid [13].

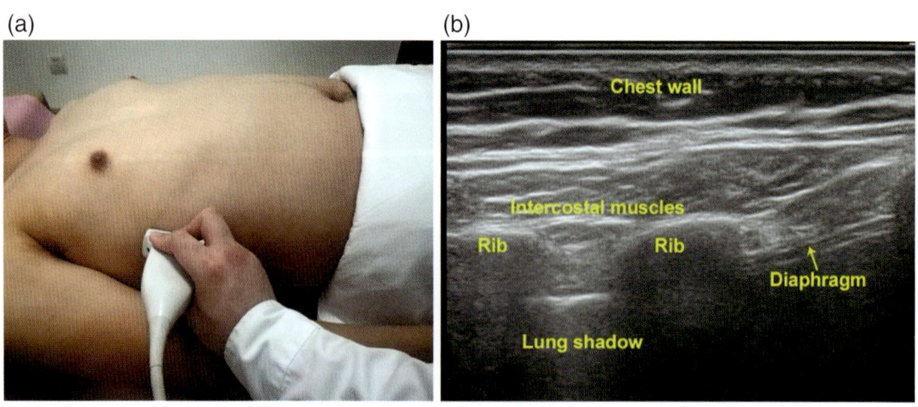

FIGURE 3.5 (a) The image shows that the transducer is placed intercostally through the 9th intercostal space in the anterior axillary line (a vertical line through the anterior axillary wrinkle wall). (b) B-mode image shows the corresponding tissues (skin, chest wall, intercostal muscle, ribs, and lung) along the direction of the sound beam.

Lymph Nodes Often, lymph nodes are not palpable, especially lymph nodes located in the chest. However, superficial lymph nodes can be assessed with ultrasound. Benign lymph nodes typically have an oval shape with a smooth, well-defined margin. Lymph nodes that are also lobulated, hyperechoic, and uniformly thin (cortex measuring 3 mm or less) have a high negative predictive value of metastasis [14]. Characteristics indicative of malignancy include round shape, focal cortical thickness >3 mm, and absence of a fatty hilum [15].

Muscle The primary feature of chest musculature in the long axis on imaging is parallel, hypoechoic muscle fibers separated by hyperechoic striation bands [16]. Their attachments and involvement with the surrounding structures are variable, but knowing their structure and function plays an important role in the identification of any pathology associated with respiratory function and daily activities.

Diaphragm The diaphragm is the central muscle of respiration, and its dysfunction can be life-threatening [17]. It also serves as a passageway for the great vessels between the chest and abdomen, as well as conducting nervous and lymphatic flow through one of its three main hiatuses. On ultrasound, it can be assessed from a subxiphoid view with the transducer pointed upwards, in a transverse view with the 5th intercostal space on the right mid-clavicular line during maximum exhalation (Fig. 3.6).

Two methods are typically used to assess the diaphragm: Evaluation of the thickness of the diaphragm during inspiration and the analysis of dome excursion with M-mode approach [18]. Markedly thinned (<2.3 mm for men, 1.7 mm for women) right hemidiaphragm and decreased right hemidiaphragm excursion (<19 mm) are suggestive of muscle wasting associated with various forms of muscular dystrophy [15, 16], prolonged mechanical ventilation [17], and neuromuscular disorders [19–22].

Assessing excursion of the diaphragm is done from the mid-clavicular subcostal view. A 3–5 MHz transducer can be used to obtain views through either the hepatic window (right side is generally easier to image) or the splenic window (left side) (Fig. 3.7). On M-mode image, the pleural line should be a hyperechogenic line during the respiratory cycle. An excursion of >25 mm during normal quiet breathing or diaphragmatic thickening on inhalation of >30% has been shown to increase a

(a) (b)

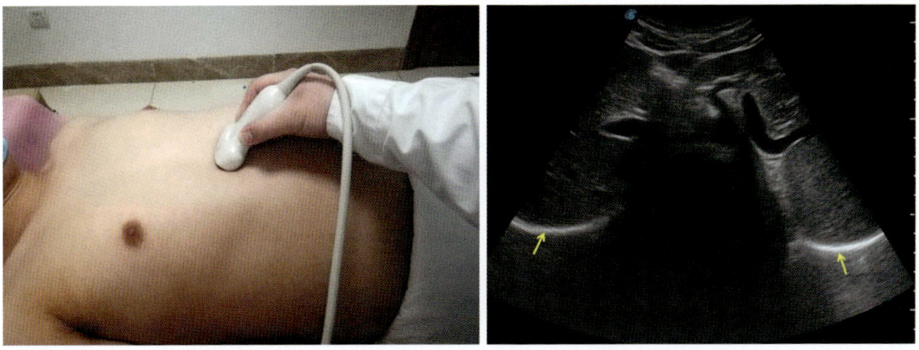

FIGURE 3.6 (a) Demonstrates the transducer placement for the subxiphoid view of the diaphragm. (b) is a B-mode ultrasound image showing both hemidiaphragms (yellow arrows) simultaneously through the subxiphoid view.

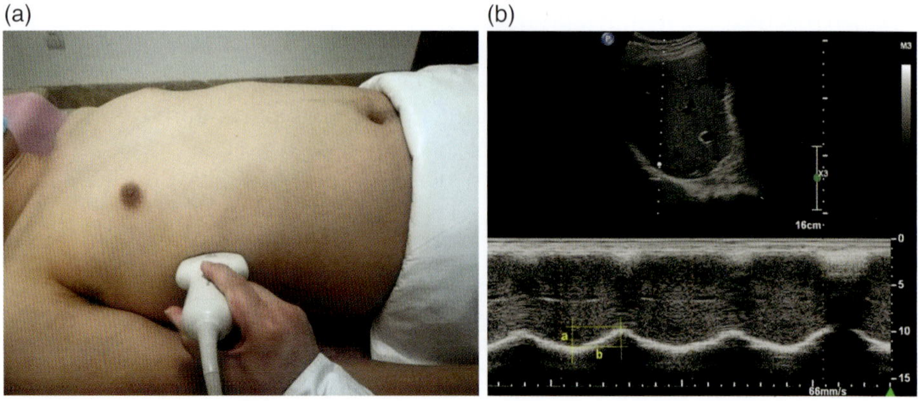

FIGURE 3.7 (a) Demonstrates the transducer placement. (b) is a M-mode image of diaphragm motion. "a" represents the amplitude of excursion during deep breathing, and "b" represents the time frame used for diaphragm contraction, which is used to calculate the velocity of the diaphragm movement. Velocity = "a" cm/"b" seconds.

ventilated patient's chance of success on a spontaneous breathing trial after being on a mechanical ventilator [23, 24].

Bone and Cartilage Bone and ribs can be recognized easily by their periosteal hyperechogenic qualities along with posterior shadowing. Cartilage, on the other hand, is often hypoechoic due to its high-water content [25]. Specific evaluation of bone and cartilage will be further discussed in the dedicated section about rib fractures.

Tendons/Ligaments Tendons and ligaments are hyperechoic and differ from muscle by anatomical location, tissue echogenicity, and character of anisotropy [26]. Anisotropy has a stronger tendency for nerves and tendons to appear more hypoechoic than they really are when the transducer is not perpendicular to the nerve or tendon, compared to muscles. This artifact tends to interpret a false positive for tears or rupture. Tendons tend to be more echogenic and densely striated than muscles when the transducer is perpendicular to tissues [27, 28].

Pleura: Under normal conditions, it is unusual to see the details of the pleura in conventional B-mode ultrasound. In pathological situations, such as pleural effusion, pleura appear clearly.

Common Pathologies

Pneumothorax

A pneumothorax occurs when air enters the pleural space. As air enters, the visceral pleura of the lung separates from the parietal pleura inside the lung cavity, resulting in complete or partial atelectasis, or lung collapse [29, 30]. Upon physical exam, a pneumothorax will present with decreased or absent lung sounds in that area. Causes of a pneumothorax include traumatic, iatrogenic, primary spontaneous, and secondary spontaneous.

B-mode ultrasound is best used to rule out the presence of a pneumothorax by observing lung sliding, which is present in healthy individuals [10]. The probe of choice is a high-frequency linear probe. To visualize the pneumothorax, the image depth is commonly set to about 4 cm. The image depth can be adjusted for pediatrics and patients with obesity [31].

Start with the patient supine, and the probe is placed at the mid-clavicular line on the right side or anterior axillary line on the left side. Beginning at the third or fourth intercostal space is ideal [31].

A "lung pulse" is an artifact caused by the heartbeat that, when present, can verify that the lung pleura are intact. A "lung pulse" will be identified on M-mode as a pulse that aligns with the electrocardiogram. The presence of the "seashore sign", B-lines, and the "lung pulse" is not visualized in patients with pneumothorax [10].

Lung sliding on B-mode real-time ultrasound is absent in patients with pneumothorax. A typical "Barcode sign" in M-mode is observed in patients with pneumothorax (Fig. 3.2). There will be a point where lung sliding is present and where it is not. This point can be identified with ultrasound and is called the "lung point." This is a unique feature of a pneumothorax and can be used to confirm the diagnosis [10]. Using the borders of the lung identified by the "lung point," the affected region of the pneumothorax can be estimated [31].

Hydrothorax (Pleural Effusion)

Hydrothorax is commonly caused by congestive heart failure (CHF), renal failure, and low-protein states. Some patients with mild hydrothorax are completely asymptomatic [32].

As mentioned previously, to evaluate for a pleural effusion, the patient is supine if the patient is unstable (or trauma) or upright position if the patient tolerates. Using a microconvex, phased-array, or convex transducer, scan the posterior axillary line, just above the splenic and hepatic windows. With a normal lung, a reflection of the spleen or liver (depending on your window) will be visible as a mirror image artifact above the diaphragm. Anechoic appearance commonly indicates simple pleural effusion. Fluid with internal fine echoes may present inflammatory or hemorrhagic hydrothorax (Fig. 3.8). A diagnostic thoracentesis can help to determine the histology analysis of the pleural effusion.

Empyema

Empyema, or pyothorax, is a type of infected pleural effusion that is potentially life-threatening. It is typically loculated and can mimic a peripheral pulmonary abscess; however, computer tomography is helpful to differentiate. On thoracic ultrasound, the appearance of empyema depends on the composition of the collection (Fig. 3.9) [33].

Hemothorax

Hemothorax is the collection of blood within the pleural cavity in patients with trauma. Hemothorax is easily identified with a chest evaluation for pleural fluid in patients with a high suspicion of trauma (Fig. 3.10). The effectiveness of thoracic

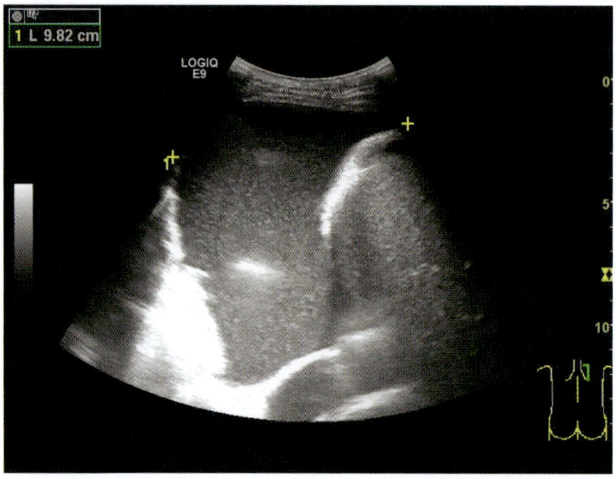

FIGURE 3.8 A 65-year-old male suffered from dyspnea and fever. B-mode ultrasound showed a large amount of right hydrothorax containing internal fine echoes. Hydrothorax with infection was confirmed as yellow turbid liquid by diagnostic thoracentesis.

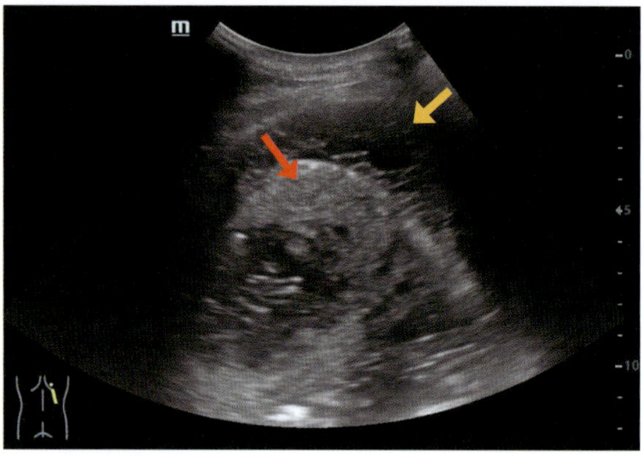

FIGURE 3.9 A 62-year-old male patient showing loculated pyothorax (yellow arrow) and pulmonary consolidation (red arrow).

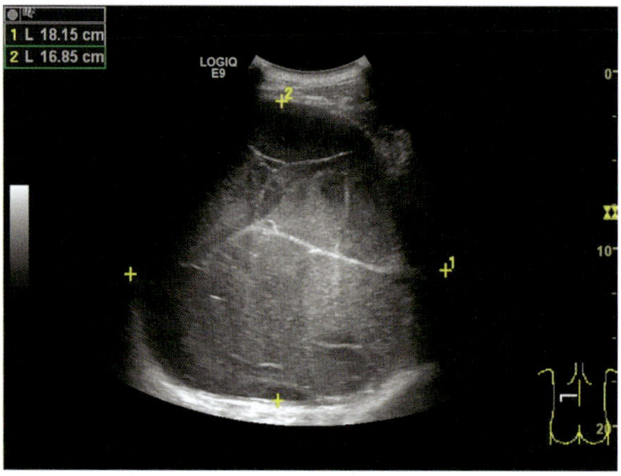

FIGURE 3.10 A 55-year-old male suffered from shortness of breath after a blunt trauma. Ultrasound examination showed a large amount of hypoechoic area in the left thorax, with the longitudinal diameter of 20.6 cm, the anteroposterior diameter of 16.9 cm, and the transverse diameter of 18.2 cm. It was confirmed as a hemothorax by thoracentesis.

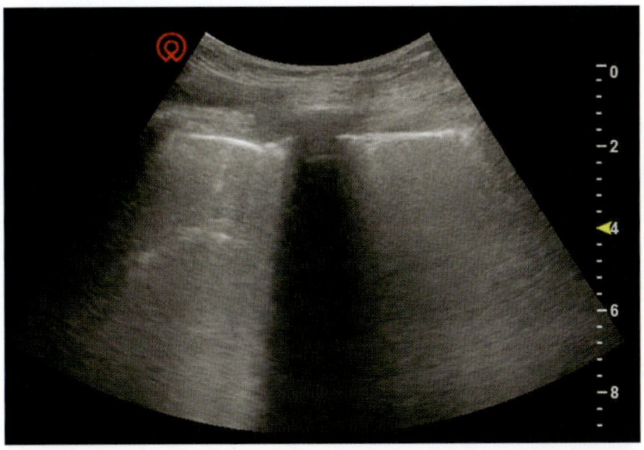

FIGURE 3.11 A 74-year-old male suffered from both lung infections. B-mode ultrasound showed heterogeneous distribution of B-lines and pleural line modifications.

ultrasound has been found to be similar to chest radiography in the detection of hemothorax [34]. It is common to note the coexistence of hemothorax and pneumothorax in trauma patients [35].

Pulmonary Edema

Bedside Lung Ultrasound in Emergency (BLUE) is the most popular lung-specific protocol to explore the immediate diagnosis of acute respiratory failure. Pulmonary edema, pulmonary embolism, pneumonia, chronic obstructive pulmonary disease (COPD), asthma, and pneumothorax yield specific profiles. These applications require the mastery of 10 signs indicating normal lung surface (bat sign, lung sliding, A-lines), pleural effusions (quad and sinusoid sign), lung consolidations (fractal and tissue-like sign), interstitial syndrome (lung rockets), and pneumothorax (stratosphere sign and the lung point). These signs have been assessed in adults, with diagnostic accuracies ranging from 90% to 100%, allowing consideration of ultrasound as a reasonable bedside gold standard [36].

Pulmonary edema can be divided into cardiogenic pulmonary edema and non-cardiogenic pulmonary edema. Sonographic appearance of cardiogenic pulmonary edema is characterized by homogeneous distribution of B-lines. Non-cardiogenic pulmonary edema shows heterogeneous distribution of B-lines with spared areas, pleural line modifications (increase in the thickness of pleural line), and lung consolidations (Fig. 3.11) [37].

Special Cases

Chest Wall Mass

Ultrasound is sensitive to localize chest wall mass and is most beneficial to assess its echotexture (cystic or solid) and guide biopsy of chest wall lesions [38, 39].

Lipomas are fat-containing masses that can be seen on the chest wall as a lobular hyperechoic mass (Fig. 3.12) without vascularization [39]. They are typically diagnosed with CT or T1-weighted MRI [39]. Uncommon malignant

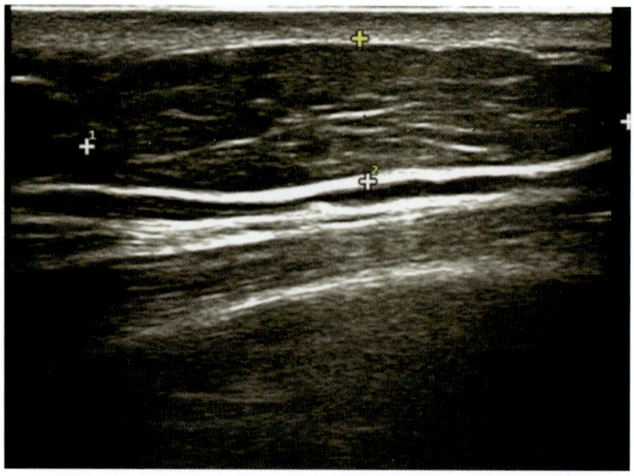

FIGURE 3.12 B-mode ultrasound image shows a chest wall lipoma (outlined by two pairs of "+").

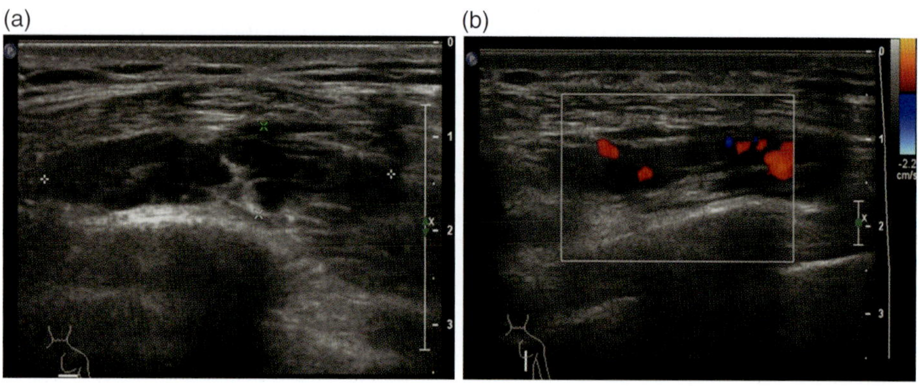

FIGURE 3.13 **(a, b)** A chest wall hemangioma (outlined by two pairs of "+") appears on B-mode image (a) and color flow imaging (b).

tumors such as rhabdomyoma or leiomyosarcoma can be seen as hypoechoic tumors invading the chest wall [40].

Hemangiomas are benign neoplasms that originate from the vasculature. Hemangiomas appear as multiple anechoic compressible lesions on B-mode ultrasound image and slow blood flow signals on color flow imaging (Fig. 3.13) [39].

Trauma-Rib Fractures

Blunt injuries to the chest account for nearly 25% of all trauma-related deaths in the United States [41]. Ultrasound is effective to identify rib fractures (Fig. 3.14); however, it doesn't improve the detection rate of fractures and may be too painful to examine the patient's thoracic wall over a suspected fracture [42, 43]. The real value of chest ultrasound over rib fractures is to assess complications secondary to the rib fracture, such as chest wall hematomas, pneumothorax, pleural effusion, and hemothorax [44].

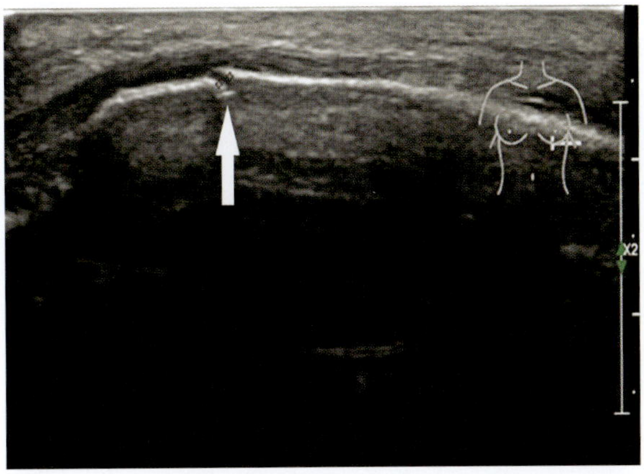

FIGURE 3.14 An 88-year-old female presented with chest trauma. US examination showed that her seventh rib cortex was discontinued with a gap of about 1.0 mm (white arrow), and the surface was slightly displaced. A rib fracture was then confirmed using X-ray.

Chest and Lung Ultrasound in Neonates

It is suggested that ultrasonography could be used in conjunction with X-ray in the diagnosis and monitoring of chest and lung diseases in neonates. When scanning neonates, a higher-frequency linear probe is selected to produce high-quality images due to their thin chest walls (Fig. 3.15). The neonate can be positioned supine, lateral, or prone [45].

Respiratory distress syndrome (RDS) is typically due to underdeveloped lungs in preterm neonates. Lack of pulmonary surfactant plays a major role in developing RDS. RDS occurs hours following birth, and patients require ventilation. On B-mode

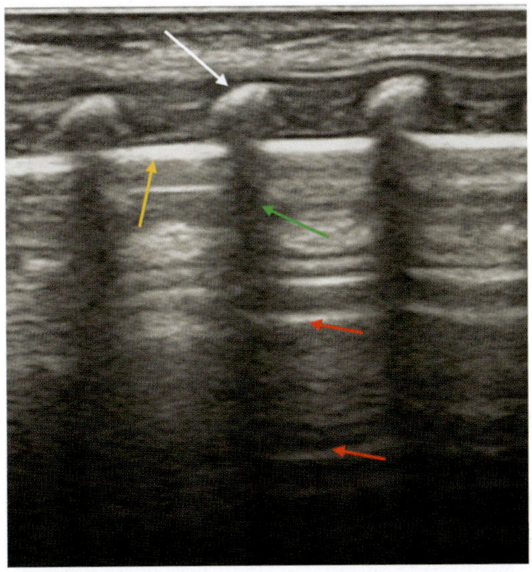

FIGURE 3.15 Normal neonatal lung on B-mode ultrasound image (yellow arrow points to pleura line, red arrows point to A-lines, white arrow points to rib, green arrow points to acoustic shadow behind the rib).

(a) (b)

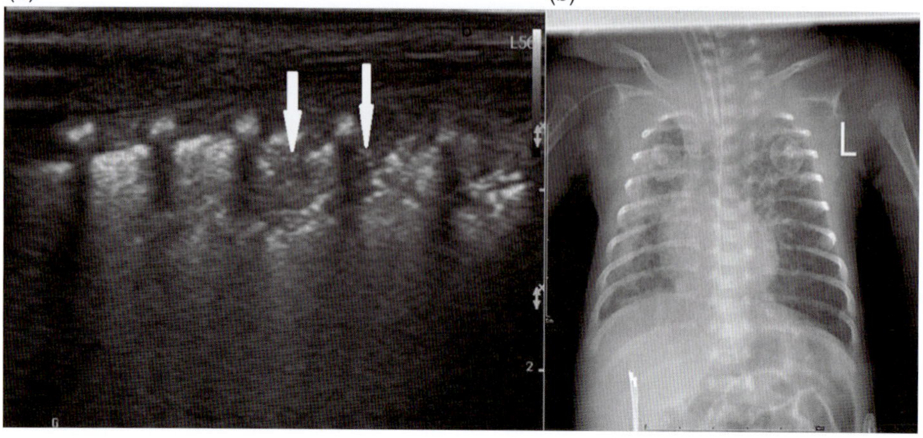

FIGURE 3.16 **(a, b)** A preterm neonate with a gestational age of 25 weeks was diagnosed with neonatal apnea, neonatal respiratory distress syndrome (RDS), and neonatal pneumonia. Lung ultrasound (a) shows pulmonary consolidation (white arrows) and compact B-lines. Chest X-ray (b) shows consolidations of the lungs (L, left).

images, the lungs will appear hyperechoic, and B-lines are compact [45]. Alveolar collapse is common in RDS and can be seen as multiple consolidations (Fig. 3.16) [46].

Transient tachypnea of newborns (TTN) is another common cause of respiratory distress in neonates. This is caused by delayed fluid clearance in neonatal lungs. Cesarean section and preterm infants are at higher risk of developing TTN. Many neonates with TTN will be in mild distress at birth, which improves significantly after 24 hours. Compact B-lines primarily appear in the inferior lung fields due to pulmonary edema and can be visualized in the superior lung fields in severe cases [45].

Pneumonia can be fatal, presenting with neonatal respiratory distress like TTN and RDS that are caused by a variety of pathogens. Pneumonia appears as irregular margins surrounded by B-lines, no lung sliding or pleural line on B-mode ultrasound [44]. Air bronchograms may be useful to assess bronchial patency, which makes atelectasis less likely [47–49].

Atelectasis in neonates can be caused by airway obstruction, compression of parenchyma, or increased surface tension. Chest radiography and CT provide the standard for diagnosing atelectasis, but there is some evidence that ultrasound can aid in the diagnosis. Lung consolidation will be present with defined borders, abnormal pleural B-lines (an increase in the number of B-lines), and possible absence of lung sliding [45].

Summary

Ultrasound, with its advantages of high availability, portability, accuracy, no radiation exposure, and low cost, overcomes its limitations (poor penetration into air-filled lungs) to diagnose chest and pleural diseases, especially for patients in critical care and emergency rooms. Its development has the potential to be used in rural areas and developing countries where other imaging modalities (e.g. CT and X-ray) are not available.

Review Questions

1. A 25-year-old male presents to your neurology office with a complaint of clumsiness and progressive weakness in his upper and lower limbs for the last 2 years. He denies any trauma. His family history is significant for a cousin who has amyotrophic lateral sclerosis (ALS). He has drool down his lip as he talks, and his speech is slurred. Deep tendon reflexes (DTR) are diminished in all posts. He also has significant foot drop during his gait. What muscle(s) play(s) an important prognostic indicator in his disease process, and what is the ultrasound image mode and appropriate window best used to check it's movement?
   a. Diaphragm, A-mode, subxiphoid
   b. Muscle, M-mode, mid-clavicular subcostal
   c. Diaphragm, M-mode, mid-clavicular subcostal
   d. Muscle corset, B-mode, anterior axillary line
   e. Diaphragm, B-mode, posterior axillary line
2. A 19-year-old female military recruit presents to your office complaining cough with productive green sputum. She also has a fever and dyspnea. The symptoms last for 3 days after getting wet in the rain. What BLUE protocol profile would you expect to find on an ultrasound evaluation?
   a. Nude profile
   b. B-profile
   c. A′-profile
   d. C-profile
   e. A-no-V-PLAPS-profile
3. A 49-year-old male presents to your emergency room following a serious motor vehicle accident. He is unconscious, and his breathing is labored. You want to assess a rib fracture. What is the best reason to use ultrasound to identify rib fractures?
   a. It allows the assessment of complications secondary to the rib fracture
   b. It is better at visualizing tiny rib fracture when X-ray is not available
   c. It is much easier to perform an ultrasound examination than a chest X-ray.
   d. A and B are correct
   e. All of the above
4. A neonate with a body weight of 4000 g was born at 35 weeks of gestation through c section. Compact B-lines and echoic lungs appear in both the superior and inferior anterior lung fields on B-mode ultrasound images. What is the best answer for the main cause of those ultrasound findings?
   a. Pulmonary embolism
   b. Pulmonary edema
   c. Transient tachypnea
   d. Asthma
   e. Spontaneous tension pneumothorax

5. A 28-year-old male presents with difficulty breathing for the last two hours after being tackled during a football game. On B-mode ultrasound images, lung sliding is absent on the left side, and lung point is between the 5th and 6th rib in the mid-clavicular line. What findings can be observed on the M-mode ultrasound of his left lung?
   a. Barcode sign
   b. Seashore sign
   c. B-lines
   d. Lung pulse
   e. PLAPS points

Correct answers: 1. c; 2. d; 3. d; 4. b; 5. a.

References

1. Gargani L, Volpicelli G. How I do it: lung US. *Cardiovasc US* 2014; 12: 25. https://doi.org/10.1186/1476-7120-12-25.
2. Shah VP, Tunik MG, Tsung JW. Prospective evaluation of point-of-care ultrasonography for the diagnosis of pneumonia in children and young adults. *JAMA Pediatr* 2013; 167: 119–125.
3. Tardella M, Gutierrez M, Salaffi F, et al. US in the assessment of pulmonary fibrosis in connective tissue disorders: correlation with high-resolution computed tomography. *J Rheumatol* 2012; 39: 1641–1647.
4. Volpicelli G, Elbarbary M, Blaivas M, et al. International evidence-based recommendations for point-of-care lung US. *Intensive Care Med* 2012; 38: 577–591.
5. Mayo PH, Beaulieu Y, Doelken P, et al. American College of Chest Physicians/La Société de Réanimation de Langue Française statement on competence in critical care ultrasonography. *Chest* 2009; 135: 1050–1060.
6. Lichtenstein D, Goldstein I, Mourgeon E, et al. Comparative diagnostic performances of auscultation, chest radiography, and lung ultrasonography in acute respiratory distress syndrome. *Anesthesiology* 2004; 100: 9–15.
7. Koh DM, Burke S, Davies N, Padley SPG. Transthoracic US of the chest: clinical uses and applications. *RadioGraphics* 2002; 22(1): e1. https://doi.org/10.1148/radiographics.22.1.g02jae1e1.
8. Lee RK, Griffith JF, Ng AWH, Sitt JCM. Sonography of the chest wall: a pictorial essay. *J Clin US* 2015; 43: 525–537.
9. Liu J, Copetti R, Sorantin E, et al. Protocol and guidelines for point-of-care lung US in diagnosing neonatal pulmonary diseases based on international expert consensus. *J Visualized Exp* 2019; 6(145): e58990.
10. Piette E, Daoust R, Denault A. Basic concepts in the use of thoracic and lung US. *Curr Opin Anesthesiol* 2013; 26: 20–30.
11. Ng A, Swanevelder J. Resolution in US imaging. *Continuing Education in Anesthesia Critical Care Pain* 2011; 11: 186–192.
12. Smereczyński A, Kołaczyk K, Bernatowicz E. Chest wall – a structure underestimated in ultrasonography. Part III: neoplastic lesions. *J Ultrason* 2017; 17: 281–288.
13. O'Rourke K, Kibbee N, Stubbs A. US for the evaluation of skin and soft tissue infections. *Mo Med* 2015; 112: 202–205.
14. Shetty MK, Carpenter WS. Sonographic evaluation of isolated abnormal axillary lymph nodes identified on mammograms. *J US Med* 2004; 23: 63–71.

15. Dialani V, James DF, Slanetz PJ. A practical approach to imaging the axilla. *Insights Imaging* 2015; 6: 217–229.
16. Bianchi S, Martinoli C. US of the musculoskeletal system. Springer Science & Business Media, 2007.
17. McCool FD, Tzelepis GE. Dysfunction of the diaphragm. *N Engl J Med* 2012; 366: 932–942.
18. Faysoil A, Behin A, Ogna A, et al. Diaphragm: pathophysiology and US imaging in neuromuscular disorders. *J Neuromuscul Dis* 2018; 5: 1–10.
19. Nason LK, Walker CM, McNeeley MF, et al. Imaging of the diaphragm: anatomy and function. *RadioGraphics* 2012; 32: E51–E70.
20. Umbrello M, Formenti P. Ultrasonographic assessment of diaphragm function in critically ill subjects. *Respir Care* 2016; 61: 542–555.
21. Skaarup SH, Løkke A, Laursen CB. The area method: a new method for US assessment of diaphragmatic movement. *Crit US J* 2018; 10: 15.
22. Sarwal A, Walker FO, Cartwright MS. Neuromuscular US for evaluation of the diaphragm. *Muscle Nerve* 2013; 47: 319–329.
23. Mayo P, Volpicelli G, Lerolle N, et al. Ultrasonography evaluation during the weaning process: the heart, the diaphragm, the pleura and the lung. *Intensive Care Med* 2016; 42: 1107–1117.
24. Aliverti A. Assessment of human diaphragm function by USs. *J Acoust Soc Am* 2019; 145: 1656–1657.
25. Supakul N, Karmazyn B. US evaluation of costochondral abnormalities in children presenting with anterior chest wall mass. *AJR* 2013; 201(2): W336–W341.
26. Hodgson RJ, O'connor PJ, Grainger AJ. Tendon and ligament imaging. *Br J Radiol* 2012; 85: 1157–1172.
27. Allison SJ, Nazarian LN. Musculoskeletal US: evaluation of ankle tendons and ligaments. *AJR* 2010; 194: W514–W514.
28. An overview of point-care-US for soft tissue and musculoskeletal applications in the emergency department. *J Intensive Care* 2016; 4: 55. https://doi.org/10.1186/s40560-016-0173-0.
29. Imran JB, Eastman AL. Pneumothorax. *JAMA* 2017; 318: 974. https://doi.org/10.1001/jama.2017.10476.
30. Chan SS. Emergency bedside US to detect pneumothorax. *Acad Emerg Med* 2003; 10: 91–94.
31. Koratala A, Kazory A. An introduction to point-care-US: Laennec to Lichtenstein. *Adv Chronic Kidney Dis* 2021; 28: 193–199.
32. Qureshi NR, Gleeson FV. Imaging of pleural disease. *Clin Chest Med* 2006; 27(2): 193–213.
33. Elyashiv D, Alpert EA, Granat N. Empyema necessitans diagnosed by point-care-US. *J Emerg Med* 2020; 59(6): e221–e223. https://doi.org/10.1016/j.jemermed.2020.09.020.
34. Rahimi-Movaghar V, Yousefifard M, Ghelichkhani P, et al. Application of ultrasonography and radiography in detection of hemothorax; a systematic review and meta-analysis. *Emergency* 2016; 4: 116–126.
35. Ali HA, Lippmann M, Mundathaje U, Khaleeq G. Spontaneous hemothorax: a comprehensive review. *Chest* 2008; 134: 1056–1065.
36. Lichtenstein DA. BLUE-protocol and FALLS-protocol: two applications of lung ultrasound in the critically ill. *Chest* 2015; 147: 1659–1670.
37. Copetti R, Soldati G, Copetti P. Chest sonography: a useful tool to differentiate acute cardiogenic pulmonary edema from acute respiratory distress syndrome. *Cardiovasc Ultrasound* 2008; 6: 16.
38. Bandi V, Lunn W, Ernst A, et al. US vs CT in detecting chest wall invasion by tumor: a prospective study. *Chest* 2008; 133: 881–886.
39. Carter B, Benveniste M, Betancourt S, et al. Imaging evaluation of malignant chest wall neoplasms. *Radiographics* 2016; 36: 1285–1306.
40. Hsu PK, Hsu HS, Li AFY, et al. Non-Hodgkin's lymphoma presenting as a large chest wall mass. *Ann Thorac Surg* 2006; 81: 1214–1218.

41. Tomas X, Facenda C, Vaz N, et al. Thoracic wall trauma-misdiagnosed lesions on radiographs and usefulness of US, multidetector computed tomography and magnetic resonance imaging. *Quant Imaging Med Surg* 2017; 7: 384–397.
42. Hurley ME, Keye GD, Hamilton S. Is US really helpful in the detection of rib fractures? *Injury* 2004; 35(6): 562–566.
43. Turk F, Kurt AB, Saglam S. Evaluation by US of traumatic rib fractures missed by radiography. *Emerg Radiol* 2010; 17(6): 473–477.
44. Talbot BS, Gange CP Jr, Chaturvedi A, et al. Traumatic rib injury: patterns, imaging pitfalls, complications, and treatment. *Radiographics* 2017; 37: 628–651.
45. Liang HY, Liang XW, Chen ZY, et al. US in neonatal lung disease. *Quant Imaging Med Surg* 2018; 8: 535–546.
46. Copetti R, Cattarossi L, Macagno F, et al. Lung US in respiratory distress syndrome: a useful tool for early diagnosis. *Neonatology* 2008; 94: 52–59.
47. Copetti R, Cattarossi L. US diagnosis of pneumonia in children. *Radiol Med* 2008; 113: 190–198.
48. Liu J, Chen SW, Liu F, et al. The diagnosis of neonatal pulmonary atelectasis using lung ultrasonography. *Chest* 2015; 147: 1013–1019.
49. Hussain A, Burns B. Anatomy, thorax, wall. In: StatPearls [Internet]. Treasure Island, FL: StatPearls Publishing, 2018.

CHAPTER 4

The Heart

Anthony Tran[1], Ashna Haque[1], Ryan Brauman[1], and Li-Juan Du[2]

[1] Rocky Vista University, College of Osteopathic Medicine, Ivins, Utah, USA

[2] Department of Ultrasound, Beijing Tiantan Hospital, Capital Medical University, Beijing, China

Introduction

Cardiovascular disease is the leading cause of death worldwide. Coronary artery disease (CAD) is the most common form of heart disease, with a high death rate (about 2 in 10) in adults less than 65 years old [1]. In addition, there are an estimated 2.4 million individuals with a congenital heart defect [2]. Given the prevalence and severity of heart disease, several imaging modalities can be used to identify pathologies and assess the overall health of the heart. Of the different methods, cardiac ultrasound or echocardiography (ECHO) is a preferred technique given its ability to evaluate the heart's anatomy and functionality while also being accurate, noninvasive, and lacking radiation [3]. Comparatively, chest computed tomography (CT) and CT angiography expose the patient to radiation, and magnetic resonance imaging (MRI) has a high cost and contraindications [4]. Compared with CT and MRI, ECHO is considered a cost-effective imaging modality in the assessment of cardiac diseases [5]. Importantly, ECHO provides real-time observation of global and segmental left ventricle motion and evaluation of heart valve activities with fast results, high portability, acceptance, accuracy, and repeatability.

Anatomy of the Heart

The heart is a four-chambered organ that provides oxygenated blood for systemic circulation and reoxygenates blood via pulmonic circulation [6]. It is located within the thoracic cavity, medial to the lungs and posterior to the sternum. The heart is enclosed by a membranous structure called the pericardium that consists of two layers, an outer fibrous layer and an inner serous membrane, for the protection and lubrication of the heart [6]. The heart itself is divided into four chambers: a left atrium, a right atrium, a left ventricle, and a right ventricle. Separating the two ventricles is a thick interventricular septum that bulges to the right and lies obliquely across the heart within a coronal plane [7]. Blood first enters the right atrium through the inferior and superior vena cava (Fig. 4.1). This is where

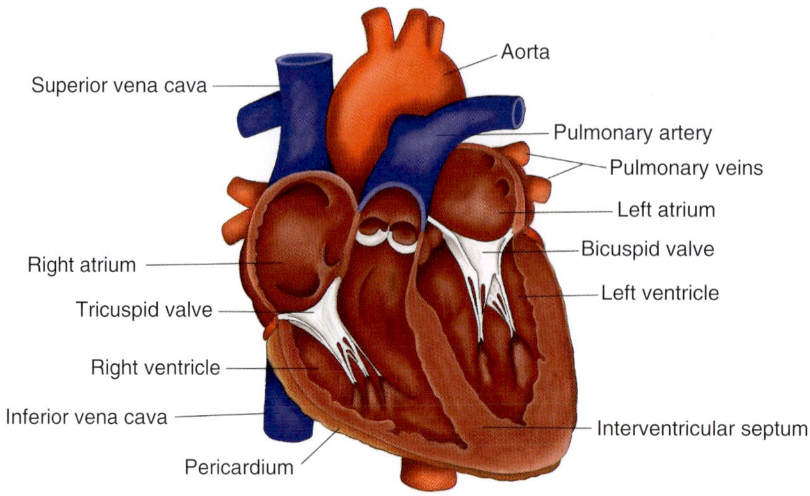

FIGURE 4.1 Anatomy of the heart.

deoxygenated blood returns to the heart, and it must travel to the lungs for reoxygenation. Other structures associated with the right atrium are the fossa ovalis and coronary sinus [6]. To reach the lungs from the right atrium, deoxygenated blood passes through the tricuspid valve in order to enter the right ventricle. The right ventricle is the anterior-most chamber and can be differentiated from the right atrium by its thicker ventricular wall and trabeculae carneae. These structures allow for the propulsion of blood superiorly through the pulmonary valves, into the pulmonary arteries, and finally into the lungs [7]. Upon arrival in the lungs, blood becomes oxygenated. Following oxygenation, blood returns to the heart via the pulmonary veins. Pulmonary veins carry oxygenated blood into the posterior-most chamber of the heart, the left atrium. The left atrium, alongside other vessels, forms the base of the heart, which is the superior most portion of the heart located by the third costal cartilage [6]. From the left atrium, blood flows into the left ventricle by first traveling through the bicuspid (mitral) valve. The left ventricle forms the apex, which is the inferior-most portion of the heart, located to the left of the sternum between the fourth and fifth ribs. It contains the thickest myocardial wall of the four chambers, allowing the left ventricle to expel blood into systemic circulation [7]. To enter systemic circulation, blood from the left ventricle will flow into the aorta by passing through the aortic valve. This oxygen-rich blood enters the organs and tissues via the arterial system. After deoxygenation, blood will drain within the venous system into the superior and inferior vena cava before returning into the heart in the right atrium, completing the circuit [6].

Ultrasound Techniques

Based on the scanning approach, the two types of ECHO examinations are transthoracic echocardiogram (TTE) and transesophageal echocardiogram (TEE), which both acquire two-dimensional grayscale and color Doppler images [8]. TTE is the most common form of ECHO used. It involves placement of the transducer at various locations on the thorax skin to produce a two-dimensional (2D) image of the heart [9]. It is easy to perform and highly acceptable for patients in all age groups. Common clinical indications for TTE are for the assessment of sustained or nonsustained atrial fibrillation, suspected complications from a myocardial infarction (MI) or ischemia, respiratory failure of unknown etiology, and for congenital heart disease [8].

Although TTE is a valuable diagnostic method, TEE can provide far superior images of posterior cardiac structures [10]. TEE is similar to a gastrointestinal endoscopy in that a flexible endoscopic probe is passed through a patient's esophagus, but the probe contains an ultrasound transducer. Because of the transducer's placement within the esophagus, the probe is located closer to the heart without air or lung obstruction compared to TTE. Therefore, the structures on the posterior side of the heart are better visualized compared to TTE, such as the mitral valve, interatrial septum, left atrium, and pulmonary veins [10]. TEE is considered moderately invasive and is typically performed with conscious sedation. As a result, TEE contains more contraindications than TTE. Absolute contraindications for TEE include perforated viscus, esophageal stricture, tumor, perforation, diverticulum, and active upper gastrointestinal bleeding. Complications from TEE include esophageal perforation, gastrointestinal bleeding, pharyngeal hematoma, and methemoglobinemia [11]. TEE is typically reserved for evaluation of cardiac pathologies that cannot be clearly assessed by TTE, such as valvular structure, infective endocarditis, small defects, and pulmonary veins because of the increased risk and patient discomfort, according to the appropriate use criteria of echocardiography [8].

B-mode Grayscale Image

ECHO is initiated with B-mode imaging to observe the anatomic morphology of the heart. The size of each chamber of the heart, thickness of ventricular walls and intraventricular septum, calcification, and vegetation of the valves can be assessed in grayscale images. In addition, dynamic movement of the left ventricular wall and activity (opening and closure) of the cardiac valves can be observed in real-time images. The presence and severity of a pericardial effusion are also assessed in a B-mode grayscale image. Notably, a high-frequency transducer can acquire an image with high resolution, whereas a low-frequency transducer can deepen the penetration of the sound beam when performing grayscale imaging [9].

M-Mode

Motion mode (M-Mode) produces one-dimensional images using a sampling rate of over 1800 frames per second, compared to a frame rate of 30–60 per second in two-dimensional and three-dimensional grayscale images. This allows for the identification of thin moving structures such as the ventricular endothelium and heart valves [10]. M-Mode is primarily performed in parasternal long- and short-axis views to measure the aortic root, ejection fraction, and heart chamber dimensions, to quantify aortic valve separations, and to identify valve vegetations [12]. In addition to the standard two-dimensional images that TTE and TEE provide, M-mode assists in specific diagnosis or identification of valve pathologies [10].

Color Flow Imaging/Spectral Doppler

The Doppler techniques in ECHO are color flow imaging and spectral Doppler, which can be used to determine the direction and velocity of blood flow [12]. In color-coded flow imaging, red and blue colors represent blood flowing toward the transducer and blood flowing away from the transducer, respectively. This technique is also useful to determine whether the flow of blood is laminar or turbulent based on the brightness of the color and mixed variable colors in the region of interest, which may indicate a hemodynamic abnormality, such as seen in stenosis, regurgitation, and shunts [13]. The rapid visualization of blood flow provides qualitative data, making it an exceptional tool for screening and assessing valve stenosis and regurgitation. Although color Doppler provides qualitative data, it is useful to guide further quantitative assessment [11].

Unlike color Doppler, spectral Doppler provides quantitative information regarding the hemodynamic properties of the heart [13]. Spectral Doppler is capable of accurately measuring the amount of blood (velocity, m/s) ejected from the heart or passing through a cardiac valve, the velocity of the blood, and its direction. These measurements are then used to calculate stroke volume, which is useful in evaluating hemodynamic abnormalities of the heart and quantifying the severity of regurgitation, stenosis, and shunt [10].

Stress Echocardiography

Stress ECHO is performed by comparing pre- and post-exercise measurements of chamber dimensions, wall thickness, and left ventricular function [14, 15]. These measurements are used to detect early-stage or subclinical CAD, preoperative risk assessment, and evaluation after revascularization [16]. As standard of care, a stress ECHO should be performed under the supervision of a cardiologist [17].

Examination Protocols

When performing a standard two-dimensional TTE, there are four common ultrasound windows for transducer placement: parasternal, apical, subcostal, and suprasternal windows (Fig. 4.2). The views that can be obtained through those ultrasound windows include long-axis, short-axis, four-chamber, and five-chamber [11]. Generally, a phased array probe with a frequency of 3.5 MHz for adults (5 MHz or higher for pediatrics) would be most appropriate, and the ultrasound machine with presettings for cardiac ultrasound can be selected. Water-based ultrasound gel should be placed between the transducer and skin at the site of scanning to improve ultrasound transmission into the body. There aren't any special preparations required for ECHO. Electrocardiography (ECG) tracking is standard in performing ECHO for determining cardiac cycle of systole and diastole [13].

Parasternal Window

To obtain an image at the parasternal window, the patient should be lying in the left lateral decubitus position if tolerated. The transducer should then be placed in the left parasternal region on the third or fourth left intercostal space [13].

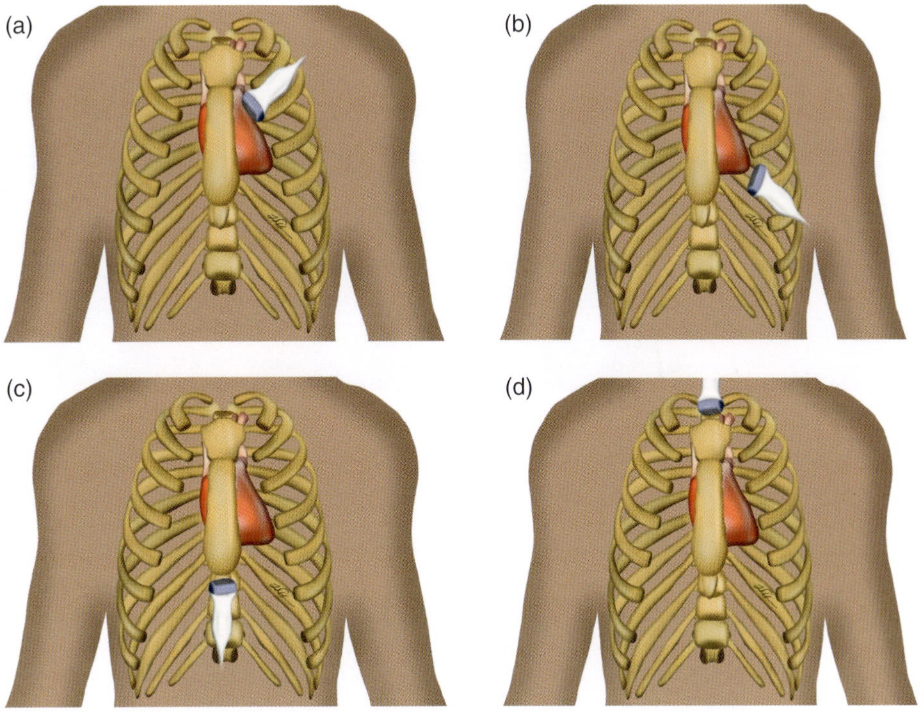

FIGURE 4.2 Illustration of four windows: parasternal (a), apical (b), subxiphoid (c), and suprasternal (d).

Parasternal Long-Axis View 2D grayscale image: Align the sound beam parallel to the long axis of the heart by placing the transducer lateral to the sternum in the third or fourth intercostal space. Ensure that the indicator is pointed superiorly. Sweep the transducer until the ascending aorta is relatively horizontal in orientation. If viewed properly, the image obtained will be of a sagittal section of the heart, and the following structures will be viewed (Fig. 4.3).

M-mode: M-mode will be activated when a grayscale parasternal long-axis view is displayed. It is important to ensure the M-mode cursor is perpendicular to the structure of interest [10].

Aortic root, aortic valve, and left atrium – M-mode records the left atrium and aortic root by placing the cursor perpendicular to the aortic root and left atrium. The aortic root should be measured at the end of diastole and before the onset of the QRS complex based on ECG tracing [12]. The typical average diameter of the ascending aorta is $3.0\,\text{cm} \pm 0.4$ in males and 2.7 ± 0.4 in females [18]. The left atrium will appear posterior to the aorta and fill during atrial diastole while emptying during atrial systole. The cycle of filling and emptying of the left atrium is the cause of the anterior and posterior motion of the aortic root and can be indicative of increased filling and emptying or decreased filling and emptying if the rate of movement increases or decreases [10]. The dimension of the left atrium in normal subjects is similar to the diameter of the aorta [9]. The last structure that can be identified in this view is the aortic leaflet, which is visualized as a thin line during diastole that separates immediately during systole and looks like an "open box" (Fig. 4.4). If the leaflets do not open completely or close abruptly after opening, this can be an indication of a stenosis [19].

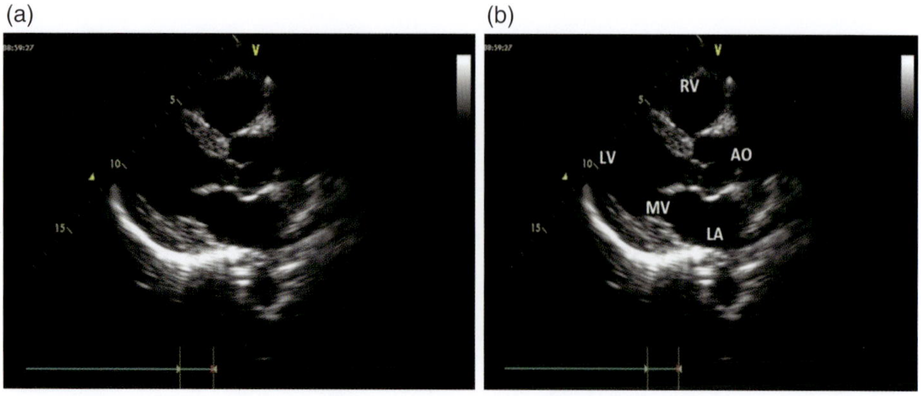

FIGURE 4.3 B-mode ultrasoundimage of the parasternal long axis of the heart. AO, aortic root and aortic valves – ; LA, left atrium – posterior-most chamber; LV, left ventricle – largest chamber furthest to the left; MV, mitral valve - thin structure separating the left ventricle and left atrium; RV, right ventricle – anterior-most chamber.

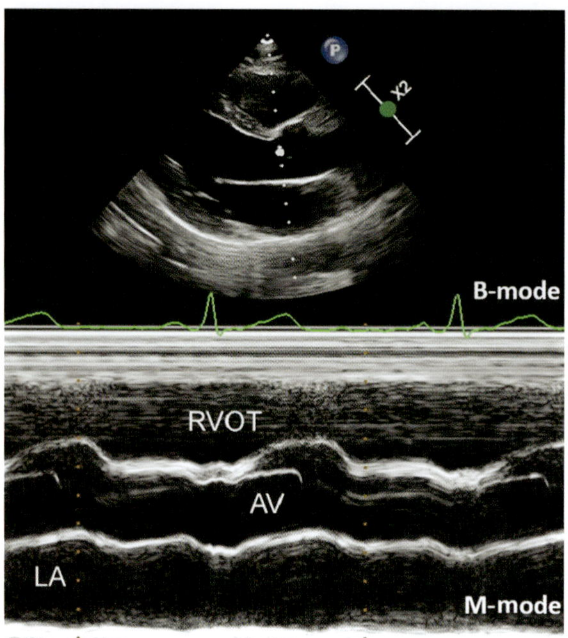

FIGURE 4.4 M-mode image of the aortic root, aortic valve (AV), left atrium (LA), and right ventricle outflow tract (RVOT) in the parasternal long-axis window with all measurements. The upper is B-mode image, and the bottom is M-mode image.

Left ventricle – To identify and measure the left ventricle in M-Mode, ensure the cursor is perpendicular to the mitral valve/papillary muscle. In M-mode, the chamber of the left ventricle (Fig. 4.5) will appear as the large chamber on the screen, posterior to the right ventricular chamber. The narrowest diameter of the chamber represents the end of systole, and the largest diameter represents the end of diastole.

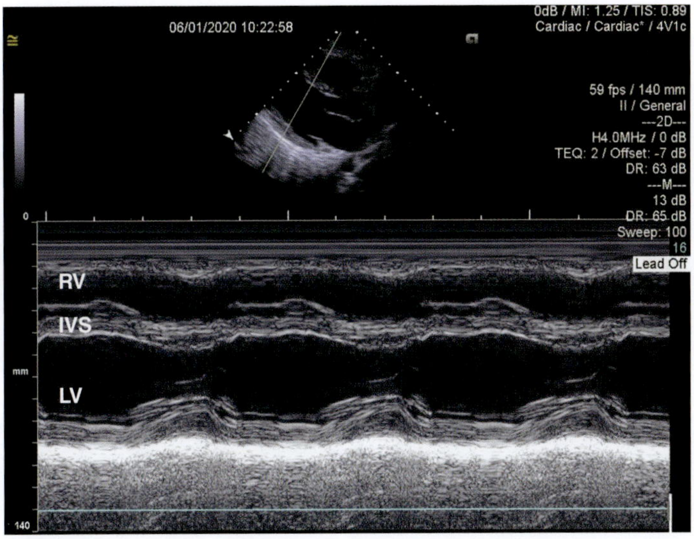

FIGURE 4.5 M-mode image of the left ventricle in parasternal long axis. IVS, interventricular septum; LV, left ventricle; RV, right ventricle.

Measurements of the dimensions of the left ventricle are taken at the end of diastole and end of systole. Measurements of the left ventricular wall thickness are taken only at the end of diastole [12]. The end-diastolic volume of the left ventricle is normally 106 mL ± 22 for males and 76 ± 15 for females, and the end-systolic volume is normally 41 ± 10 in males and 28 ± 7 in females [18]. Using the diameter of the left ventricle at the end of systole and diastole, the ejection fraction can also be calculated [12]. A normal left ventricular ejection fraction (LVEF) is between 52% and 72% in males and 54–74% in females [18].

Mitral valve – To obtain mitral valve images, place the cursor perpendicular to the long axis of the left ventricle and the tip of mitral leaflet [12]. During systole, the mitral valve will move slightly anteriorly, and during diastole, the leaflets separate widely [9].

Parasternal Short-Axis View From the parasternal long-axis view, rotate the transducer 70°–110° clockwise to place the transducer perpendicular to the plane of the long axis of the left ventricle. The operator should fan the transducer posteriorly from the right shoulder to the left hip to record the cross section of the short axis of the heart (Fig. 4.6). This view will provide cross-sectional views of the heart from the base to the apex [10, 20].

Apical Window

Obtaining an apical image requires the patient to lie in the left lateral decubitus position with the transducer placed at or in the immediate vicinity of the point of maximal impulse. The point of maximal impulse is the point within the chest wall where the maximal cardiac impulse is felt [10].

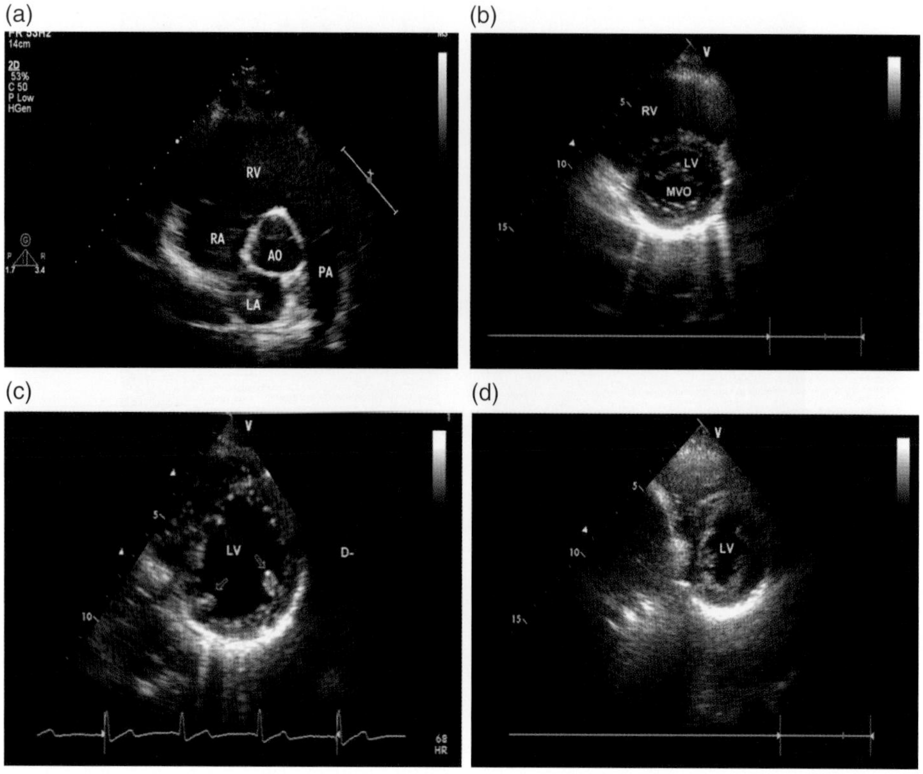

FIGURE 4.6 B-mode ultrasound images in parasternal short axis: (a) the base of the heart at aortic valve level; (b) mitral valve level; (c) papillary muscle (green arrows) level of the left ventricle; (d) the apex of the left ventricle. AO, aortic root and valves; MV, mitral valve; MVO, mitral valve orifice; LV, left ventricle; PA, pulmonary artery; RA, right atrium; RV, right ventricle.

Four-Chamber View 2D grayscale image: A four-chamber view requires the ultrasound beam to be directed superiorly and medially toward the patient's right scapula. When scanning properly, all four chambers of the heart (Fig. 4.7), interventricular septum, and interatrial septum should be seen [9]. This view provides information on the size of all ventricles and atria and gross estimation of left ventricle contractility. In addition, an abnormal movement of atrioventricular valves can also be observed in the real-time grayscale image [10, 20].

Color Flow Imaging Color flow imaging is commonly performed from the apical four-chambered window to visualize blood flow direction and mean velocity. Given that the transducer is placed at the apex of the heart, the trajectory of the blood that flows from the left atrium to the left ventricle will be toward the transducer (Fig. 4.8). The pattern of blood flow appears red in color during left ventricular filling [21]. As the ventricles contract, blood flows from the left ventricle to the aorta away from the transducer. The blood flow during left ventricle ejection away from the transducer and flow pattern will appear blue on the screen. Upon assessment, ensure that the flow of blood appears laminar and uniform. Turbulent flow appearing as mixtures of red and blue during ventricular ejection or filling may indicate stenosis or regurgitation. It should be noted on

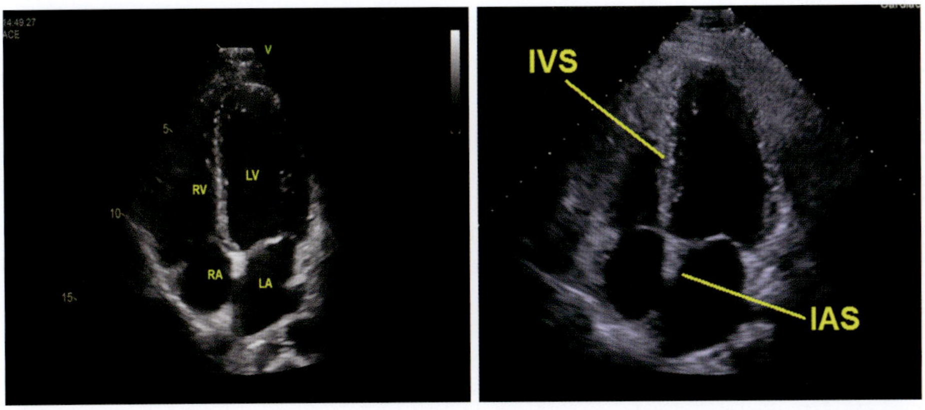

FIGURE 4.7 B-mode image of apical four-chamber view of the heart. IAS, interatrial septum; IVS, interventricular septum; LA, left atrium; LV, left ventricle; RA, right atrium; RV, right ventricle.

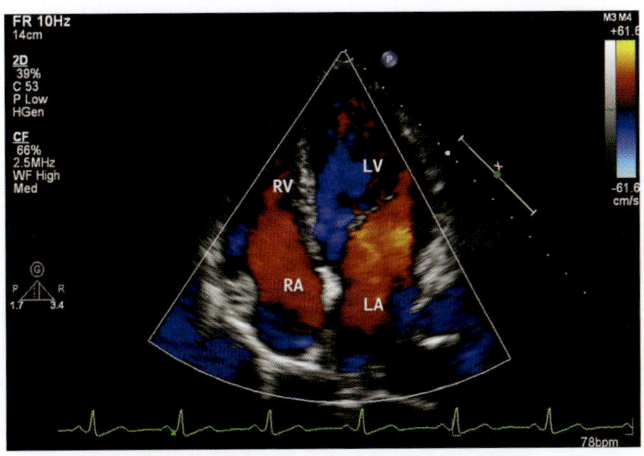

FIGURE 4.8 Color flow imaging of the apical four-chamber view. LA, left atrium; LV, left ventricle; RA, right atrium; RV, right ventricle.

color flow imaging and evaluated further by conducting a quantitative evaluation with spectral Doppler [22].

Spectral Doppler Spectral Doppler is an ideal tool for quantitative measurements of left ventricular flow by placing the cursor through the mitral valve and tricuspid valve to trace trans-valve flow velocity. The notion is that the maximum velocity is measured when the Doppler angle between the direction of emission of the sound beam and the direction of blood flow is zero degrees. However, Doppler angle correction of less than 60° is acceptable (Chapter 1, Doppler). Spectral Doppler can also be used to assess blood flow direction. The spectrum will be above the baseline if the blood flows toward the transducer, and the spectrum will be below the baseline if the blood is flowing away from the transducer [21]. To obtain the stroke volume, multiply the area under the blood flow curve by the cross-sectional area. To obtain the value for cardiac output, multiply the previously calculated stroke volume by the heart rate [10].

Apical Two-Chamber and Five-Chamber Views

Two-Chamber View 2D grayscale image: A two-chamber view requires the transducer to be rotated 60° counterclockwise on the basis of the four-chamber view. When viewed properly, the image shows the left atrium, MV, and left ventricle (Fig. 4.9).

Color Flow Imaging The MV should be interrogated using an apical two-chamber view. To demonstrate the stenotic or regurgitant jets through the MV, the valve should be positioned in the center of the sector to ensure that the entire valve is included in the color box. In the apical four-chamber view, which is most parallel to inflow, forward flow is best demonstrated. However, in the apical two-chamber, the flow partially directed toward the lateral wall of the left ventricle can be found.

Spectral Doppler In the apical two-chamber view, spectral Doppler is used to characterize the patterns of forward diastolic flow across the MV, and continuous wave Doppler is used to record the regurgitant flow of mitral regurgitation (MR).

Five-Chamber Views

2D grayscale image: From the apical four-chamber view, the apical five-chamber view is obtained by tilting the transducer anteriorly until the left ventricular outflow tract (LVOT), AV, and the proximal ascending aorta come into view (Fig. 4.10). The key point in this view should focus on the LVOT, AV, and MV.

(a) (b)

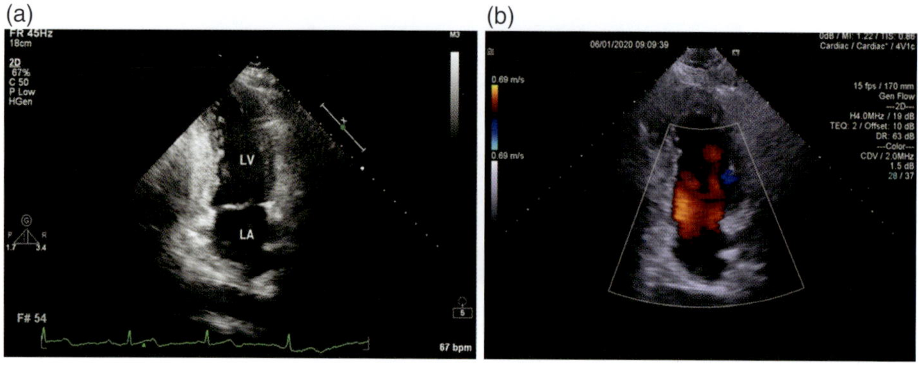

FIGURE 4.9 B-mode (a) and color flow imaging (b) of apical two-chamber view are important to depict mitral valve stenosis and regurgitation. LA, left atrium; LV, left ventricle.

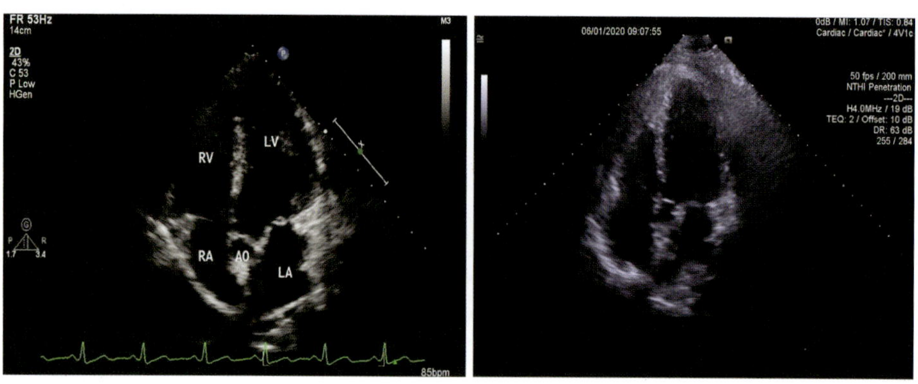

FIGURE 4.10 B-mode image of apical five-chamber: AO, aortic valve/root; IVS, interventricular septum; MV, mitral valve; LA, left atrium; LV, left ventricle; LVOT, left ventricular outflow tract; RA, right atrium; RV, right ventricle.

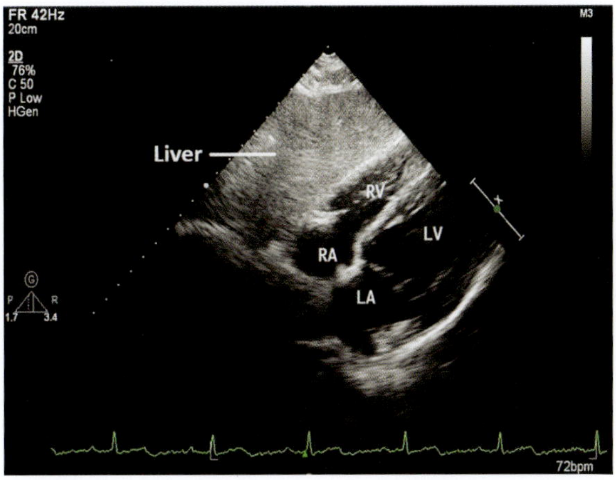

FIGURE 4.11 B-mode subxiphoid (subcostal) image of the heart. LA, left atrium; LV, left ventricle; RA, right atrium; RV, right ventricle.

Color Flow Imaging The LVOT and AV can be evaluated by the view of apical five-chamber. The laminar versus turbulent forward flow in systole and the turbulent regurgitant flow patterns in diastole across the AV can be evaluated. If turbulence is noted in the LVOT, using color flow imaging combined with M-mode imaging is of considerable value to characterize the timing of events.

Spectral Doppler In the apical five-chamber views, pulse Doppler is used to obtain velocity in the LVOT. If high velocity or turbulent flow is present on color flow imaging, pulse Doppler should be used to depict the highest velocity by tracing trans-valve flow velocity from the LV apex to the AV. As the aortic regurgitant jet is frequently eccentric on color flow imaging, which is used to guide continuous wave Doppler to measure the peak velocity and pressure half-time.

Subxiphoid (Subcostal) Window

A subcostal image is performed on individuals with chronic obstructive lung disease or emphysema due to obstruction of the normal sites by hyperinflated lungs [13]. It is also a part of trauma ultrasound to assess potential pericardial effusion in emergency medicine (Fig. 4.11). The patient will lie supine with their knees bent in order to relax the abdominal muscles. The transducer will be placed horizontally below or to the right of the xiphoid process. This view allows for visualization of the four chambers of the heart, interventricular septum, interatrial septum, left ventricular walls, and pericardium [10, 20].

Common Cardiac Pathologies

ECHO is a valuable diagnostic tool to assess not only the anatomy of the heart but also its physiological properties and function. It is the first line imaging study in the assessment of cardiac pathologies in adults and pediatric populations [20]. Common cardiac pathologies that can be identified using ECHO are left ventricular hypertrophy

(LVH), aortic valve stenosis, aortic valve insufficiency (regurgitation), mitral valve stenosis/regurgitation, myocardial infarction, pericardial effusion, rheumatic cardiac disease, Marfan syndrome, atrial septal defect (ASD), and ventricular septal defect (VSD) [10].

Left Ventricle Hypertrophy

LVH occurs as end-organ damage due to long-standing hypertension. Reversal of LVH can lead to improvement of patient outcomes, and therefore, early identification is necessary for management of hypertension [22]. LVH is defined as an increase in LV mass $>134\,g/m^2$ for men and $>110\,g/m^2$ for women when indexed for surface area. The thickness of the anterior septum and posterior wall, as well as end-diastolic dimension, can be obtained using the parasternal 2D long-axis view (Fig. 4.12). Left ventricular mass is calculated using the intraventricular septal thickness (IVST), posterior wall thickness (PWT), and left ventricular end-diastolic volume (LVED): $0.8\ (1.04\ (IVST + PWT + LVED)^3 - LVED)^3 + 0.6\,g$. The left ventricular mass index is calculated by dividing left ventricular mass by body surface area [23].

Aortic Valve Stenosis

Aortic valve stenosis is a progressive and life-threatening condition that has a poor prognosis if left untreated. Aortic stenosis is often the result of left ventricular outflow obstruction and usually requires valve replacement for long-term treatment [24]. Ultrasound can be used to aid in the clinical diagnosis of aortic stenosis, as well as determine the severity of the stenosis, which is important for physicians to make treatment plans [25]. The aortic leaflets can be viewed in the parasternal long-axis window using M-mode to monitor movement during systole and diastole. If the leaflets do not open completely or close abruptly after opening, this can be an indication of stenosis [26]. Continuous wave Doppler can be used to record the peak systolic velocity of blood flow through the aortic valve and the mean pressure gradient across

(a) (b)

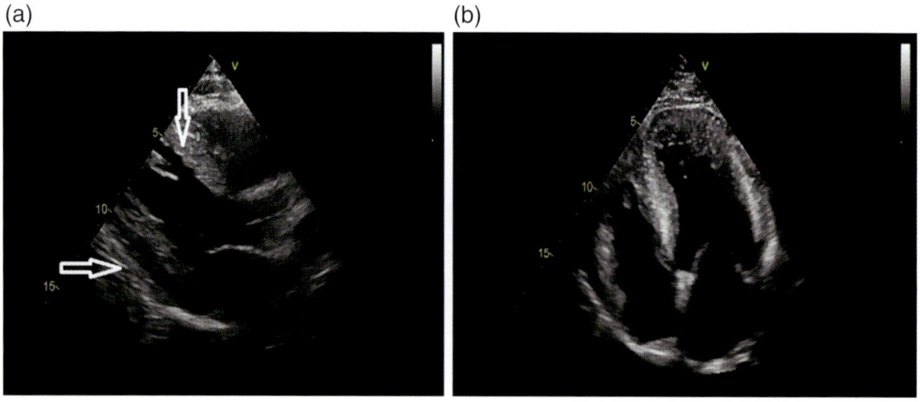

FIGURE 4.12 Parasternal long-axis (a) and apical four-chamber (b) views show increased thickness of interventricular septum and posterior wall (arrows) of the left ventricle in a patient with LVH.

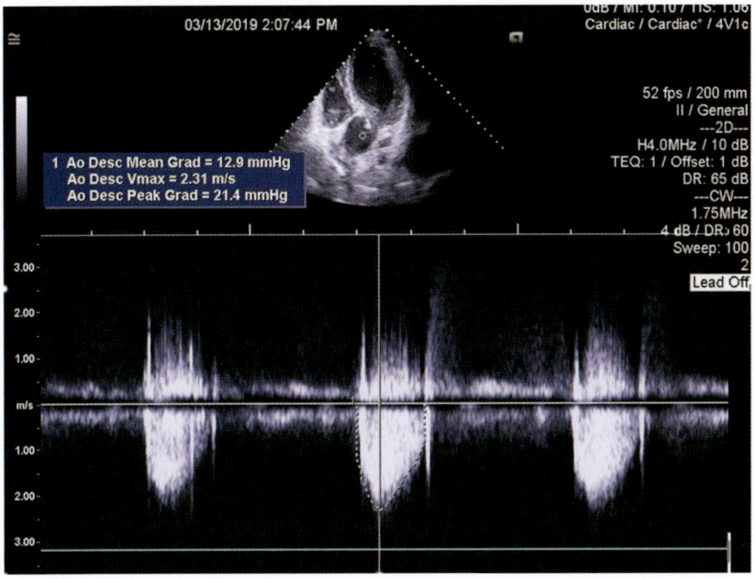

FIGURE 4.13 Continuous wave Doppler of left ventricle outflow tract (LVOT) to measure trans-aortic valve velocity for grading the severity of aortic valve stenosis.

the aortic valve (Fig. 4.13). These measurements, combined with a calculation of aortic valve area on B-mode image, can provide insight into the severity of the disease and subsequent progression [24].

Aortic Insufficiency

Aortic insufficiency (regurgitation) has a variety of etiologies (Fig. 4.14). It is often caused by rheumatic disease in developing countries, whereas it is commonly the result of congenital abnormalities or degenerative disease in Western Europe and

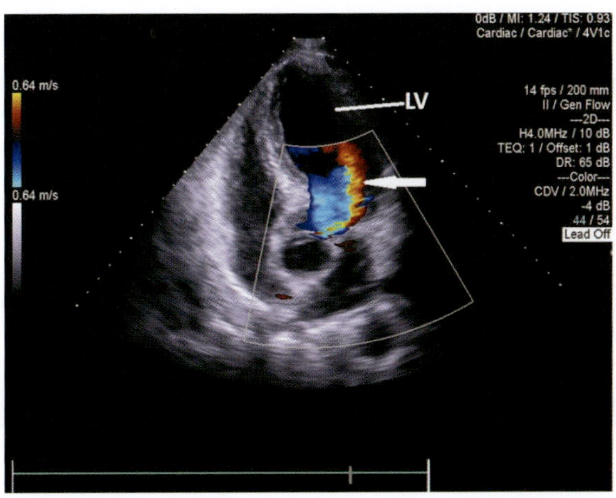

FIGURE 4.14 Aortic valve regurgitation (arrow, red color) is detected using color flow imaging through the apical five-chamber view. LV, left ventricle.

North America. In the diagnosis and monitoring of aortic regurgitation, Doppler ultrasound is performed via parasternal and suprasternal views of the heart to assess reversal of flow at the aortic valve. Long-term and severe aortic insufficiency may lead to a reduction in left ventricular function and/or dilated left ventricular hypertrophy. LVEF can indicate the prognosis of a disease, and a diminished LVEF below 50–55% can be a sign of a reduced prognosis even among asymptomatic patients. The ability to measure LVEF if a disease state is suspected can lead to early diagnosis and early initiation of treatment [27].

Mitral Valve Stenosis

Mitral valve stenosis (MS) has numerous etiologies, most commonly presenting in developing countries due to rheumatic heart disease, as well as congenital malformations or degenerative disease. It is due to the hardening of the mitral valve, obstructing blood flow from left atrium to left ventricle. If left untreated, this can lead to a variety of serious complications, such as pulmonary hypertension alongside right heart failure [28].

Mitral stenosis can be evaluated in the apical or parasternal views. B-mod ultrasound can be used to assess the extent of diastolic doming and classic "hockey-stick" shape to the anterior mitral leaflet, whereas the posterior mitral leaflet will often present with decreased mobility. Color flow imaging and spectral Doppler (Fig. 4.15) in the parasternal long-axis or apical four-chamber view can be used to assess the degree of turbulence of blood flow through the valve [29].

Mitral Valve Regurgitation

Mitral regurgitation (MR) is one of the most common valvular pathologies in North America, and it is often diagnosed and monitored via ECHO. Color flow imaging is especially helpful in observing reversal flow through the mitral valve during systole (Fig. 4.16). MR can be diagnosed in a similar way to the evaluation of mitral valve stenosis. Using a parasternal long-axis and apical four-chamber views of the mitral

(a) (b)

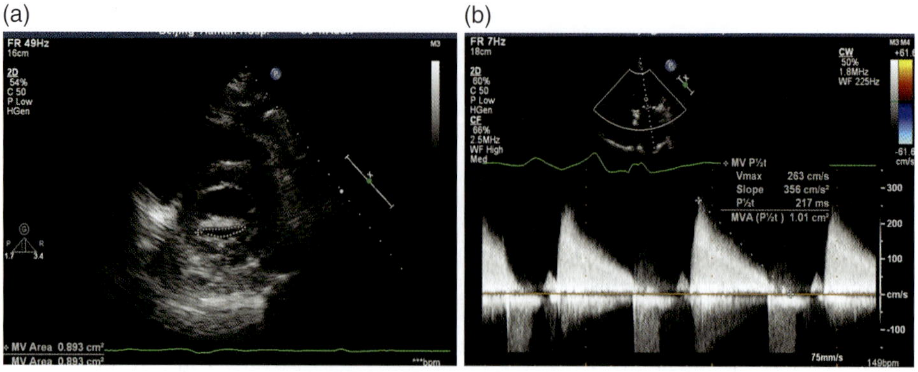

FIGURE 4.15 Parasternal short axis of mitral valve orifice shows thickened MV leaflets and decreased opening in diastole in B-mode ultrasound (a). Continuous wave Doppler (b) measures trans-MV velocity to assess the area of MV opening (MVA) for grading the severity of MV stenosis (via apical two-chamber or four-chamber view).

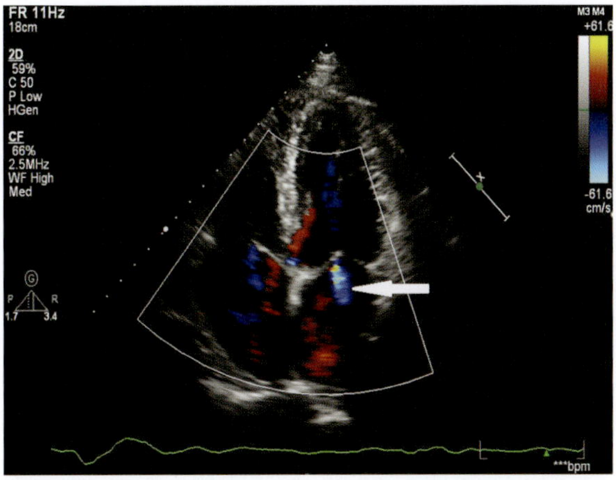

FIGURE 4.16 Mild mitral valve regurgitation (arrow) is observed on color flow imaging of the apical four-chamber view.

valve, backflow into the left atrium through the mitral valve during systole is an indication of MR. MS can precipitate MR and should be taken into consideration as an etiology of MR if observed during ultrasound examination [30].

Myocardial Infarction

An acute myocardial infarction (MI) is an emergency, and being able to recognize the clinical symptoms of an acute MI presenting in a patient is imperative for providing proper treatment. Diagnosis is often made via troponin levels and certain ECG findings (ST elevation or depression, left bundle branch block, etc.). Ultrasound imaging can be used to quickly assess for left ventricle motion abnormalities in MI, and if monitoring early, can even be used to detect cardiac abnormalities before ECG changes or in asymptomatic patients. The major electrocardiographic change that can be observed in an MI includes areas of abnormal cardiac wall movement due to local ischemia. This observation is often best seen initially in grayscale, and it is especially helpful to establish the location, extent, and severity of the ischemic regions. Cardiac ultrasound may also be utilized to reassess post-MI patients during a low-dose dobutamine stress test, again looking for areas of akinesia or dyskinesia within the myocardium, to assess the extent of the damage not already remedied by treatment [31].

Pericardial Effusion

Pericardial effusion is a condition where there is excess fluid between the heart and pericardium (Fig. 4.17). The effusion itself can be observed as an anechoic stripe in the pericardial space. A pericardial effusion can be viewed using any of the standard cardiac views. Besides trauma, while not always emergent, it can be an indication of more severe pathology, such as ventricular interdependence, where the increase in volume of one ventricle decreases the volume in the other ventricle. The best way to assess pericardial effusion is from a subcostal and an apical four-chamber view [31].

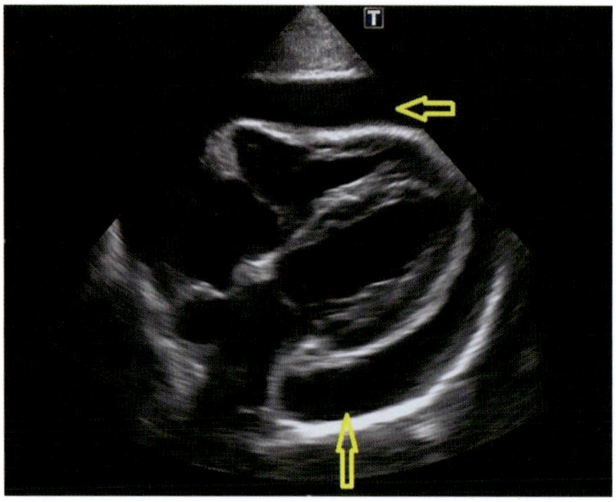

FIGURE 4.17 Fluid (yellow arrows) appears in the pericardium, indicating pericardial effusion.

Rheumatic Cardiac Disease

Rheumatic cardiac disease is caused by valvular damage following an immune response to group A streptococcal infection. The early detection of valvular damage after the successful treatment of a group A streptococcal infection is important for long-term management of patient care. Monitoring of rheumatic cardiac disease would include techniques used to identify MR, structural changes of the MV, AR, and structural changes of the AV. This focused exam should include parasternal long- and short-axis views, as well as apical views, to visualize affected valves. Grayscale image may be used to observe structural changes (vegetation, Fig. 4.18), while color flow imaging is useful in observing regurgitation across valves [32].

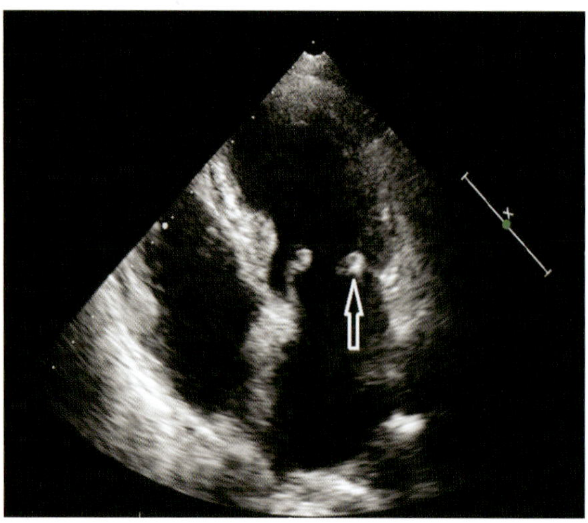

FIGURE 4.18 Vegetation (arrow) on the tip of mitral valve leaflets in a patient with rheumatic cardiac disease.

Marfan Syndrome

Marfan syndrome in adult patients often presents with cardiac manifestations of the disease later in life. Common pathologies include aortic root dilatation, mitral prolapse, aortic regurgitation, and various other valve pathologies. Ultrasound is an accurate tool that can be used to either screen for or monitor the listed cardiac abnormalities in a patient with Marfan syndrome to aid in the management of this disease. Aortic root dilatation can be diagnosed by visualizing the aortic root on a parasternal view and measuring an aortic diameter greater than 3.0 cm [33]. In pediatric patients with Marfan syndrome, aortic dilatation is of the most concern with regard to cardiac complications. Pediatric patients present more often with valvular defects, and these tend to cause more morbidity among pediatric patients with Marfan syndrome [34].

Pediatric ASD and VSD

ASDs are common heart defects that can be diagnosed postpartum in infants. There are four different types of ASDs, the most common being a patent foramen ovale, known as an ostium secundum ASD. A small defect normally resolves, but large defects can remain patent and eventually contribute to pathology as the patient ages. ASDs can be diagnosed via a four-chamber view of the atrial wall. Color Doppler can be used to observe flow between atria, indicating a defect in the atrial walls (Fig. 4.19) [35].

A VSD is the most common congenital cardiac defect with differing levels of severity. There are three types of VSD: membranous, muscular, and supracristal, the latter being the least commonly found. Most VSDs spontaneously close within the first year of life, often depending on their size and location. A four-chamber view of the fetal heart and a lateral view can be used to diagnose a VSD, whereas color flow imaging can be used to distinguish any areas of bidirectional flow, indicating a VSD (Fig. 4.20). A five-chamber view of the fetal heart can be more beneficial in diagnosing a membranous defect. A defect that is greater than the aortic diameter is considered a large defect [35].

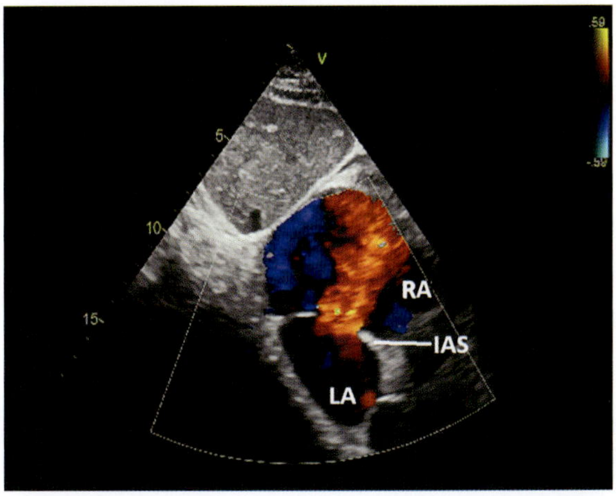

FIGURE 4.19 Cardiac subcostal view of color flow imaging shows left-to-right shunt, as blood flow from left atrium to right atrium (red color) in a patient with ASD. IAS, interatrial septum; LA, left atrium; RA, right atrium.

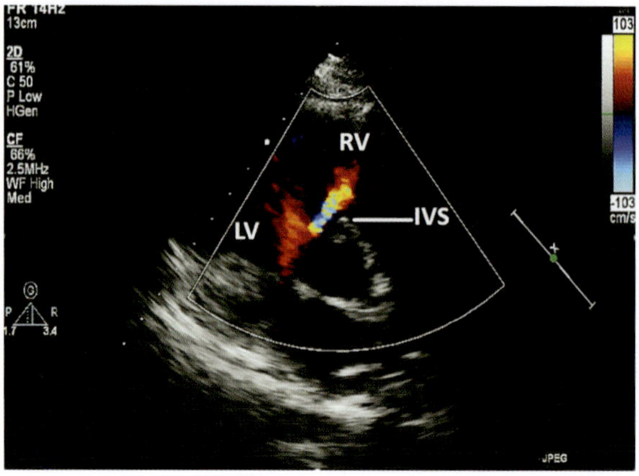

FIGURE 4.20 Parasternal view of color flow imaging shows the communication between the left and right ventricles. IVS, interventricular septum; LV, left ventricle; RV, right ventricle.

Summary

Ultrasound of the heart is an integration in primary care and medicine in other specialties. This is largely due to its high accuracy, accessibility, noninvasiveness, and low cost. Some indications for cardiac ultrasound include atrial fibrillation, acute chest pain, surveillance of moderate or severe valvular stenosis/regurgitation, and pulmonary embolism. The two most common forms are TTE and TEE, with the latter providing far superior but being more invasive. Adequate images of B-mode, color flow, and spectral Doppler can be obtained through the parasternal long axis, parasternal short axis, apical four-chamber, and subcostal approach. Given the prevalence of heart disease in developed countries and elderly, the usage of cardiac ultrasound will continue to grow.

Review Questions

1. Flow between the atrium and ventricle on both left and right can be identified using color flow imaging at which transthoracic cardiac ultrasound window?
   - **a.** Apical four-chamber
   - **b.** Parasternal long axis
   - **c.** Parasternal short axis
   - **d.** Subcostal
2. What imaging technique would be most appropriate to visualize the posterior structures of the heart in a young child?
   - **a.** Transthoracic echocardiography (TTE)
   - **b.** Transesophageal echocardiography (TEE)

c. CT of the heart

d. X-ray plan files of the heart

3. Which of the following is not an indication for cardiac ultrasound?

   a. Acute chest pain with suspected acute myocardial infarction

   b. Suspected cardiovascular source of embolus

   c. Pneumonia

   d. Routine surveillance of moderate or severe valvular regurgitation

4. How is the patient positioned during a parasternal long-axis view?

   a. Prone

   b. Supine

   c. Left lateral decubitus

   d. Standing

5. Which of the following is not used to measure left ventricular hypertrophy?

   a. Intraventricular septal thickness

   b. Left ventricular end-systolic volume

   c. Posterior wall thickness

   d. Left ventricular end-diastolic volume

6. Which view below is most commonly used to view the aortic or mitral leaflets in aortic or mitral stenosis?

   a. Subcostal

   b. Parasternal long axis

   c. Parasternal short axis

   d. Apical four-chamber

7. Which of the following is not a common pathology associated with Marfan syndrome?

   a. Aortic root dilation

   b. Mitral regurgitation

   c. Ventricular septal defect

   d. Aortic regurgitation

8. Ultrasound was performed on a 2-year-old female. In the apical four-chamber view with color flow imaging, flow was seen communicating between the posterior two chambers. What defect does the patient most likely have?

   a. Ventricular septal defect

   b. Pulmonary stenosis

   c. Aortic regurgitation

   d. Atrial septal defect

9. A 1-year-old male presents with rapid breathing, poor eating, and failure to thrive. Four-chamber view of the heart on color flow imaging shows bidirectional flow in the ventricles, and the defect is greater than the aortic diameter. How will the patient be treated?

   a. Wait for spontaneous closure

   b. Diuretic and ACE inhibitor

   c. Surgery or catheter procedure to close the defect

   d. Supportive care until symptoms worsen, then catheter procedure

10. Patient presents with chest pain and dyspnea. Subxiphoid ultrasound shows an anechoic strip surrounding the heart. What is the most likely diagnosis?

a. Pericardial effusion

b. Myocardial infarction

c. Ventricular septal defect

d. Marfan syndrome

Correct answers: 1. a; 2. b; 3. c; 4. c; 5. b; 6. c; 7. c; 8. d; 9. c; 10. a.

References

1. Benjamin EJ, Muntner P, Alonso A, et al. Heart disease and stroke statistic – 2019 update: a report from the American Heart Association. *Circulation* 2019; 139: e56–e528.
2. Gilboa SM, Devine OJ, Kucik JE, et al. Congenital heart defects in the United States: estimating the magnitude of the affected population in 2010. *Circulation* 2016; 134: 101–109. https://doi.org/10.1161/CIRCULATIONAHA.115.019307.
3. Patel A. Echocardiography essentials: physics and instrumentation. Up-to-date, 2019. https://www.uptodate.com. Accessed: February 21, 2021
4. Mettler FA Jr, Huda W, Yoshizumi TT, Mahesh M. Effective doses in radiology and diagnostic nuclear medicine: a catalog. *Radiology* 2008; 248: 254–263.
5. Gardner BI, Bingham SE, Allen MR, et al. Cardiac magnetic resonance versus transthoracic echocardiography for the assessment of cardiac volumes and regional function after myocardial infarction: an intrasubject comparison using simultaneous intrasubject recordings. *Cardiovasc Ultrasound* 2009; 7: 38. https://doi.org/10.1186/1476-7120-7-38.
6. Moore KL, Dalley AF, Agur AMR. Clinically oriented anatomy. 7th ed. Baltimore, MD: Lippincott Williams & Wilkins, 2014.
7. Whitaker RH. Anatomy of the heart. *Medicine* 2014; 42: 406–408. https://doi.org/10.1016/j.mpmed.2014.05.007.
8. American College of Cardiology Foundation Appropriate Use Criteria Task Force; American Society of Echocardiography; American Heart Association et al. ACCF/ASE/AHA/ASNC/HFSA/HRS/SCAI/SCCM/SCCT/SCMR 2011 Appropriate Use Criteria for Echocardiography. A report of the American College of Cardiology Foundation Appropriate Use Criteria Task Force, American Society of Echocardiography, American Heart Association, American Society of Nuclear Cardiology, Heart Failure Society of America, Heart Rhythm Society, Society for Cardiovascular Angiography and Interventions, Society of Critical Care Medicine, Society of Cardiovascular Computed Tomography, and Society for Cardiovascular Magnetic Resonance endorsed by the American College of Chest Physicians. *J Am Coll Cardiol* 2011; 57: 1126–1166. https://doi.org/10.1016/j.jacc.2010.11.002.
9. Patel A. Transthoracic echocardiography: normal cardiac anatomy and tomographic views. Up-to-date, 2019. https://www-uptodate-com.proxy. Accessed: February 21, 2021
10. Otto C. Textbook of clinical echocardiography. 6th ed. Philadelphia, PA: Elsevier, 2018.
11. Szyszka A, Plońska-Gościniak E. Transesophageal echocardiography. *J Ultrason* 2019; 19(76): 62–65. https://doi.org/10.15557/jou.2019.0009.
12. Mangion J. Essential echocardiography: companion to Braunwald's heart disease. 1st ed. Philadelphia, PA: Elsevier, 2019; 16–26.

13. Oh J, Seward J, Tajik A. The echo manual. 3rd ed. Philadelphia, PA: Lippincott Williams & Wilkins, 2006.
14. Marwick TH. Stress echocardiography. *Heart* 2003; 89: 113–118. https://doi.org/10.1136/heart.89.1.113.
15. Pellikka PA, Arruda-Olson A, Chaudhry FA, et al. Guidelines for performance, interpretation, and application of stress echocardiography in ischemic heart disease: from the American Society of Echocardiography. *J Am Soc Echocardiogr* 2020; 33(1): 1–41.e8. https://doi.org/10.1016/j.echo.2019.07.001.
16. Sicari R, Cortigiani L. The clinical use of stress echocardiography in ischemic heart disease. *Cardiovasc Ultrasound* 2017; 15: 7. https://doi.org/10.1186/s12947-017-0099-2.
17. Pinto FJ. Stress echocardiography-refining the diagnosis of coronary artery disease. *Eur Cardiovasc Dis* 2007; 3: 52–53.
18. Lang RM, Badano LP, Mor-Avi V, et al. Recommendations for cardiac chamber quantification by echocardiography in adults: an update from the American Society of Echocardiography and the European Association of Cardiovascular Imaging. *J Am Soc Echocardiogr* 2015; 28: 1–39. https://doi.org/10.1016/j.echo.2014.10.003.
19. Foster E. Echocardiographic evaluation of the aortic valve. Uptodate, 2019. https://www-uptodate-com.proxy. Accessed: February 10, 2022
20. Patel A. Principles of Doppler echocardiography. Uptodate, 2020. https://www-uptodate-com.proxy. Accessed: December 20, 2022
21. Cikes M, Kalinic H, Baltabaeva A, et al. The shape of the aortic outflow velocity profile revisited: is there a relation between its asymmetry and ventricle function in coronary artery disease? *Eur J Echocardiogr* 2009; 10: 847–857.
22. Możdżan M, Wierzbowska-Drabik K, Kurpesa M, et al. Echocardiographic indices of left ventricular hypertrophy and diastolic function in hypertensive patients with preserved LVEF classified as dippers and non-dippers. *Arch Med Sci* 2013; 2: 268–275. https://doi.org/10.5114/aoms.2013.34534.
23. Vourvouri EC, Poldermans D, Schinkel AF, et al. Left ventricular hypertrophy screening using a hand-held ultrasound device. *Eur Heart J* 2002; 23: 1516–1521.
24. Kurtz CE, Otto CM. Clinical aspects of diagnosis and management, with 10 illustrative case reports from a 25-year experience. *Medicine* 2010; 89: 349–379.
25. Berthelot-Richer M, Pibarot P, Capoulade R, et al. Discordant grading of aortic stenosis severity: echocardiographic predictors of survival benefit associated with aortic valve replacement. *JACC Cardiovasc Imaging* 2016; 9: 797–805.
26. Foster E. Echocardiographic evaluation of the atria and appendages. Uptodate, 2019. https://www-uptodate-com.proxy.rvu.edu/contents/echocardiographic-evaluation-of-the-atria-and-appendages. Accessed: January 25, 2021
27. Maurer G. Aortic regurgitation. *Heart* 2006. https://www.ncbi.nlm.nih.gov/pmc/articles/PMC1860728.
28. Shah SN and Sharma S. Mitral Stenosis. Treasure Island (FL): StatPearls Publishing; 2025. https://www.ncbi.nlm.nih.gov/books/NBK430742/ Accessed: January 20, 2021.
29. Ganesan G. How to assess mitral stenosis by echo – a step-by-step approach. *J Indian Acad Echocardiogr Cardiovasc Imaging* 2017; 1(3): 197–205.
30. Grigioni F, Russo A, Pasquale F, et al. Clinical use of Doppler echocardiography in organic mitral regurgitation: from diagnosis to patients' management. *J Cardiovasc Ultrasound* 2015; 23: 121–133.
31. Singhapricha T, Taylor T, Meer J. Emergency ultrasound: pericardial effusion and tamponade: making the diagnosis at bedside with point-of-care echocardiography. *Emerg Med* 2017; 49: 517–519.
32. Mirabel M, Bacquelin R, Tafflet M, et al. Screening for rheumatic heart disease: evaluation of a focused cardiac ultrasound approach. *Circ Cardiovasc Imaging* 2015; 8(1): e002324. https://doi.org/10.1161/CIRCIMAGING.114.002324.

33. Brown OR, DeMots H, Kloster FE, et al. Aortic root dilatation and mitral valve prolapse in Marfan's syndrome: an echocardiographic study. *Circulation* 1975; 52: 651–657.
34. Bravo-Valenzuela NJ, Peixoto AB, Junior EA. Prenatal diagnosis of congenital heart disease: a review of current knowledge. *Indian Heart J* 2018; 70: 150–164.
35. Moore C. Current issues with emergency cardiac ultrasound probe and image conventions. *Acad Emerg Med* 2008; 15: 278–284. https://doi.org/10.1111/j.1553-2712.2008.00052.x.

CHAPTER 5

Gastroenterology

Abigail Limov[1], Edwin Seldon Davis[1], Dale Woodbury[1], and Man Zhang[2]

[1] Rocky Vista University, College of Osteopathic Medicine, Ivins, Utah, USA

[2] Department of Radiology, University of Michigan, Ann Arbor, Michigan, USA

Introduction

Ultrasound is a widely accessible and essential medical imaging tool for assessment of intra-abdominal organs such as the liver, gallbladder, bile ducts, pancreas, spleen, and gastrointestinal system [1]. Studies have shown a variety of ultrasound applications for the abdomen, including the evaluation of gallstones, liver parenchyma disease, acute abdomen, pediatric abdomen, inflammatory or parasitic intestinal diseases, and much more [2–6]. Importantly, ultrasound is safe, mobile, less expensive than other imaging modalities, and offers real-time imaging to evaluate the morphology and blood flow of the abdominal organs [7]. Given these advantages, many specialties such as gastroenterologists, family medicine, emergency, and critical care physicians have been using abdominal ultrasound in their daily patient care [7, 8].

This chapter will cover the gastrointestinal ultrasound indications, anatomy, scanning protocols, and common pathologies for the liver, gallbladder, pancreas, spleen, and intestines.

General Anatomy of the Abdomen

The abdomen is divided into four quadrants that are delineated by a vertical line from the xiphoid process to the pubic symphysis and a horizontal line through the umbilicus [9]. The separation of the abdomen into quadrants aids in the identification of organs within the abdomen (Fig. 5.1). The right upper quadrant (RUQ) contains the gallbladder, right hepatic lobe, right kidney, hepatic flexure of the colon, proximal transverse colon, and the head of the pancreas [9]. The left upper quadrant contains the left hepatic lobe, stomach, left kidney, spleen, distal transverse colon, splenic flexure, and the remainder of the pancreas [9]. The left lower quadrant contains the descending colon, sigmoid colon, small intestine, and the left ureter. The right lower quadrant contains the appendix, ascending colon, cecum, small intestine, and right ureter [9]. Knowledge of the abdominal anatomy is critical to guide the appropriate placement of the transducer when assessing a target organ or structure.

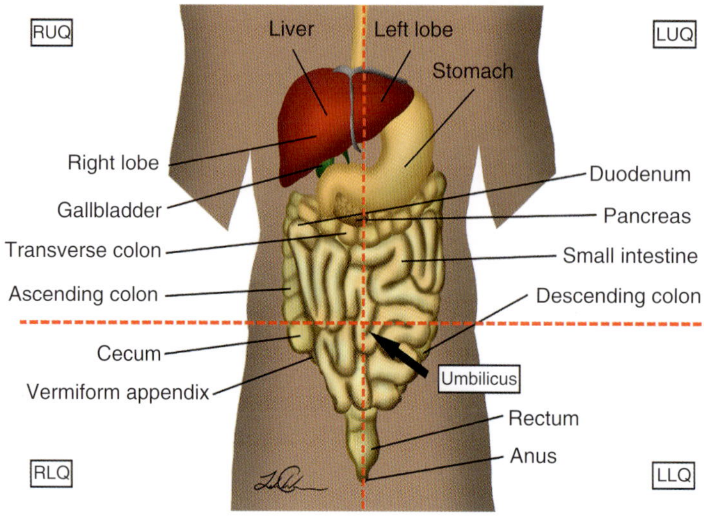

FIGURE 5.1 Illustration of the abdominal anatomy.

Ultrasound Techniques

Fasting for six hours prior to an abdominal ultrasound is routinely requested. Ultrasound techniques performed in the abdomen consist of grayscale imaging, color, and spectral Doppler. Emerging ultrasound elastography and contrast-enhanced ultrasound (CEUS) are only available on high-end ultrasound machines. Abdominal ultrasonography scan in adults is usually performed using a curved linear or phased array transducer. A higher-frequency transducer or probe has better image resolution; however, it comes with a tradeoff of decreased depth penetration [10]. For pediatric patients, it is preferred to use a probe with a frequency of 5 MHz or higher [11]. Adult abdominal ultrasound is best performed in a frequency range of 4–6 MHz for the liver, but a higher frequency may be needed when assessing the abdominal wall and bowel [10]. It is important to use a low-frequency transducer to improve beam penetration in order to visualize the deeper structures, even though the image resolution may decrease.

Common Indications for Abdominal Ultrasound

Abdominal ultrasound is a noninvasive imaging method to screen and/or diagnose various liver, gallbladder, pancreatic, splenic, and intestinal diseases. The indications for abdominal ultrasound include acute and chronic abdominal pain, palpable masses, jaundice, abnormal laboratory values, or follow-up abdominal organ pathologies identified by other imaging studies [8]. Ultrasound is also valuable for hepatocellular cancer surveillance, evaluation and follow-up of liver cirrhosis and its sequelae of portal hypertension, and abdominal organ transplantation. In addition, ultrasound is often used to guide abdominal procedures such as intra-abdominal organ biopsy, hepatocellular cancer ablation, paracentesis, and drainage of intra-abdominal fluid collection [8].

Common Abdominal Ultrasound

Liver

Anatomy

The liver is the largest solid organ in the body and predominantly sits just below the right hemidiaphragm. The liver consists of four lobes: right, left, quadrate, and caudate lobes [12]. Using the Couinaud classification, the liver is further divided into eight segments [9].

The intrahepatic biliary tree is an outflow network of various channels that carry bile in the liver (Fig. 5.2). Despite a large amount of variation reported on the branching and draining of bile in the hepatic parenchyma, the left hepatic duct is consistently superior to the hepatic portal vein. The left hepatic duct is longer and more horizontal compared to the right hepatic duct, which is shorter and vertical. The common bile duct (CBD) most frequently crosses anteriorly over the right hepatic artery. However, 25% of CBD will travel posterior to the right hepatic artery in the hilum of the liver [13].

The liver receives a dual blood supply from the portal vein and the hepatic artery. The hepatic artery supplies oxygen-rich blood to the liver. The portal vein supplies nutrient-rich blood from the gastrointestinal tract. The liver can process the nutrients from the blood and filter out any toxic substances it contains before the blood goes back into general circulation [14]. The hepatic arterial system can have a variety of branching patterns, with the most common being the right and left hepatic artery branching off the proper hepatic artery and the middle hepatic artery branching off the right or left hepatic artery [14].

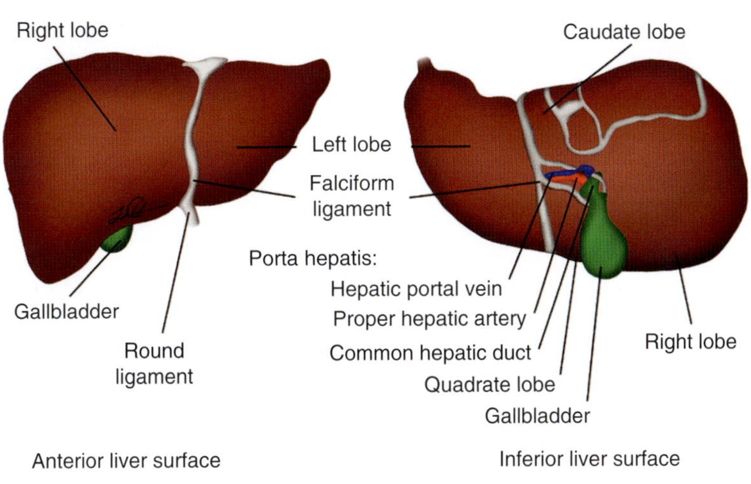

FIGURE 5.2 Illustration of the liver anatomy.

At the entrance to the liver, the portal vein bifurcates into the right and left portal veins that subsequently branch into segmental branches, which follow the hepatic arteries throughout the liver. The most common anatomical variation of the portal vein is a trifurcation into the left portal vein, anterior and posterior right portal veins [14]. Three large hepatic veins – the left, middle, and right hepatic veins drain deoxygenated blood from the liver into the inferior vena cava (IVC) [15].

Ultrasound Imaging of the Normal Liver

The liver should be imaged in the transverse and longitudinal axes; specifically, the longitudinal axis is used to measure the size of the liver [16]. The echogenicity of a normal liver should be similar to that of the cortex of the right kidney. In addition, normal liver parenchyma is diffusely homogeneous in echotexture without a focal lesion [17].

The major lobes of the liver, left, right, and caudate lobes (Fig. 5.3a,b) should be visualized, including the capsular surface, to assess surface nodularity. The vascular elements of the liver also need to be analyzed (Fig. 5.3c,d), which consist of the hepatic arteries, hepatic veins, main portal vein, and right and left branches of the intrahepatic portal vein. Color and spectral Doppler techniques are used to assess

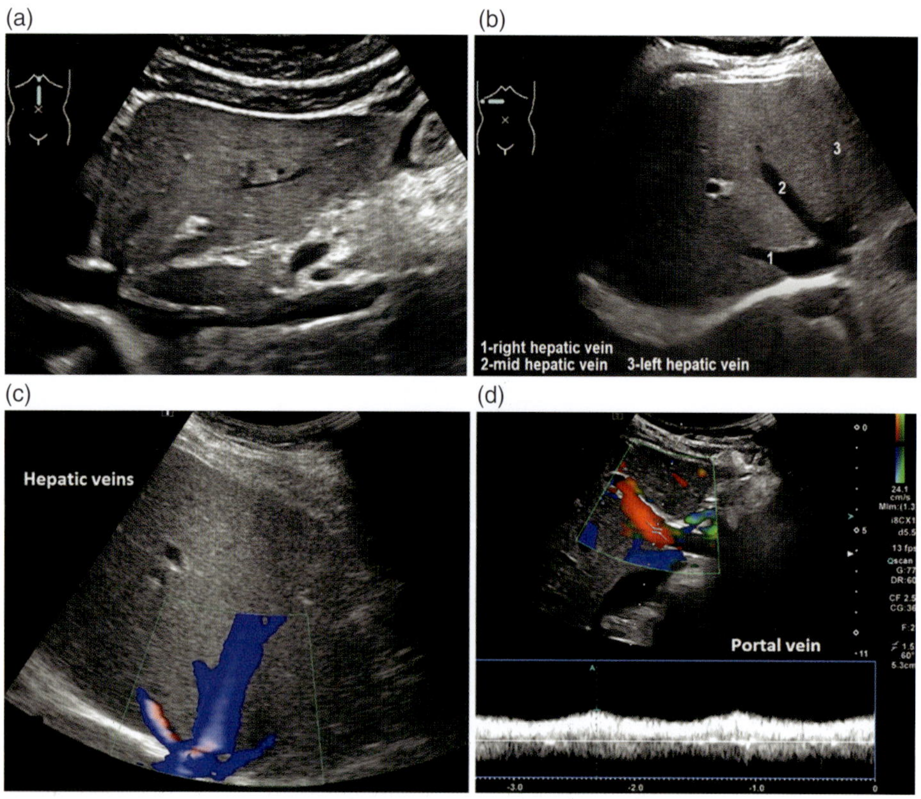

FIGURE 5.3 (a) B-mode ultrasound images of a normal left lobe (longitudinal plane); (b) left and right lobes (transverse plane) of the liver; (c) color flow imaging of the hepatic veins; (d) color and spectral Doppler demonstrate hepatopetal flow in the portal vein.

the hepatic vascular structures, including the patency of the vessels, and the velocity and direction of blood flow [17].

Common Pathology of the Liver

Benign Liver Cysts and Hemangiomas Liver cysts occur in a range from 2.5% to 18% of the general population. The incidence of liver cysts increases with age and is characterized by an epithelial cell lining with a fluid-filled space [18]. Besides simple cysts, hepatic cystic lesions can appear in amebic infection, echinococcal infection, hematoma, biloma, and necrotic/cystic neoplasms. Ultrasound-guided intervention in patients with confirmed cysts is only recommended if they are symptomatic. In B-mode ultrasound image, a simple cyst appears anechoic with posterior acoustic enhancement (Fig. 5.4a) and has no Doppler signal in color flow imaging (Fig. 5.4b). Internal echoes may be present in a cyst with hemorrhage or infection [18]. Another common benign focal liver lesion is a hemangioma. Either single or multiple liver hemangiomas appear as a hyperechoic structure with well-defined borders (Fig. 5.4c,d) [18].

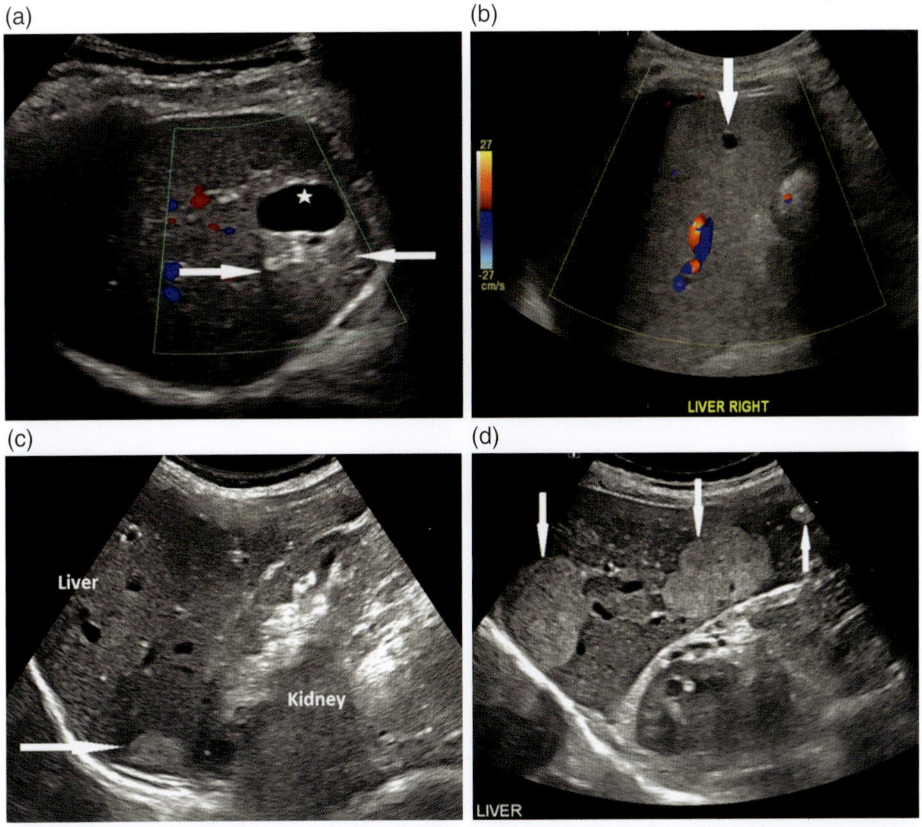

FIGURE 5.4 (a) Most liver cysts appear as anechoic structures (*) with posterior acoustic enhancement (arrows) in B-mode image, (b) no color signal (no blood flow) appears within the cyst (arrow) in color flow imaging. (c, d) Liver hemangioma (white arrows) is a common benign incidental finding on abdominal ultrasound. It can be a single (c) or multiple (d) in the liver.

Liver Abscesses Liver abscesses may mimic anechoic cysts on ultrasound. However, patients with liver abscess commonly present with fever, malaise, anorexia, and RUQ pain [19]. Hepatic abscesses may also appear as avascular hypoechoic lesions from suppuration. Other ultrasonographic features include internal septation, debris, and a range of wall thickness [20].

Metabolic Dysfunction-Associated Steatotic Liver Disease Nonalcoholic fatty liver disease (NAFLD) is a hepatic manifestation of metabolic syndrome, which is characterized by hepatic steatosis with minimal alcohol intake (<49 g/ wk) [21]. The new name for NAFLD is metabolic dysfunction-associated steatotic liver disease (MASLD), which was adopted in 2023 to reduce stigma and better reflect the metabolic origins of the disease, rather than focusing on a lack of alcohol as the defining factor [22].

MASLD is diagnosed by having greater than 5% hepatocytes containing fat. MASLD is the leading cause of chronic liver disease worldwide [22]. The current gold standard for diagnosis of MASLD is liver biopsy, which is invasive and can have complications or sampling errors [23]. The liver ultrasound for screening MASLD uses an intercostal approach [24]. Grayscale ultrasound is used to assess mild, moderate, and severe steatosis of the liver (Fig. 5.5). Mild steatosis is visualized by a mild diffuse

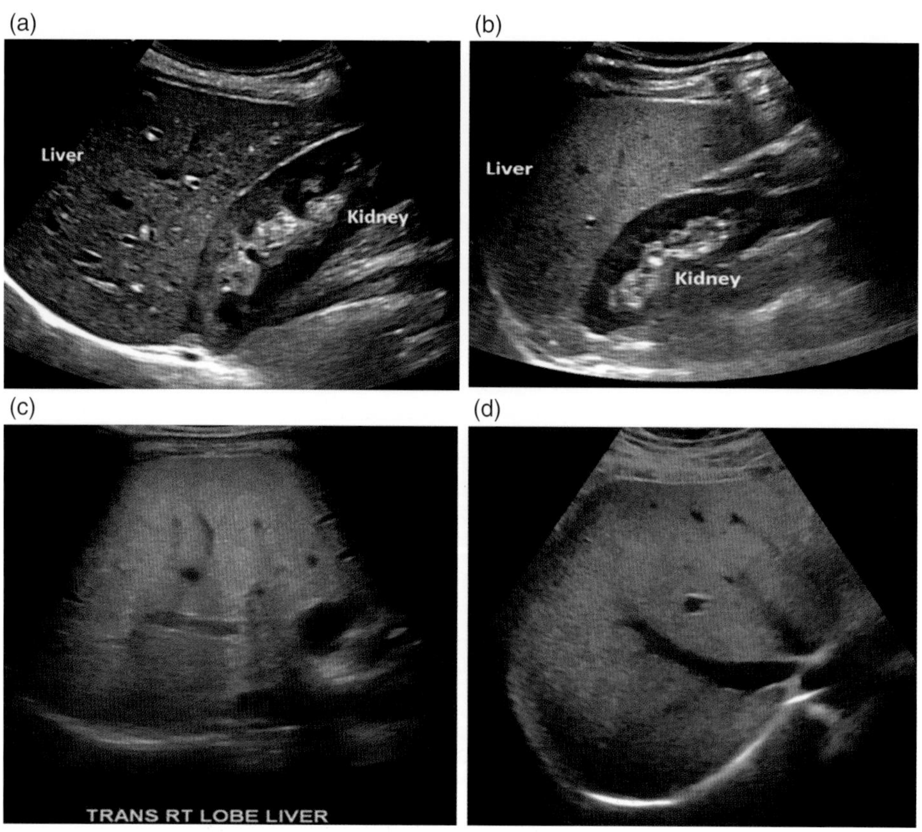

FIGURE 5.5 Based on echogenicity, intrahepatic vessels, and visibility of the diaphragm, conventional B-mode ultrasound is used to assess normal liver (a) and the liver with mild (b), moderate (c), and severe (d) steatosis.

increase in echogenicity of the liver. Moderate steatosis is seen with moderate diffuse echogenicity and mild impairment of view of the intrahepatic vessels and the diaphragm. Severe steatosis appears with a marked increase in echogenicity, with poor penetration of the posterior right lobe and little to no view of the liver vessels and diaphragm [25].

Acute and Chronic Hepatitis Chronic hepatitis is characterized by progressive liver fibrosis; therefore, early diagnosis is key to treatment. Chronic hepatitis is considered when acute hepatitis lasts longer than six months. The treatment of the disease depends on the cause, such as viral or metabolic [26]. Ultrasound provides a way to diagnose and follow the morphological changes associated with liver fibrosis in chronic hepatitis patients, with or without confirmatory liver biopsy. In many cases of chronic hepatitis, the liver has a normal morphology on grayscale ultrasound; therefore, a normal-appearing liver on conventional grayscale ultrasound image will not rule out chronic hepatitis [27].

Acute hepatitis on the other hand will present swollen hepatocytes, which leads to decreased echogenicity of the hepatic parenchyma and increased brightness of the portal triads due to the increased lymphocytes and monocyte infiltration. Hepatomegaly can also occur in acute hepatitis [27].

Cirrhosis and Portal Hypertension Ultrasound is the first-line modality to monitor cirrhosis. Patients with a history of alcoholism, chronic viral hepatitis, MASLD and steatohepatitis, autoimmune liver diseases, iron and copper overload, and drug toxicity have a higher risk of cirrhosis [28]. Cirrhosis can be observed on ultrasound as coarse parenchymal echotexture and surface irregularity (nodularity). The spectral Doppler waveform of the hepatic artery may appear as the pattern of increased resistance flow in individuals with cirrhosis [29].

Normal portal venous spectral waveform is seen as a mild undulating pattern above the baseline on spectral Doppler. There is a decreased portal venous flow velocity upon the development of portal hypertension. As portal hypertension becomes more severe, the portal venous flow will start to reverse – from the liver to the portal vein as "hepatofugal – non-forward portal flow" (Fig. 5.6). This can be assessed by color and spectral Doppler imaging [30]. In addition to a decrease in portal venous flow velocity and/or hepatofugal flow direction, an enlarged spleen, ascites, and upper abdominal varices, including patent paraumbilical vein, can be observed in grayscale ultrasound in a patient with severe portal hypertension (Fig. 5.6).

Gallbladder

Gallbladder Anatomy

The gallbladder is an oblong, pear-shaped sac that lies on the inferior surface of the liver in the gallbladder fossa, suspended by the mesentery [13, 31]. The gallbladder is a reservoir for the storage and concentration of bile, with a maximum capacity of 50 mL. It is divided into a fundus, body, and neck. The fundus of the gallbladder projects beyond the anterior margin of the liver and sits posterior to the 9th rib costal

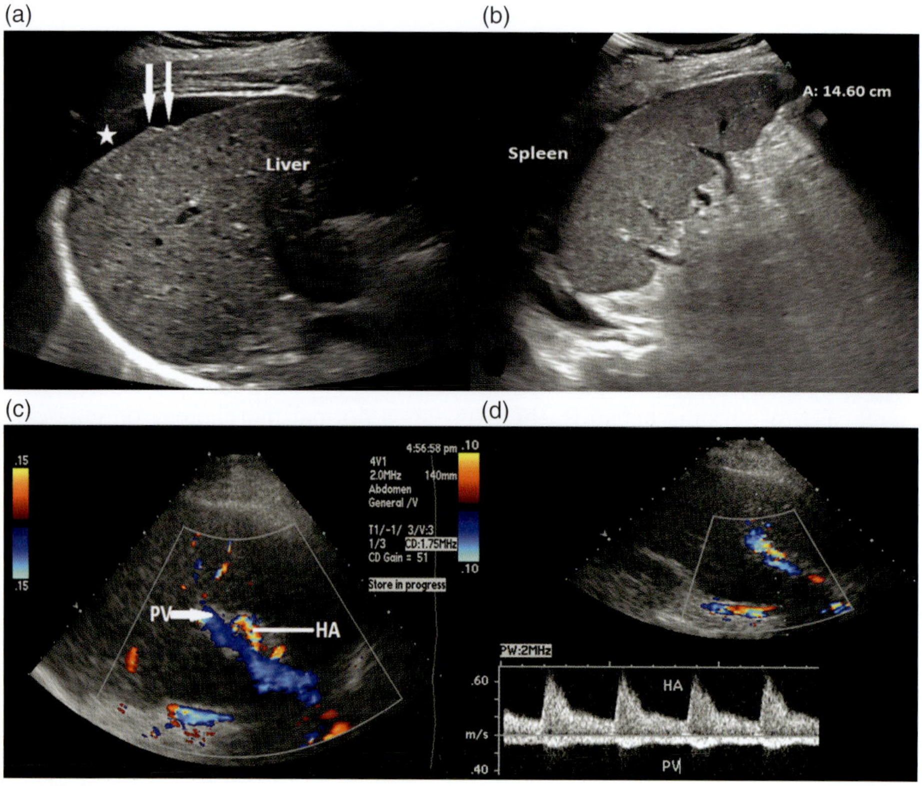

FIGURE 5.6 In a patient with cirrhosis and portal hypertension, heterogeneous liver parenchyma with nodular contour (a, white arrows), peritoneal ascites (a, *), and splenomegaly (b, spleen measures 14.60 cm) can be observed in B-mode image. In addition, color (c, blue color) and spectral Doppler (d, spectrum below the baseline) demonstrate forward flow (above the base line) in the hepatic artery and hepatofugal flow (below the base line) in the portal vein. HA, hepatic artery; PV, portal vein.

cartilage. The body and neck extend posterior, superior, and medial toward the spine [31]. The cystic bile duct and the common hepatic duct form the CBD, which drains through the Ampulla of Vater into the duodenum [13].

The CBD is 7.5–11 cm in length with a diameter of 0.6–0.8 cm that increases with age. The Ampulla of Vater opens into the duodenum via the major duodenal papilla through the sphincter of Oddi. The sphincter is normally closed unless stomach contents enter the duodenum, which then stimulates the release of cholecystokinin. Cholecystokinin leads to gallbladder contraction and relaxation of the sphincters, allowing bile and pancreatic secretions to be released into the duodenum [31].

Imaging of the Gallbladder and Biliary Tree

On grayscale ultrasound, a normal gallbladder lumen appears anechoic. In the fasting state, the gallbladder is distended with the thin gallbladder wall, measuring no more than 3 mm in thickness (Fig. 5.7). In the non-fasting state, the gallbladder may be contracted, and the wall tends to be thicker than that in fasting [13]. The gallbladder should be imaged with moderate distension for appropriate visualization

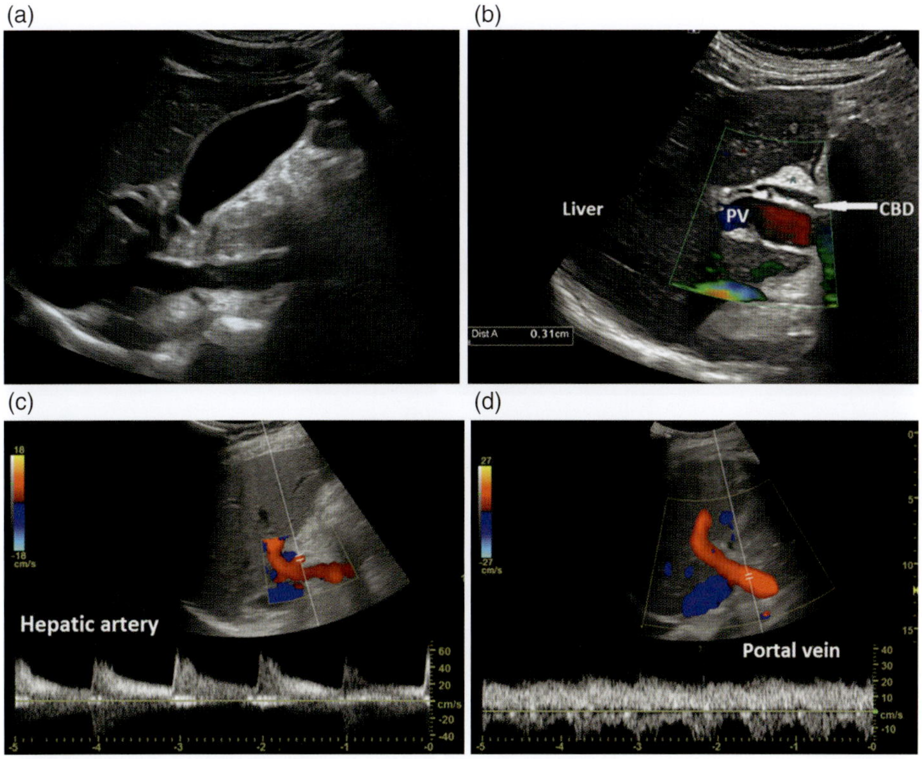

FIGURE 5.7 Normal gallbladder in B-mode image. (a) B-mode (b), color flow (c), and spectral Doppler (d) are useful to assess the common bile duct (CBD), hepatic artery (c), and portal vein (PV).

of structures. Distention can be induced by fasting six hours before the ultrasound scan. In children, the fasting period needs to be adjusted to their age. If they are unable to fast for the period needed, the gallbladder will appear smaller and more difficult to visualize [10]. The gallbladder should be imaged in longitudinal and transverse planes, with the patient in the supine and/or upright or lateral decubitus positions.

Doppler ultrasound can be used to differentiate between the bile duct, portal veins, and hepatic arteries (Fig. 5.7c,d). The bile ducts should be assessed for wall thickening, dilation, and intraluminal abnormalities. The diameter of the common duct at the porta hepatis should be reported, and if possible, the CBD behind the pancreatic head should also be measured [10]. The common duct usually measures 6 mm or less in diameter adjacent to the right hepatic artery at the porta hepatis. However, in elderly patients, the CBD can measure up to 8–9 mm without any associated pathology [13].

Gallbladder Pathology

Cholelithiasis Cholelithiasis, or gallstones, is a common disease with a prevalence of 10% in the general population, with ⅔ of patients being asymptomatic [32]. On grayscale ultrasound, a gallstone appears as a hyperechoic structure within the

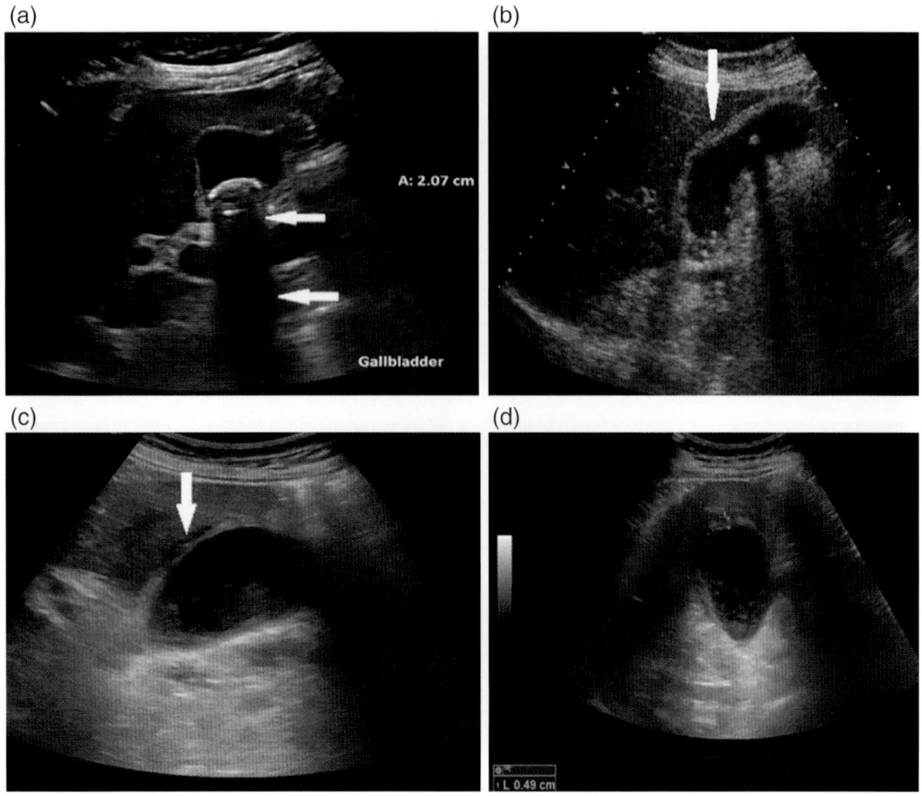

FIGURE 5.8 A Gallstone appears as an echogenic structure (a, size of gallstone: $A = 2.07\,\text{cm}$) with acoustic shadowing (a, white arrows) in B-mode ultrasound image. Gallstones can be single (a) and multiple (b). Gallstones (c), pericholecystic fluid (c, white arrow), thickened gallbladder wall (d, the anterior wall of the gallbladder measures 4.9 mm), and sludge (b–d, internal echoes in the gallbladder) are observed in patients with acute cholecystitis.

gallbladder lumen with posterior acoustic shadowing if the stone is greater than 3 mm in size (Fig. 5.8). For the detection of gallstones, it is preferred to use a high-frequency transducer so that the shadowing from the stone is maximized, allowing for greater visualization [33]. A change in position from supine to lateral decubitus or upright position may help evaluate the mobility of gallstones and distinguish small gallstones from polyps.

Cholecystitis Acute cholecystitis, characterized by the inflammation of the gallbladder, is commonly seen in patients with an acute abdomen. The physiopathology of cholecystitis is the obstruction of the gallbladder at the neck, leading to luminal distension, inflammation, ischemia, and necrosis of the gallbladder [34]. Clinically, patients present with RUQ or epigastric pain as well as fever, leukocytosis, increased serum bilirubin, and serum alkaline phosphatase. Findings on ultrasound include thickening of the gallbladder wall (>3 mm), distension of the gallbladder lumen (>4 cm in transverse dimension), gallstones (may or may not be impacted in the neck of the gallbladder), pericholecystic fluid (Fig. 5.8c), positive sonographic Murphy sign, and a hyperemic gallbladder wall on color flow imaging [27, 35].

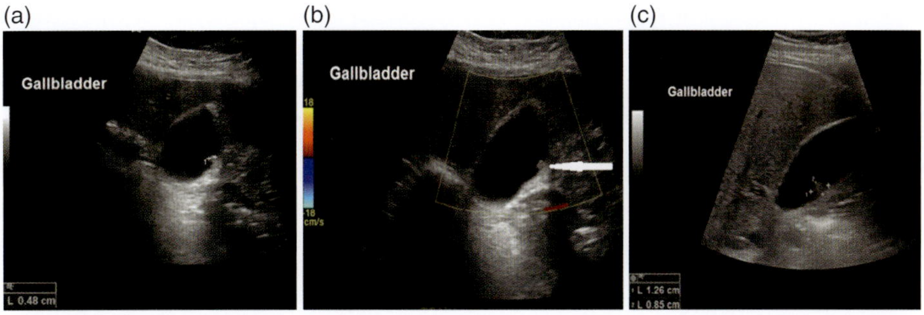

FIGURE 5.9 Gallbladder polyps appear as echogenic foci (4.8 mm) without acoustic shadowing (a). No color Doppler signal is observed in small (<8 mm) polyps (b). The size of gallbladder polyps ranges from 2 mm to more than 10 mm (c) in diameter.

Gallbladder Polyps The presence of polyps in the gallbladder is associated with the presence of cholesterolosis, or the buildup of lipids within macrophages in the gallbladder. The risk factors for cholesterolosis are the same as those seen with cholelithiasis; however, the diseases are rarely seen together [36]. Upon grayscale ultrasound, there may be one or multiple nonmobile non-shadowing lesions on the wall of the gallbladder [36]. The size of polyps ranges from 2 mm to more than 10 mm (Fig. 5.9). Some of the gallbladder polyps, especially the large ones, may have a vascular stalk on color flow imaging [37].

Gallbladder Cancer Compared to small benign polypoid lesions in the gallbladder, malignancies in the gallbladder are usually more than 10 mm in diameter [38]. The most common gallbladder malignancy is gallbladder adenocarcinoma, which accounts for the majority of gallbladder carcinoma in western population [39]. Primary gallbladder adenocarcinoma is seen as a large solid mass along the base of the gallbladder on ultrasound. However, it can look like thickening of the gallbladder wall or have a polypoid appearance [38]. Gallbladder metastatic mass from malignant melanoma appears as a vascular hyperechoic polypoid mass [40]. Another type of gallbladder metastasis is from gastric cancer, which is seen as a diffuse infiltrative cancer on ultrasound [41]. Increases in internal vascularity on color flow imaging may suggest malignancy. Ultrasound is a complementary imaging tool in the early detection of gallbladder carcinoma by identifying changes in polyps or gallbladder wall during surveillance [38].

Pancreas

Pancreas Anatomy

The pancreas is an elongated, slender organ located posterior to the inferior half of the stomach. Anatomically, the pancreas is divided into the head, uncinate process, neck, body, and tail. The typical length of this gland in a healthy adult is 14–18 cm long, 2–9 cm wide, and 2–3 cm thick, with the greatest mass concentrated in the head of the pancreas [42]. The head, or the widest and thickest part of the pancreas, can be found posterior to the stomach and duodenum. The body makes up much of the pancreatic parenchyma and extends toward the left side while tapering superiorly with the greater curvature of the stomach. The tail proceeds to be roughly adjacent to the spleen. Since the pancreas is posterior to the stomach and duodenum, the majority of the pancreas may be obscured from an anterior abdominal approach [42].

Pancreas divisum, seen in 10% of the general population, is a common congenital anomaly of the pancreas. Other congenital anomalies include pancreatic agenesis, hypoplasia, annular pancreas, and ectopic pancreatic tissue, which may also occur [43]. In up to 25% of patients with recurrent idiopathic pancreatitis, the underlying etiology may arise from pancreas divisum, or a secondary lack of fusion of the dorsal and ventral pancreatic ducts. The secretin stimulation test is used in patients with an increase of duct size and can be used to differentiate between chronic pancreatitis (CP) and a functional ductal obstruction [44].

The pancreatic ducts begin in the tail and progressively merge to form the main passage that meets with the CBD. At this junction, pancreatic secretions are deposited into the hepatopancreatic Ampulla of Vater, which further descends into the duodenum [42]. The opening of the orifice into the duodenum is known as the major duodenal papilla and is usually located 8–10 cm distal to the pylorus. Some individuals have a secondary/accessory pancreatic duct supplemental to the main pancreatic duct, usually found 2 cm from the main duct [45].

The pancreas has a rich arterial and venous supply required for its endocrine and exocrine functions, as well as its own perfusion. Any obstruction to flow in the aorta, the celiac trunk, the superior mesenteric artery, or any of its branches places the patient at higher risk for ischemia of the pancreas [45]. Venous drainage from the pancreas travels into the portal system through the portal vein, formed from the junction of the splenic and superior mesenteric veins. The portal vein is directly posterior to the neck of the pancreas, but venous drainage typically has more variation than arterial vasculature [45].

The pancreas has an extensive lymphatic drainage; however, the lymphatics are not particularly prominent unless exaggerated due to a pathological condition. The greatest potential for fluid and particulate drainage via lymphatics is evident in pancreatitis, which presents as edema or hemorrhage. Lymphatic channels typically parallel the blood vessels traversing the pancreas properly [45]. The pancreaticosplenic nodes, found along with the splenic artery, are the nodal drainage for the pancreatic body and tail [46]. Other peripancreatic lymph nodes, like the pancreaticoduodenal nodes, are usually grouped based on location. These nodes are anterior or posterior to where the pancreatic head curves around the duodenum [45]. The pancreaticoduodenal nodes may either drain inferiorly to the superior mesenteric nodes or superiorly to the hepatic nodes. The pancreatic head also has some direct lymphatic drainage through the subpyloric nodes and the hepatic nodes [46]. These nodes drain through the intestinal lymphatic trunk into the cisterna chyli and ultimately the thoracic duct or the left subclavian vein. These various lymphatic connections are extensive and important in consideration of the location of metastases from a pancreatic adenocarcinoma [45].

Ultrasound Imaging of the Pancreas

The pancreas is commonly scanned with the patient in the supine position. To increase the visualization quality, the investigator may ask the patient to drink water to fill the stomach [10]. All parts of the pancreas, including the main duct, head, uncinate process, neck, body, and tail, should be imaged (Fig. 5.10). Upon imaging,

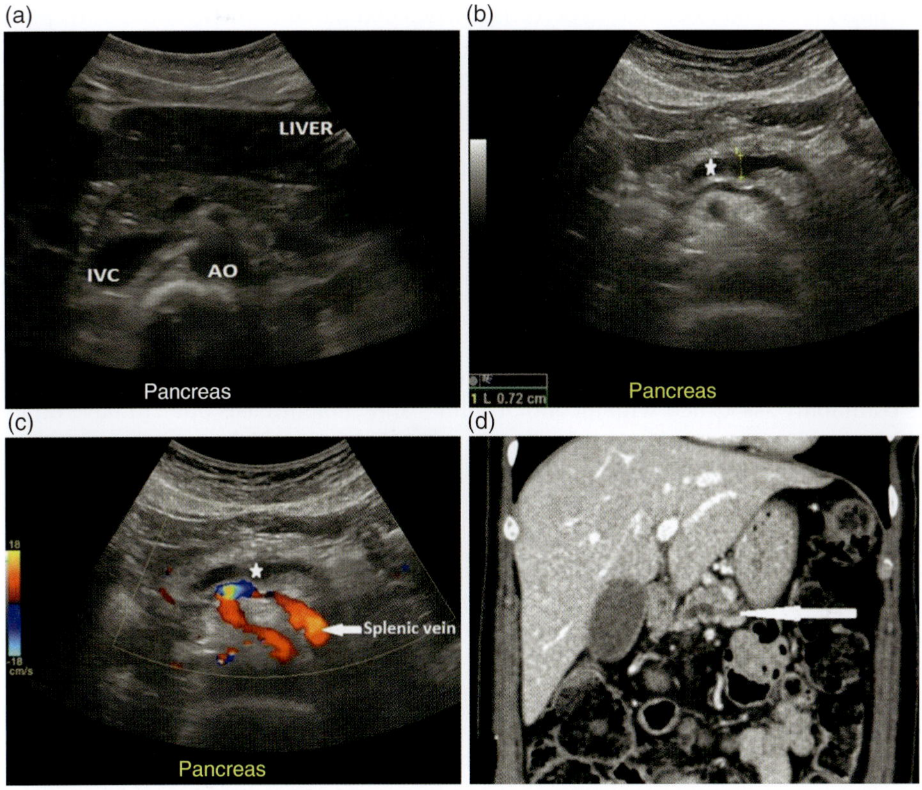

FIGURE 5.10 (a) B-mode ultrasound image of a normal pancreas. AO, aorta; IVC, inferior vena cava. Pancreatic duct dilatation is visualized in B-mode image (b, *), color flow imaging (c, *), and abdominal CT (d, arrow) in a patient with pancreatic (head) cancer and the dilatation of the main pancreatic duct (b–d).

evaluate the pancreas by looking for parenchymal abnormalities (masses or calcium deposition), the CBD near the head of the pancreas, the pancreatic duct for dilation or abnormalities, and the peripancreatic region for adenopathy or fluid [10].

Ultrasound allows studying the pancreas in detail in real-time at the patient's bedside. Ultrasound can also be an important aid for guiding pancreatic percutaneous procedures such as biopsy, ablation, or drainage. However, given the retroperitoneal location of the organ, visualizing the full extent of the pancreas can be difficult. The tail of the pancreas is sometimes referred to as a "blind area" due to gas in the stomach, making visualization difficult [47]. CT and MRI are superior to US for full visualization of the pancreas, as well as for demonstrating its relations with surrounding structures. It is also worth noting that graded compression is particularly useful for visualizing the pancreas and may be necessary to displace the overlying hollow organs [10], and the application of tissue harmonic imaging [44].

Pancreatic Pathology

The pancreas is normally located at the level of the L2 vertebrae, but this position is variable with respect to respiration. Texture, size, contour, and all anatomic portions of the pancreas should always be evaluated. A normal pancreas should appear homogeneous and isoechoic/hyperechoic when compared to the liver in adults [44]. Lipomatosis/fat deposition will occur in the pancreatic parenchyma, which may cause the gland to appear like peripancreatic fat associated with obesity and aging [48]. The size of the pancreas also depends upon the patient's body habitus and age. The main pancreatic duct appears as a thin hypoechoic line bordered by two echogenic margins. The upper limit of a normal main duct measures 4 mm in the head of the pancreas. The dilatation of the main pancreatic duct (Fig. 5.10b,c,d) may be present in patients with neoplasms, stones in the distal duct region. An accessory pancreatic duct can be visualized occasionally [44].

Acute Pancreatitis Defined as an acute inflammatory process of the pancreas, the diagnosis is usually based on serum lipase and amylase levels. Acute pancreatitis is commonly associated with alcohol, trauma, and cholelithiasis but can have other etiologies. There are two types of acute pancreatitis – interstitial edematous pancreatitis and necrotizing pancreatitis [44].

Ultrasound findings in patients with mild acute interstitial edematous pancreatitis may be unremarkable, while in more severe forms, the inflamed pancreas will appear more hypoechoic than the liver due to the inflammatory process causing edema and necrosis [44]. The presentation can be either diffuse or focal, with focal presenting as a heterogeneous appearance of the pancreas. When differentiating pancreatitis from a tumor, power Doppler may aid in showing increased vasculature associated with the hyperemic inflammatory process following pancreatitis [44]. Other complications of acute pancreatitis such as acute peripancreatic fluid collections, abscesses, hemorrhage, pseudocysts, or walled-off necrosis can also be present and must be taken into consideration when performing this exam [44, 46].

Pancreatic Abscesses/Necrosis and Pseudocysts Pancreatic necrosis is defined as a focal or diffuse area of nonviable pancreatic parenchyma. Computed tomography is the typical standard imaging modality [49]. A pancreatic pseudocyst is the most common pancreatic cystic lesion seen clinically, requiring immediate attention if rupture and subsequent hemorrhage of the cyst occur. On ultrasound, the pancreatic pseudocyst appears as a well-defined, anechoic or hypoechoic structure with posterior acoustic enhancement. The shape of a pancreatic pseudocyst is typically spherical or round [50]. A pancreatic walled-off necrosis, if occurring as a complication of necrotizing pancreatitis, usually occurs four weeks after acute onset, and may present as a heterogeneous structure containing debris in grayscale imaging. The debris may consist of pus, cellular infiltrates, or gas bubbles. These necrotic collections typically require percutaneous drainage or surgical debridement, and as previously stated, ultrasound can be the modality to guide a percutaneous drainage [44].

Chronic Pancreatitis Chronic Pancreatitis (CP) denotes chronic inflammation of the pancreas, leading to scarring and diminished function. The diagnosis of CP is usually based upon medical history, clinical findings, laboratory evaluations of pancreatic function, and morphologic changes. The sensitivity of ultrasound in diagnosing CP is variable, yet most studies provide a value of 60–70% [44]. This can be increased if ultrasound is utilized following a secretin stimulation test in which the pancreatic duct does not respond by increasing in size. With chronic pancreatitis, the pancreas is usually hyperechoic and atrophic because much of the pancreatic parenchyma has been replaced by adipose tissue, fibrosis, and local calcifications [44].

Pancreatic Adenocarcinoma Pancreatic adenocarcinomas represent most pancreatic cancers and have a very poor prognosis. Earlier diagnosis is associated with higher rates of full recovery and resectability if tumors are small, typically less than 1 cm, and limited to the epithelium of the duct, as considered an early stage. Pancreatic adenocarcinomas commonly present in the pancreatic head (Fig. 5.11a, b) and as a hypoechoic mass in grayscale imaging [44]. Color flow imaging can be utilized when assessing the extent of pancreatic adenocarcinoma, as it can help determine the extent of portal vein/peripancreatic artery vascular involvement. Since the outflow vasculature may be compromised by the tumor, a narrow vessel lumen with decreased flow velocities may present [44]. As such, B-mode and Doppler imaging can assist in assessing intra- and extrahepatic biliary dilatation resulting from pancreatic head tumor obstruction (Fig. 5.11c,d), and in assessing tumor resectability by evaluating hepatobiliary system, vasculature involvement, lymphadenopathy, or peritoneal metastases. Intraductal ultrasound is one of the more sensitive techniques for the detection of smaller pancreatic adenocarcinomas and may offer improved detection of papillary proliferation of the ductal epithelium, a common characteristic of carcinomas and adenomas. However, CT is considered superior to ultrasound in the assessment of pancreatic malignancy [51].

Cystic Neoplasms In addition to pancreatic pseudocyst, there are three common types of pancreatic cystic neoplasms: intraductal papillary mucinous neoplasm (IPMN), serous cystic neoplasm (SCN), and mucinous cystic neoplasm (MCN), among which SCN is the only tumor without malignant potential. SCN can be differentiated

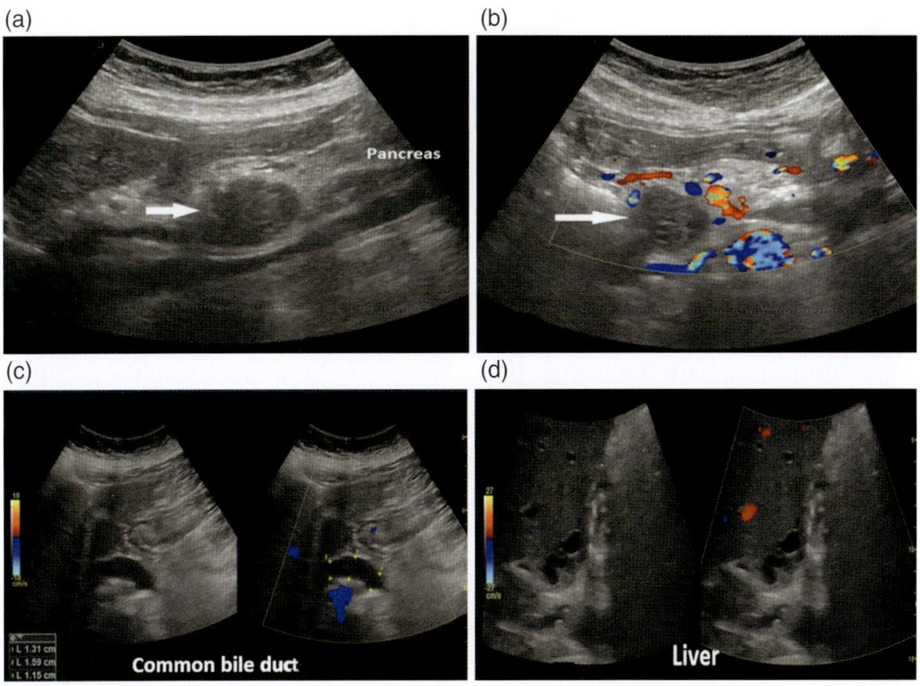

FIGURE 5.11 Pancreatic neoplasm (a, b, white arrow) with biliary obstruction on ultrasound (c, d). B-mode and color flow imaging show the dilatation of the common bile duct (c, CBD, common bile duct measures 12–16 mm) and intrahepatic ducts (d).

from a pancreatic adenocarcinoma based on echogenicity, as the adenocarcinoma will appear hypoechoic frequently, while the SCN will appear hyperechoic [52]. SCNs are commonly present in the head of the pancreas, while MCNs are usually present in the body or tail of the pancreas [44]. MCN usually appears as a unilocular cystic lesion that will not be as hyperechoic as the SCNs. Uncommon types of pancreatic cystic neoplasms include solid pseudopapillary neoplasm and cystic degeneration of neuroendocrine tumors [44].

Spleen

Anatomy of the Spleen

The spleen is a soft, highly vascular, ovoid organ situated in the left upper quadrant of the abdomen, lateral to the stomach and inferior to the left hemidiaphragm, protected by the 9th to 11th ribs [53, 54]. The spleen typically measures up to 12–13 cm in length in adults, although size varies with age, body habitus, and underlying pathology [55]. The spleen is suspended within the peritoneal cavity by the gastrosplenic and splenorenal ligaments, which also transmit the splenic vessels [53].

The spleen has convex diaphragmatic and concave visceral surfaces. The hilum is located on the visceral surface, providing entry and exit points for the splenic artery, vein, nerves, and lymphatic vessels [53, 54]. Structurally, the spleen is divided into the white pulp, which is lymphatic tissue involved in immune surveillance, and the red pulp, which is responsible for filtration and removal of senescent red blood cells [56]. Approximately 10–30% of individuals possess accessory splenic tissue (splenule), most commonly at the hilum or pancreatic tail [57].

Ultrasound Imaging of the Spleen

On grayscale ultrasound, the spleen is typically homogeneous with a fine, low-to-mid level echotexture that is slightly more hypoechoic than the liver [54, 58]. Ultrasound evaluation of the spleen is usually performed in both longitudinal and transverse planes, with the patient in a supine or right lateral decubitus position. Deep inspiration can improve the acoustic window by moving the spleen inferiorly, below the ribs [54, 59].

A low-frequency (2–5 MHz) curvilinear transducer is ideal for assessing the adult spleen, providing penetration and optimal resolution. In pediatric patients, a higher-frequency (5–7.5 MHz) transducer can be used for better resolution [59]. Spleen length is measured along the longest axis, extending from the dome to the inferomedial tip. The spleen should be evaluated for contour, echotexture, size, vascularity, and the presence of focal lesions or perisplenic fluid [55].

Color flow imaging is used to assess splenic vascularity, detect splenic vein thrombosis, and differentiate splenic vessels from adjacent bowel loops [60]. The splenic artery and vein can often be seen at the splenic hilum, with the splenic vein coursing toward the portal vein [59, 60].

Spleen Pathology

Ultrasound is a safe, portable, and effective imaging modality for evaluating the spleen, providing valuable information about its size, morphology, and pathology. Recognizing the normal anatomy and typical sonographic features of common splenic diseases is crucial for prompt diagnosis and guiding clinical management.

Splenomegaly Splenomegaly is defined sonographically as a craniocaudal length >12–13 cm in adults. Etiologies include portal hypertension, hematologic disease, infection, and infiltrative disorders [55, 61]. On ultrasound, the spleen appears enlarged but typically maintains its homogenous texture unless complicated by other pathology [55, 58] (Fig. 5.12). Marked enlargement raises suspicion for chronic disease or malignancy [55].

Splenic Trauma The spleen is the most frequently injured intra-abdominal organ in blunt abdominal trauma [62]. Ultrasound findings depend on the injury's type and severity and may include subcapsular hematoma (crescentic hypoechoic or anechoic collection), laceration (linear or wedge-shaped hypoechoic defect), or parenchymal hematoma (heterogeneous or hypoechoic focal lesion) [62]. Free intraperitoneal fluids may be seen in cases of rupture [62]. More details of splenic trauma can be found in Chapter 12 of this book.

Focal Splenic Lesions Splenic cysts/pseudocysts appear as well-defined, anechoic lesions with posterior acoustic enhancement, thin walls, and no internal vascularity [63]. Complex cysts/pseudocysts may have septations or internal debris (Fig. 5.13).

Splenic abscesses are rare, usually presenting as complex masses with irregular margins and internal echoes. Gas within an abscess can produce reverberation or ring-down artifacts [64] (Fig. 5.14).

Splenic hemangiomas are the most common benign primary neoplasm, presenting as well-circumscribed, usually hyperechoic lesions (Fig. 5.15), though less commonly these can be isoechoic [65].

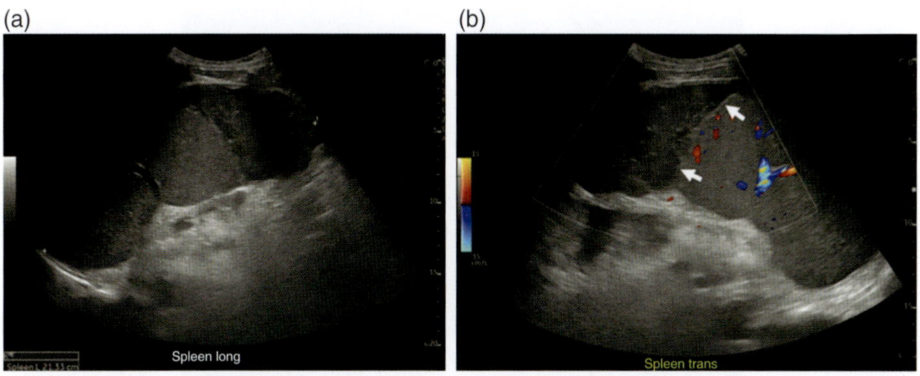

FIGURE 5.12 Longitudinal ultrasound (a) demonstrates splenomegaly (spleen length 21.3 cm). A wedge-shaped hypoechoic, avascular area in the spleen (arrows), consistent with splenic infarction (b).

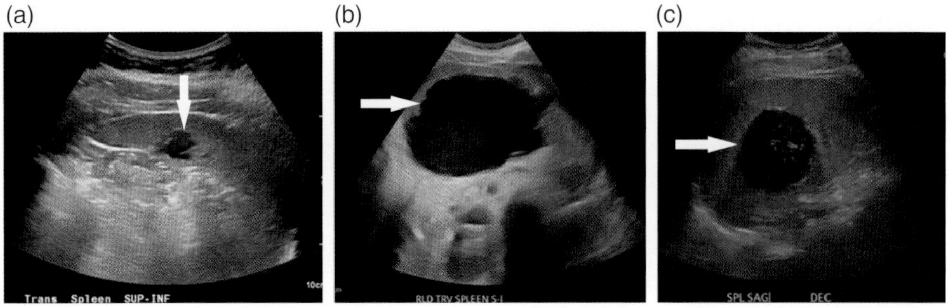

FIGURE 5.13 Splenic cyst (a), pseudocyst from recent trauma (b), and hematoma (c) on B-mode ultrasound images (arrows).

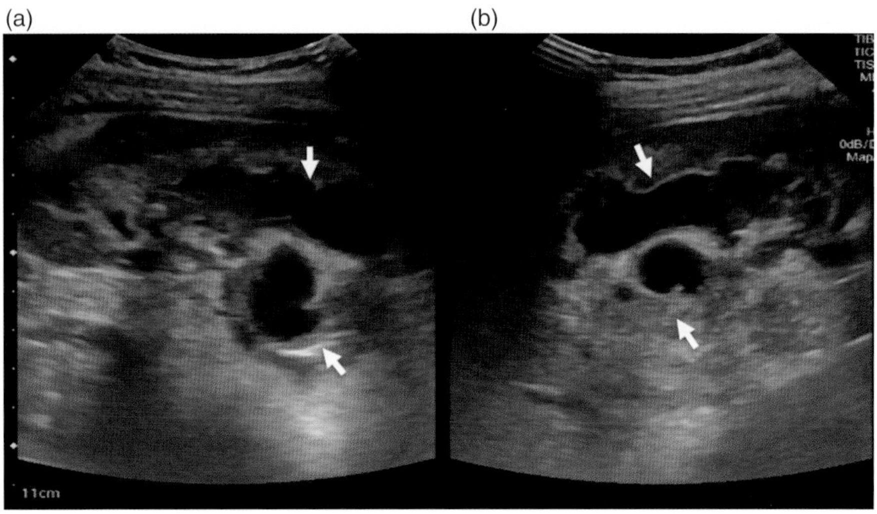

FIGURE 5.14 Transverse and longitudinal images (a, b) of multifocal splenic abscesses (arrows) on B-mode images.

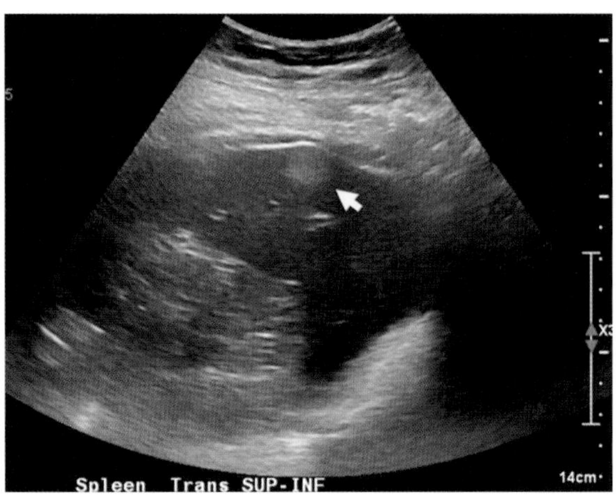

FIGURE 5.15 A well-circumscribed hyperechoic splenic hemangioma (white arrow) on B-mode ultrasound image.

Calcified granulomas in the spleen are usually the sequelae of prior granulomatous infections. On ultrasound, they appear as small, discrete, well-defined hyperechoic foci within the splenic parenchyma (Fig. 5.16), often with posterior acoustic shadowing. Calcified granulomas are usually asymptomatic incidental findings, reflecting remote and inactive disease.

Malignant lesions such as lymphoma (Fig. 5.17) or metastatic disease often present as hypoechoic, solitary, or multiple nodules; lymphoma can occasionally cause diffuse splenic enlargement without discrete masses, referred to as lymphomatous involvement of the spleen [66].

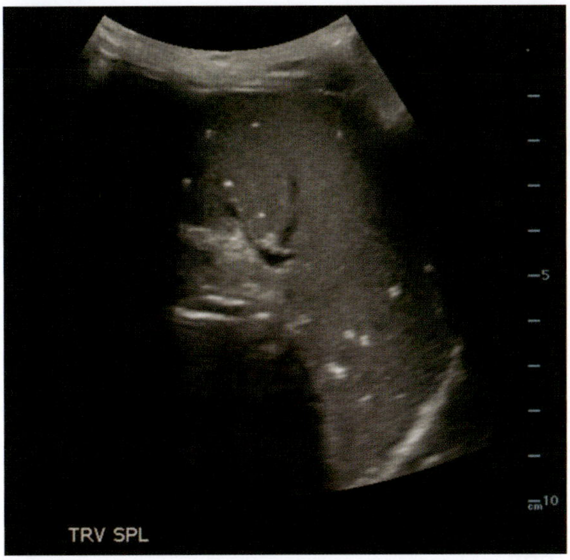

FIGURE 5.16 Multiple punctate subcentimeter splenic calcified granulomas on B-mode ultrasound image. SPL, spleen; TRV, transverse plane.

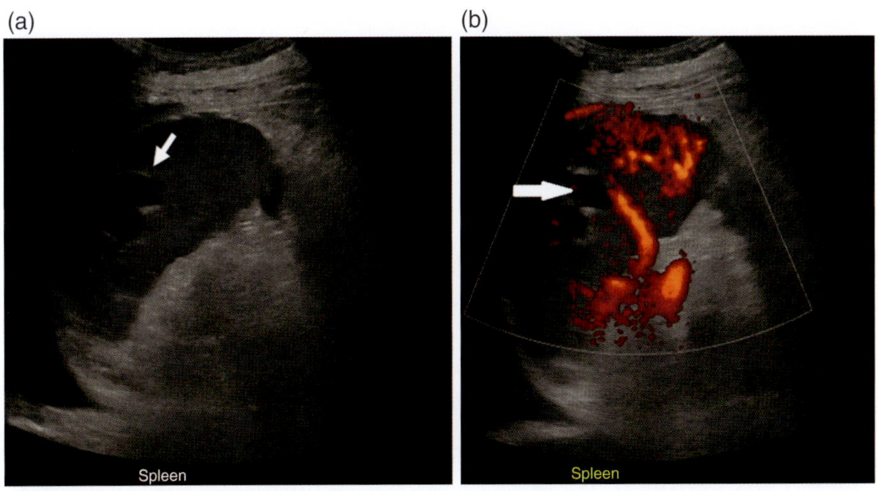

FIGURE 5.17 Hypoechoic splenic lesions (white arrow) on B-mode ultrasound image (a) and the power Doppler image (b).

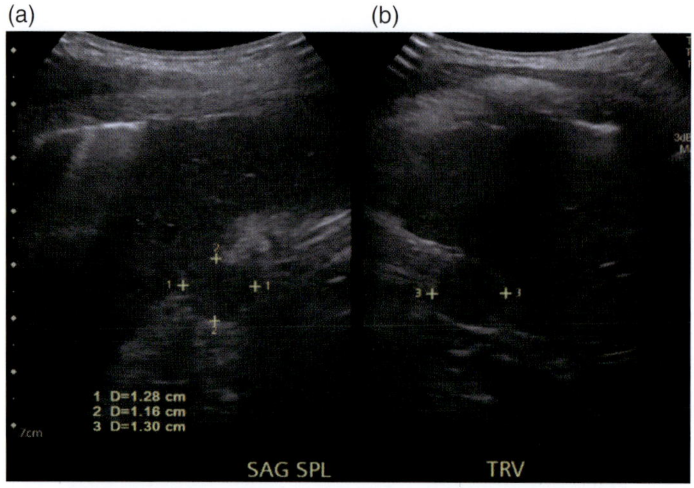

FIGURE 5.18 A small accessory spleen (between calipers) at the splenic hilum on B-mode ultrasound images. D, diameter; SAG, sagittal plane (a); SPL, spleen; TRV, transverse plane (b).

Vascular Pathology Splenic infarction results from occlusion of the splenic artery or branches and typically appears as a peripheral, wedge-shaped hypoechoic area with the base toward the capsule and apex toward the hilum. Chronic infarcts become more echogenic and may retract, creating contour deformities [67]. Splenic vein thrombosis can be visualized as echogenic material within the vein and a lack of flow on color flow imaging [68].

Accessory Spleen Accessory spleens are small (usually <2 cm), round structures with the same echotexture as the main spleen and are most often located at the splenic hilum or pancreatic tail (Fig. 5.18). They are usually of no clinical significance but can become hypertrophic after splenectomy and may be mistaken for lymphadenopathy or neoplasm [57, 69].

Gastrointestinal Tract

Anatomy of the Stomach

The stomach is the widest portion of the GI tract and is continuous with the esophagus and the small intestine. The stomach's arterial supply is usually derived from its embryological origin as the foregut; as a result, the stomach is perfused by the celiac trunk/artery [70]. Much of the stomach organ is mainly located in the left hypochondrial region, shielded partially by the rib cage, while the remaining distal parts of the organ exist in the epigastric region [46]. The stomach is highly distensible with an average capacity of 1.5 L in a grown adult; hence, its location may vary. The stomach has two curvatures, the greater curvature and the lesser curvature, which form the inferior and superior margins. The stomach also has two main orifices/apertures [71]. The superior/proximal opening drains the esophageal contents and

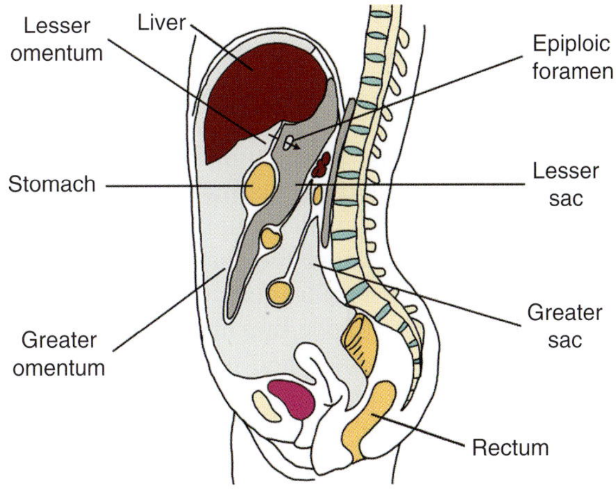

FIGURE 5.19 Illustration of the anatomy of the stomach, small intestine, and large intestine.

is known as the gastroesophageal sphincter, while the inferior/distal opening allows access to the duodenum, the first section of the small intestine, and is known as the pyloric sphincter [46]. The stomach proper is further broken down into the fundus, body, and pyloric regions, each with its own physiological and histological differences [71]. Immediately surrounding the stomach are several spaces, such as the omental bursa/lesser sac, the greater sac/general peritoneal cavity, and the epiploic foramen/foramen of Winslow [46]. These spaces may undergo pathologic changes such as filling with fluid or metastases, which may be depicted by imaging. Posteriorly, the stomach is surrounded by the omental bursa (Fig. 5.19), as well as several other structures that make up the "stomach bed." The anterior stomach borders the left hemidiaphragm while the superior lateral region of the greater curvature is adjacent to the medial border of the spleen [46].

The stomach has a rich blood supply solely arising from the celiac trunk due to its foregut origin. The celiac trunk diverges into three branches: the splenic artery, the common hepatic artery, and the left gastric artery. All three contribute to the stomach's perfusion through two connecting arterial arcades, located along the greater and lesser curvatures, providing the stomach with the majority of its blood supply [70]. Venous drainage corresponds to the arteries supplying the stomach, ultimately draining to the portal vein and the liver [46]. Lymphatic drainage for the stomach occurs through a rich network of anastomosing vessels located within the stomach's submucosa [70]. From these channels, lymph drains into the superior or inferior gastric lymph nodes, eventually passing their contents to the celiac group of preaortic lymph nodes [46].

Anatomy of Small Intestine and Large Intestine

Small Intestine The small intestine originates with the duodenum at the pyloric sphincter. The duodenum progresses until the duodenojejunal flexure, where its contents are propelled into the jejunum and then the ileum by peristaltic motion [46]. Each section of the small intestine helps to digest food and absorb its nutrients, electrolytes, and vitamins. To perform its functions, the small intestine requires an equally extensive vascularization [70]. The superior portion of the duodenum lies above the pancreatic head at the level of the first lumbar vertebrae [46]. Immediately behind the superior duodenum, the gastroduodenal artery and CBD can be found, with the IVC even more posteriorly [70]. Anteriorly, the liver and the neck of the gallbladder border the superior duodenum. The descending duodenum exists immediately lateral to the head of the pancreas and anterior to the right renal hilum and posterior to the transverse colon [46]. The main pancreatic duct and CBD share an opening into the posteromedial wall of the descending duodenum, at the major duodenal papilla. The duodenum continues its C-shaped course as the descending duodenum flows into the horizontal duodenum and then the ascending duodenum, with close relations to the muscles, organs, and surrounding vasculature [70].

The ascending duodenum continues directly as the jejunum at the duodenojejunal flexure. In contrast to the duodenum, the jejunum and ileum have a mesenteric attachment and are mobile within the abdominal cavity [70]. This mesenteric attachment is a fan-shaped, double-layered sheet of peritoneum attached to the posterior abdominal wall within a distinct divot [46]. The attachment line anchors posteriorly to the left of midline at the level of the 2nd lumbar vertebrae and proceeds across the midline toward the right iliac fossa and is known as the root of the mesentery. The root of the mesentery contains the superior mesenteric artery, vein, and lymph nodes [46]. The entire jejunum, ileum, and small intestine mesentery are in the infracolic compartment of the peritoneal cavity, inferior to the attachment of the transverse mesocolon [46]. The jejunum contains a thick and wide wall. As the jejunum transitions into the ileum, the thickness of the intestinal wall gradually decreases. The jejunum is typically more vascular than the ileum, and its loops can be found in the upper left region of the infracolic compartment, while the loops of ileum are usually located in the lower part of the abdominal cavity [46].

The small intestine typically receives its arterial flow from the superior mesenteric artery via its inferior pancreaticoduodenal, jejunal, and ileal branches. The venous drainage corresponds with and mirrors the arterial flow but will generally feature more variation than the arterial vasculature [46]. The proximal half of the duodenum receives its arterial supply from the celiac trunk, while the more distal half of the duodenum receives its arterial supply from the superior mesenteric artery, similar to the jejunum and ileum [72]. The corresponding venous drainage progresses to the superior mesenteric vein alongside the artery within the root of the mesentery [46]. Lymphatic vessels accompany these blood vessels and filter lymph into a series of nodes located between the layers of the small bowel mesentery. The mesenteric nodes eventually drain into the preaortic lymph nodes located at the origin of the superior mesenteric artery [72].

Large Intestine The ileum terminates at the ileocecal valve; this anatomical location delineates the origin of the large intestine in the right lower quadrant of the abdomen. The large intestine then runs from the cecum and appendix to the anus while acting as a frame for the small intestine on all sides [46]. Divisionally, the large intestine features the cecum, colon, rectum, and anus (Fig. 5.19). The ileocecal valve controls the flow of chyme from the ileum into the cecum, opening superomedially to the aperture of the appendix [46]. The cecum then blends into the ascending colon, as chyme is pushed superiorly by peristaltic forces. This superior path terminates at the inferior surface of the liver as the ascending colon bends to form the right colic (or hepatic) flexure, and progresses after this right angle from the right to the left as the transverse colon [46]. The transverse colon then progresses into another right-angle turn at the left colic (or splenic) flexure just inferior to the spleen. Chyme then descends from the splenic flexure to the descending colon, which enters the pelvis inferiorly to become the S-shaped sigmoid colon [46]. The colon flows in and out of the peritoneal cavity, and these anatomical relationships must be considered when performing an ultrasound to isolate pathological findings regionally. The rectum, ascending and descending colons are all located retroperitoneally, while the transverse and sigmoid colons are anchored to the posterior abdominal wall by the mesocolon. Chyme progresses from the sigmoid colon into the rectum near the third sacral vertebrae [46].

Ultrasound of the Gastrointestinal Tract

Ultrasound can be used to evaluate bowel wall thickening, hypertrophy, masses, dilatation of the bowel loops, vascularity, and other abnormalities of the bowel. For example ultrasound is valuable in evaluating the pylorus and its surrounding structures in an infant with non-bilious projectile vomiting, while graded compression sonography allows for higher quality assessment of the appendix [10]. It should be noted that color or power Doppler imaging may also be of use in suspected vascular abnormalities, such as hypervascular malignancy or ischemic changes due to vessel thrombosis or torsion [10].

Ultrasound for acute gastrointestinal pathologies is typically performed using graded compression, with pressure comparable to gentle palpation of the abdomen. Graded compression is essential to displace and compress bowel loops, decrease the distance between the structure of interest and the transducer, and to assess for rigidity. Compression of bowel loops allows for minimization of the erroneous influence of bowel contents such as gas or feces, as well to bring the high-frequency transducer closer to the structure of interest, allowing for higher image quality [73]. The rigidity felt from compression maneuvers can be utilized to differentiate between normal or soft intra-abdominal fat, inflamed, noncompressible fat, as well as to reproduce symptoms for diagnostic clarity [73]. The amount of compression applied is determined based on patient comfort, as pain from ultrasonography should never exceed the pain experienced in a given physical examination. Endocavity ultrasound is also useful for evaluating gastrointestinal conditions, such as detecting early rectal cancer and staging, visualizing sigmoid diverticulitis, or an inflamed appendix if located in an abnormally low position [74].

Both high- and low-frequency transducers should be used, as the location of the bowel and any related pathologies can be more superficial than expected, especially when using graded compression [73]. However, given their fixed retroperitoneal locations, the ascending and descending colons can reliably be visualized. A posterolateral position for scanning is recommended when attempting to scan gas-filled structures, such as an empyema of the appendix, an abscess, or a dilated loop of bowel, as the gas can affect the imaging quality in other positions such as the decubitus. If ultrasound results are inconclusive, a CT scan is indicated for further evaluation [74].

Gastrointestinal Tract Pathology

Hypertrophic Pyloric Stenosis Hypertrophic pyloric stenosis (HPS) is a common surgical condition in infants that typically occurs between 6 and 12 weeks of age. This condition is characterized by the idiopathic thickening of pyloric musculature and failure to relax the pyloric canal, resulting in progressive gastric outlet obstruction. Infants with HPS present with non-bilious projectile vomiting. In some cases, hypertrophied pylorus may be palpable as an olive-sized epigastric mass.

Ultrasound is the modality of choice in clinical settings as it provides a noninvasive and nonionizing dynamic study and allows direct visualization of the pyloric morphology and function. Ultrasound is performed with a small, high-frequency linear or curvilinear transducer in a supine or right posterior oblique position. Transverse images in the epigastric region identify the gastric pylorus to the left of the gallbladder and anteromedially to the right kidney.

An easy technique is to find the gallbladder first and then turn the probe obliquely to identify pylorus longitudinally. A small amount, approximately 20–30 mL, of clear fluid may be administered orally or by a nasogastric tube to fill the gastric antrum, acting as an acoustic window when the stomach is empty [75].

The hypertrophic muscular layer is hypoechoic on ultrasound, and the central mucosa is hyperechoic (Fig. 5.20). The dynamic assessment is also vital for the diagnosis of HPS. HPS can be confirmed by the observation of

1. Fixed thickened and elongated pyloric muscle over time
2. Frequent but ineffective peristalsis
3. Failure of the pylorus to open

The main diagnostic criterion is based on the thickness of the muscular layer. An abnormal cutoff value of 3 mm in thickness is commonly accepted (Table 5.1). Sonographic signs of HPS include antral nipple sign, cervix sign, and target sign.

(a) (b) (c)

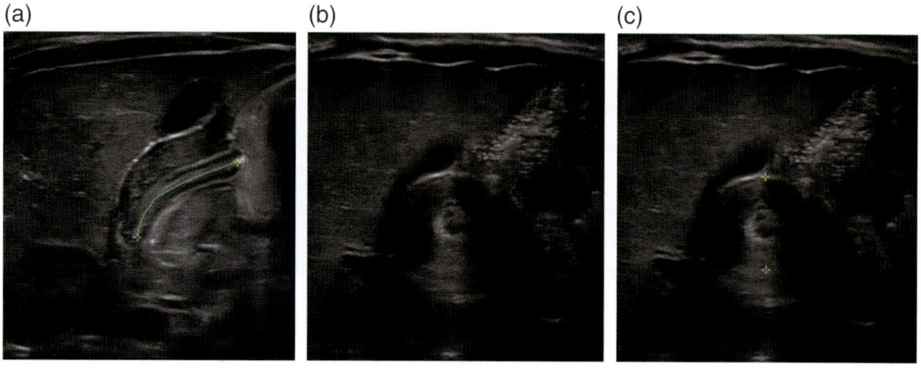

FIGURE 5.20 The length (a, 23 mm), muscle thickness (b, 4.8 mm), and width (c, 15 mm) of the pylorus are measured to assess pyloric stenosis using B-mode ultrasound image.

TABLE 5.1 **Grayscale ultrasound of normal pylorus and hypertrophic pyloric stenosis.**

	NORMAL PYLORUS	HYPERTROPHIC PYLORIC STENOSIS
Pyloric length (mm)	<15	≥16
Pyloric width (mm)	<11	≥11
Muscle thickness (mm)	<2.5	≥3

Source: Data from [75].

Sensitivity and specificity of ultrasound for the diagnosis of HPS have been reported over 97% in expert hands. It should be noted that if clinical suspicion persists after a negative ultrasound, a repeat study may be performed in two days to exclude an evolving pyloric stenosis [75].

The etiologies of pyloric stenosis in adults include tumor invasion, inflammation and infection, chronic fibrosis, et al., which are beyond the scope of this book.

Crohn's Disease and Ulcerative Colitis In Crohn's disease, the bowel walls of the terminal ileum and the cecum may appear thickened, and mesenteric lymphadenopathy may be present on ultrasound. Colonoscopy can be used to assess Crohn's disease. However, CT and MR enterography are the first-line imaging modalities for the diagnosis and surveillance of Crohn's disease. Ultrasound may be useful for early bedside evaluation, especially when colonoscopy, CT, or MR enterography are not appropriate or available [76].

Chronic inflammation in either of these conditions will result in adipose tissue depositing in the submucosal layer of the bowel wall, producing an increased echogenicity on grayscale image [77]. Doppler imaging of any actively inflamed bowel loops may demonstrate an increased vascularity, and this can be used to distinguish between active versus remission states [77, 78]. The diagnostic role of ultrasound with ulcerative colitis is less established than with Crohn's disease, but findings are similar, showing the increased submucosal echogenicity due to fat deposition [77]. In addition to grayscale and Doppler ultrasound, CEUS and ultrasound elastography may contribute to the evaluation of bowel wall stiffness and the response to medical therapy [77].

Bowel Perforations and Free Air Most patients with a perforated peptic ulcer will present with free air, seen on the erect chest or abdominal radiographs or CT, which establishes the diagnosis. Ultrasound can be useful for early diagnosis as it may reveal the true cause of abdominal pain through direct demonstration of pathology. In the case of a perforated duodenal ulcer, gastric contents would descend along the paracolic gutter toward McBurney's point. The presence of extraluminal gas, characterizing with echogenic area with "dirty shadowing," may be noted in grayscale ultrasound [78, 79]. Air within the peritoneal cavity can be observed with the patient in the left decubitus position, as air will accumulate lateral to the liver [80].

Bowel Obstruction Clinical suspicion of small bowel obstruction (SBO) is usually made based on patient history and classic presentation (crampy abdominal pain, distention, nausea, and vomiting), but these classic symptoms are not always present, especially early on [81]. Delay in diagnosis and management is associated with a higher risk for complications such as strangulation, bowel ischemia/necrosis, and even sepsis. While CT represents the gold standard imaging modality, point-of-care ultrasound is very useful and can be performed at the patient's bedside in an emergency setting. Ultrasound can also be used to identify other related causes of abdominal pain, such as gallstones, appendicitis, and an abdominal aortic aneurysm [62].

All abdominal quadrants should be scanned to detect free fluid, and either a high- or low-frequency probe can be used as necessary to visualize related structures. The diagnosis of bowel obstruction is made if dilated, fluid-filled small bowel loops are seen with the presence of peristaltic and parietal abnormalities [81]. Artifacts and interference may be seen as a result of gas in the distended bowel, and these can be avoided through thorough scanning in the oblique and coronal planes, or by using graded compression while moving over the abdomen in order to squeeze air away from the region of interest [81].

Appendicitis Given proficiency and ability to utilize the ultrasonography effectively, the inflamed appendix can be demonstrated most in pediatric patients [74]. Typically, an inflamed appendix can be found in the right lower abdomen as a hypervascular, aperistaltic, blind-ending structure that is incompressible (Fig. 5.21). The clinician/technician performing the scan should aim to identify an edematous cecal pole as well as a possible fecalith causing the obstruction and inflammation [77]. In acute appendicitis, the local fat surrounding the appendix will be inflamed and noncompressible and can be differentiated from lymphoid hyperplasia. Clinicians must take into consideration that with ischemic necrosis of the appendix, the Doppler signal will be absent; therefore, its presence cannot be reliably used diagnostically [79]. A common finding in acute appendicitis is secondarily enlarged mesenteric lymph nodes, especially in children. Abscesses can be visualized as "hypoechoic fluid collections with thick hyperemic walls containing low level echoes and sometimes gas" [79]. If the patient is symptomatic with pain or recurrent fever and abscesses are amenable, percutaneous drainage is recommended. Prior to drainage, a CT scan must be performed to confirm the location and size of the abscess and to establish a safe route for drainage. The lateral approach is preferred, but any approach can be used, given vital structures are avoided under ultrasound or CT guidance [80].

Rectal Carcinoma Endorectal ultrasonography (ERUS) is the method of choice for staging of early colorectal carcinomas, as it is the only imaging modality capable of differentiating all five layers of bowel wall [82]. Several studies have shown that "pre-operative endorectal ultrasound has a high level of accuracy in determining both the depth of mural invasion and the presence or absence of nodal involvement" [82]. However, as with most ultrasound uses, the accuracy of the imaging modality as an assessment of disease staging varies heavily based on operator experience. Patients are examined in the left lateral position using a multifrequency probe,

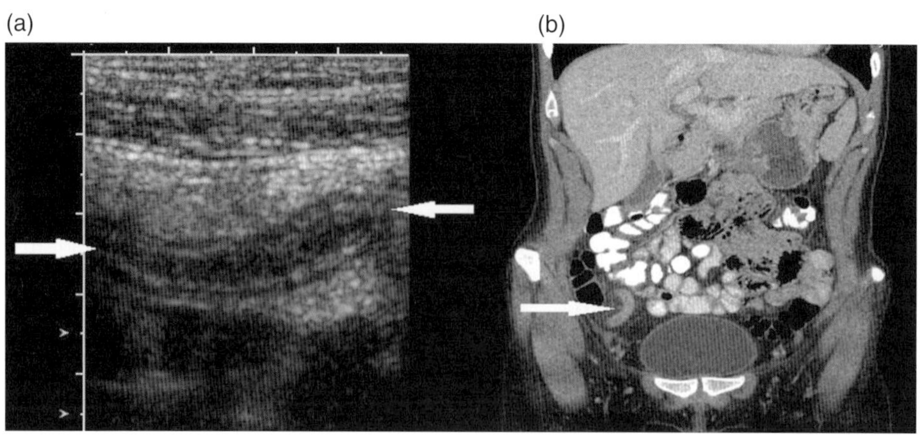

FIGURE 5.21 Appendix (white arrows) on B-mode ultrasound (a) and CT (b, coronal view).

which allows for a near circumferential image of the rectal wall. The probe may be fitted with a rubber sheath and filled with degassed water to minimize interference. ERUS allows for observation of all five layers of bowel wall, which will aid in accurate diagnosis and staging of early malignancy confined to the colorectal wall [82]. Of note, the fourth layer (2nd hypoechoic muscularis propria) may appear as two layers, reflecting the circular and longitudinal portions of the muscularis propria on ERUS [83].

Summary

In review, ultrasound is a real-time, widely available, cost-effective, and safe modality, which is used to image a variety of gastrointestinal pathologies. To make the best use of abdominal ultrasound techniques, we need to understand and get familiar with the anatomical layout of the gastrointestinal system and its surrounding structures. In particular, ultrasound has been a highly effective imaging tool for the assessment of the hepatobiliary system. The proper training and knowledge of abdominal ultrasound imaging is the key to the use of this technology.

Review Questions

1. What type of transducer and scanning frequency should be used in an adult abdominal ultrasound?
   a. 3–5 MHz, curvilinear transducer
   b. 10–20 MHz, phased array transducer
   c. 10–20 MHz, linear array transducer
   d. 20–30 MHz, linear array transducer
2. Which axis of the liver is used for measuring the size of the liver on B-mode ultrasound?
   a. Longitudinal axis
   b. Transverse axis
   c. Oblique axis
   d. Coronal axis
3. How do you differentiate between the cystic duct and surrounding cystic artery and hepatic arteries?
   a. Increased pressure with the probe
   b. Scanning the probe toward the liver and away from the gallbladder
   c. Following the cystic duct from the common bile duct
   d. Using color flow imaging to differentiate cystic duct from vessels with blood flow
4. Upon imaging of the gallbladder, there is an echogenic round structure in the gallbladder with acoustic shadowing. What is this echogenic structure present?
   a. Gallbladder polyps
   b. Gallstone
   c. Gallbladder cancer
   d. Pancreatic duct blockage

5. What pathology does hepatofugal flow in the portal vein indicate in a patient with 20 years of viral hepatitis?
   a. Cholecystitis
   b. Liver hemangioma
   c. Portal hypertension
   d. Hepatic artery occlusion
6. The most common patient's position for imaging pancreas is_______.
   a. Supine
   b. Prone
   c. Upright
   d. Lateral decubitus
7. Ultrasound examination of the pancreas should be performed after a minimum fast of how many hours?
   a. Fasting is not necessary
   b. 6 hours
   c. 12 hours
   d. 24 hours
8. What is the best ultrasound technique to assess spleen infarction?
   a. B-mode ultrasound with static image
   b. B-mode ultrasound with real-time image
   c. M-mode ultrasound
   d. Color flow imaging

Correct answers: 1. a; 2. a; 3. d; 4. b; 5. c; 6. a; 7. b; 8. d.

References

1. Gandolfi L, Torresan F, Solmi L, Puccetti A. The role of ultrasound in biliary and pancreatic diseases. *Eur J Ultrasound* 2003; 16: 141–159.
2. Holmes JF, Kelley KM, Wootton-Gorges SL, et al. Effect of abdominal ultrasound on clinical care, outcomes, and resource use among children with blunt torso trauma: a randomized clinical trial. *JAMA* 2017; 317: 2290–2296.
3. Fuster D, Garcia-Calvo X, Zuluaga P, et al. Ultrasound findings of liver damage in a series of patients consecutively admitted for treatment of alcohol use disorder. *Drug Alcohol Depend* 2018; 190: 195–199. https://doi.org/10.1016/j.drugalcdep.2018.06.012.
4. Gurien LA, Wyrick DL, Dassinger MS, et al. Use of bedside abdominal ultrasound to confirm intestinal motility in neonates with gastroschisis: a feasibility study. *J Pediatr Surg* 2017; 52: 715–717.
5. Kitamoto H, Inoue S, Okamoto K, Inokuma T. Scanning early catches the worm: abdominal ultrasound as a possible screening method for intestinal cestodes. *Lancet* 2019; 394(10205): 1264. https://doi.org/10.1016/S0140-6736(19)32132-4.
6. Janssen Lok M, Miyake H, Hock A, et al. Value of abdominal ultrasound in management of necrotizing enterocolitis: a systematic review and meta-analysis. *Pediatr Surg Int* 2018; 34(6): 589–612. https://doi.org/10.1007/s00383-018-4259-8.

7. Schneider M, Bloesch J, Lombardo P. Abdominal ultrasound referred by the emergency department – can sonographer findings help guide timely patient management? *Radiography* 2014; 20: 4–7.
8. Speets AM, Hoes AW, van der Graaf Y, et al. Upper abdominal ultrasound in general practice: indications, diagnostic yield and consequences for patient management. *Fam Pract* 2006; 23: 507–511.
9. Standring S. Abdomen and pelvis: overview and surface anatomy. In: Borley NR (ed.). Gray's anatomy: The Anatomical basis of clinical practice. Elsevier Limited, 2016; 1037–1045.
10. American Institute of Ultrasound in Medicine. AIUM physician training guidelines. American Institute of Ultrasound in Medicine, 2015. http://www.aium.org/resources/ptGuidelines.aspx.
11. Siegel MJ. Liver. In: Siegel MJ (ed.). Pediatric sonography. 4th ed. Philadelphia, PA: Lippincott Williams & Wilkins, 2010.
12. Juza RM, Pauli EM. Clinical and surgical anatomy of the liver: a review for clinicians. *Clin Anat* 2014; 27: 764–769. https://doi.org/10.1002/ca.22350.
13. Abou-Khalil JE, Bertens KA. Embryology, anatomy, and imaging of the biliary tree. *Surg Clin North Am* 2019; 99: 163–174. https://doi.org/10.1016/j.suc.2018.12.005.
14. Battaglia S, Fachinetti C, Draghi F, et al. Ultrasound examination of the liver: variations in the vascular anatomy. *J Ultrasound* 2010; 13: 49–56.
15. Pauli EM, Staveley-O'Carroll KF, Brock MV, et al. A handy tool to teach segmental liver anatomy to surgical trainees. *Arch Surg* 2012; 147: 692–693. https://doi.org/10.1001/archsurg.2012.689.
16. Wilson S, Gupta C, Eliasziw M, Andrew A. Volume imaging in the abdomen with ultrasound: how we do it. *AJR Am J Roentgenol* 2009; 193: 79–85.
17. Laing FC. Jaundice. In: Bluth EI, Benson CB, Ralls PW, Siegel MJ (eds). Ultrasonography in urology—a practical approach to clinical problems. Vol 35. 2nd ed. New York, NY: Thieme, 2008; 1734–1735.
18. Kaltenbach TEM, Engler P, Kratzer W, et al. Prevalence of benign focal liver lesions: ultrasound investigation of 45,319 hospital patients. *Abdom Radiol* 2016; 41: 25–32.
19. Reid-Lombardo KM, Khan S, Scalbas G. Hepatic cysts and liver abscesses. *Surg Clin North Am* 2010; 90: 679–697.
20. Mortele KJ, Segtto E, Ros PR. The infected liver: radiologic pathologic correlation. *Radiographics* 2004; 24: 937–955.
21. Rezvani M, Shaaban AM. Patterns of fatty liver disease. *Curr Radiol Rep* 2016; 4: 26.
22. Zhang GY, Brandman D. A clinical update on MASLD. *JAMA Intern Med* 2025; 185: 105–107. https://doi.org/10.1001/jamainternmed.2024.6431.
23. Nalbantoglu IL, Brunt EM. Role of liver biopsy in nonalcoholic fatty liver disease. *World J Gastroenterol* 2014; 20: 9026–9037.
24. Lin YH, Wan YL, Tai DI, et al. Considerations of ultrasound scanning approaches in non-alcoholic fatty liver disease assessment through acoustic structure quantification. *Ultrasound Med Biol* 2019; 45: 1955–1969.
25. Duvnjak M, Leroti I, Barši N, et al. Pathogenesis and management issues for non-alcoholic fatty liver disease. *World J Gastroenterol* 2007; 13: 4539–4550.
26. Yasmin D, Parvaneh L, Hamidreza S, et al. Diagnostic value of conventional and Doppler ultrasound findings in liver fibrosis in patients with chronic viral hepatitis. *J Medical Ultrasound* 2015; 23: 123–128.
27. Wilson SR. The liver. In: Gastrointestinal disease (6th series) test and syllabus. Reson, VA: American College of Radiology, 2004; 119–153.
28. Pavlov CS, Casazza G, Semenistaia M, et al. Ultrasonography for diagnosis of alcoholic cirrhosis in people with alcoholic liver disease. *Cochrane Database Syst Rev* 2016; (3): CD011602. https://doi.org/10.1002/14651858.CD011602.pub2.
29. Yeom SK, Lee CH, Cha SH, Park CM. Prediction of liver cirrhosis, using diagnostic imaging tools. *World J Hepatol* 2015; 7(17): 2069–2079.

30. Yang HR. Value of color Doppler ultrasound in diagnosis of portal hypertension liver cirrhosis merged with esophageal variceal bleeding. *J Hainan Med Univ* 2016; 22: 91–93.
31. Mahadevan V. Anatomy of the gallbladder and bile ducts. *Surgery* 2020; 38: 432–436. https://doi.org/10.1016/j.mpsur.2014.10.003.
32. Gupta SK, Shukla VK. Silent gallstones: a therapeutic dilemma. *Trop Gastroenterol* 2004; 25: 65–68.
33. Hasani SA, Faith M, Daadpey M, et al. Accuracy of bedside emergency physician performed ultrasound in diagnosing different causes of acute abdominal pain: a prospective study. *Clin Imaging* 2015; 39: 476–479.
34. Konikoff FM. Gallstones – approach to medical management. *MedGenMed* 2003; 5: 8.
35. Majeed A, Thomas W. Clinical investigation of hepatopancreatobiliary disease. In: Blumgart's surgery of the liver, biliary tract, and pancreas, 2012; 192–203. https://doi.org/10.1016/B978-1-4377-1454-8.00012-6.
36. Sun XJ, Shi JS, Han Y, et al. Diagnosis and treatment of polypoid lesions of the gallbladder: report of 194 cases. *Hepatobiliary Pancreat Dis Int* 2004; 3: 591–594.
37. Levy AD, Murakata LA, Abbott RM, Rohrmann CA. From the archives of the AFIP. Benign tumors and tumorlike lesions of the gallbladder and extrahepatic bile ducts: radiologic-pathologic correlation. Armed forces Institute of Pathology. *Radiographics* 2002; 22: 387–413.
38. Lai CH, Lau WY. Gallbladder cancer – a comprehensive review. *Surgeon* 2008; 6: 101–110.
39. Marone U, Caracò C, Losito S, et al. Laparoscopic cholecystectomy for melanoma metastatic to the gallbladder: is it an adequate surgical procedure? Report on a case and review of the literature. *World J Surg Oncol* 2007; 5: 141. https://doi.org/10.1186/1477-7819-5-141.
40. Holloway BJ, King DM. Ultrasound diagnosis of metastatic melanoma of the gallbladder. *Br J Radiol* 1997; 70: 1122–1125.
41. Yoon WJ, Yoon YB, Kim YJ, et al. Metastasis to the gallbladder: a single-center experience of 20 cases in South Korea. *World J Gastroenterol* 2009; 15: 4806–4809.
42. Mahadevan V. Anatomy of the pancreas and spleen. *Surgery* 2019; 37(6): 297–301.
43. Rana SS, Gonen C, Vilmann P. Endoscopic ultrasound and pancreas divisum. *JOP: J Pancreas* 2012; 13(3): 252–257.
44. Martínez-Noguera A, Montserrat E, Torrubia S, et al. Ultrasound of the pancreas: update and controversies. *Eur Radiol* 2001; 11: 1594–1606.
45. Bockman DE. Anatomy of the pancreas. In: Go VLW, DiMagno EP, Gardner JD, et al. (eds). The pancreas: biology, pathobiology, and disease. New York, New York, USA: Raven Press; 1–8.
46. Mahadevan V. Anatomy of the stomach. *Surgery* 2017; 35(11): 608–611.
47. D'Onofrio M, Beleù A, Gaitini D, et al. Abdominal applications of ultrasound fusion imaging technique: liver, kidney, and pancreas. *Insights Imaging* 2019; 10: 6. https://doi.org/10.1186/s13244-019-0692-z.
48. Li S, Su L, Lv G, et al. Transabdominal ultrasonography of the pancreas is superior to that of the liver for detection of ectopic fat deposits resulting from metabolic syndrome. *Medicine* 2017; 96(37): e8060. https://doi.org/10.1097/MD.0000000000008060.
49. Zhang H, Chen GY, Xiao L, et al. Ultrasonic/CT image fusion guidance facilitating percutaneous catheter drainage in treatment of acute pancreatitis complicated with infected walled-off necrosis. *Pancreatology* 2018; 18: 635–641.
50. EBSCO Information Services. DynaMed [Internet]. Ipswich, MA: EBSCO Information Services, 1995. Record No. T114770, Pancreatic Pseudocyst. https://www-dynamed-com.proxy.rvu.edu/topics/dmp~AN~T114770.
51. Yousuke N, Naminatsu T, Suguru M, et al. Current status of endoscopic ultrasound techniques for pancreatic neoplasms. *Clin Endosc* 2019; 52: 527. https://doi.org/10.5946/ce.2019.025.
52. Zhang LL, Sanagapalli S, Stoita A. Challenges in diagnosis of pancreatic cancer. *World J Gastroenterol* 2018; 24: 2047–2060.

53. Moore KL, Dalley AF, Agur AMR. Clinically oriented anatomy. 7th ed. Philadelphia, PA: Wolters Kluwer, 2014.
54. Rumack CM, Wilson SR, Charboneau JW, et al. Diagnostic ultrasound. 5th ed. Philadelphia, PA: Elsevier, 2017.
55. Benter T, Aldinger P, Teichgräber UK. Sonography of the spleen. *J Ultrasound Med* 2011; 30: 128–139.
56. Zavras N, Kosmidis EK, Maroulis I. The anatomy and function of the spleen. *Hell J Surg* 2017; 89: 81–89.
57. Halpert B, Alden ZA. Accessory spleens in or near the tail of the pancreas. *Arch Pathol* 1964; 77: 652–654.
58. Mendelson RM. Imaging the spleen. *Australas Radiol* 2004; 48: 393–404.
59. Levine CD, Rubesin SE, Laufer I. The role of ultrasound in splenic disease. *Radiol Clin North Am* 1997; 35: 121–132.
60. Sakai T, Higaki T, Okazaki M, et al. Sonographic diagnosis of splenic vein thrombosis. *J Ultrasound Med* 1990; 9: 511–514.
61. Dodd GD, Baron RL, Oliver JH 3rd, Federle MP. Enlarged spleen in patients with portal hypertension: sonographic and CT findings. *AJR* 1990; 154: 41–45.
62. Richards JR, McGahan JP. Focused assessment with sonography in trauma (FAST) in 2017: what radiologists can learn. *Radiology* 2017; 283: 30–48.
63. Morgenstern L, Shapiro SJ, Mirvis SM, et al. The clinical and diagnostic spectrum of splenic cysts. *Am Surg* 1980; 46: 569–574.
64. O'Keeffe GW, Marshall MJ. Splenic abscess: diagnostic considerations. *Postgrad Med J* 1986; 62(726): 385–388.
65. Falk S, Stutte HJ. Pathological features of splenic hemangioma: a study of 30 cases. *Arch Pathol Lab Med* 1993; 117: 711–716.
66. Riccio A, Gobbi D, Corradini C, et al. Splenic lymphoma: imaging findings. *Hematol Oncol* 2012; 30: 92–98.
67. Warshauer DM, Hall HL. Imaging of splenic infarction. *Semin Ultrasound CT MR* 2006; 27: 370–388.
68. Horton KM, Fishman EK. The spleen: update on radiologic imaging in the diagnosis and treatment of splenic disease. *Semin Ultrasound CT MR* 2002; 23: 20–44.
69. Kocaoglu M, Frush DP, Bulas DI. Pediatric spleen: normal appearances, variants, and pathologic conditions at US with pathologic correlation. *Radiographics* 2001; 21: 1119–1143.
70. Ellis H. Anatomy of the stomach. *Surgery* 2011; 29(11): 541–543. https://doi.org/10.1016/j.mpsur.2011.08.003.
71. Burdan F, Rozylo-Kalinowska I, Szumilo J, et al. Anatomical classification of the shape and topography of the stomach. *Surg Radiol Anat* 2012; 34(2): 171–178. https://doi.org/10.1007/s00276-011-0893-8.
72. Volk N, Lacy B. Anatomy and physiology of the small bowel. *Gastrointest Endosc Clin N Am* 2017; 27(1): 1–13. https://doi.org/10.1016/j.giec.2016.08.001.
73. Smereczyński A, Kołaczyk K. Pitfalls in ultrasound imaging of the stomach and the intestines. *J Ultrason* 2018; 18: 207–211. https://doi.org/10.15557/JoU.2018.0031.
74. Puylaert JBCM. Ultrasound of colon diverticulitis. *Dig Dis* 2012; 30(1): 56–59. https://doi.org/10.1159/000336620.
75. Bates J. Abdominal ultrasound – how, why, and when. 2nd ed. Edinburg, London: Churchill Livingstone, 2004.
76. Schmidt T, Hohl C, Haage P, et al. Phase-inversion tissue harmonic imaging compared to fundamental B-mode ultrasound in the evaluation of the pathology of large and small bowel. *Eur Radiol* 2005; 15: 2021–2030.
77. Lu C, Merrill C, Medellin A, et al. Bowel ultrasound state of the art: grayscale and Doppler ultrasound, contrast enhancement, and elastography in Crohn disease. *J Ultrasound Med* 2019; 38: 271–288.
78. Wilson SR, Burns PN, Wilkinson LM, et al. Gas at abdominal US: appearance, relevance, and analysis of artifacts. *Radiology* 1999; 210: 113–123.

79. Mathur M, Scoutt LM. Nongynecologic causes of pelvic pain: ultrasound first. *Obstet Gynecol Clin N Am* 2019; 46: 733–753. https://doi.org/10.1016/j.ogc.2019.07.007.
80. Gray RE, Gaddey HL. An imaging guide to abdominal pain. *J Fam Pract* 2015; 64: 286–291.
81. Tamburrini S, Lugarà M, Iaselli F, et al. Diagnostic accuracy of ultrasound in the diagnosis of small bowel obstruction. *Diagnostics* 2019; 9(3): 88. https://doi.org/10.3390/diagnostics9030088.
82. Badger SA, Devlin PB, Neilly PJD, Gilliland R. Preoperative staging of rectal carcinoma by endorectal ultrasound: is there a learning curve? *Int J Color Dis* 2007; 22: 1261–1268.
83. Mondal D, Betts M, Cunningham C, et al. How useful is endorectal ultrasound in the management of early rectal carcinoma? *Int J Color Dis* 2014; 29: 1101–1104. https://doi.org/10.1007/s00384-014-1920-0.

CHAPTER 6

Obstetrics and Gynecology

Kathryn Forneris[1], Jacquelyn Flor[1], and Yun-Yun Ren[2]

[1]Rocky Vista University, College of Osteopathic Medicine, Ivins, Utah, USA

[2]Department of Ultrasound, Obstetrics & Gynecology Hospital, Fudan University, Shanghai, China

Introduction

Ultrasound is a noninvasive technique used to monitor pregnancy and diagnose a wide range of pathologies in obstetrics and gynecology. The American Institute of Ultrasound in Medicine (AIUM) started an initiative in 2012 known as "Ultrasound First" to encourage the use of ultrasound as a first-line imaging method due to its advantages in comparison to other techniques. These include high accuracy, widespread availability, low-cost, portability, and no radiation exposure to patients. Ultrasound can be performed in major imaging centers and other clinical settings in rural areas. Another benefit is that ultrasound allows the operator to observe specific organs and vessels in real time [1]. The quality of ultrasound imaging and interpretation is highly operator-dependent and strongly dependent upon provider training and expertise. Therefore, it is important for all operators to receive proper training [2]. This chapter will provide a brief overview of female reproductive anatomy, indications for the use of ultrasound, as well as normal and common pathologic ultrasound images in obstetrics and gynecology.

General Anatomy

The vagina is a hollow, flexible tube composed of fibromuscular tissue that contains rugal folds. It is the connection between the cervix and the perineum. The shape of the vagina can be described as a trapezoid that is widest at the apex and cervix [2]. The vagina is fixed within the pelvis by several ligamentous structures and is found within the retroperitoneum [3].

The uterus is composed of the uterine corpus and the uterine cervix (Fig. 6.1). Generally, the uterus is pear-shaped. The size of the uterus varies during the lifetime of a woman and is influenced by hormones, previous pregnancies, and various pathologies. Women of childbearing age have a uterine corpus that is larger than the cervix; however, the corpus and cervix are similar in size before puberty and after menopause [4].

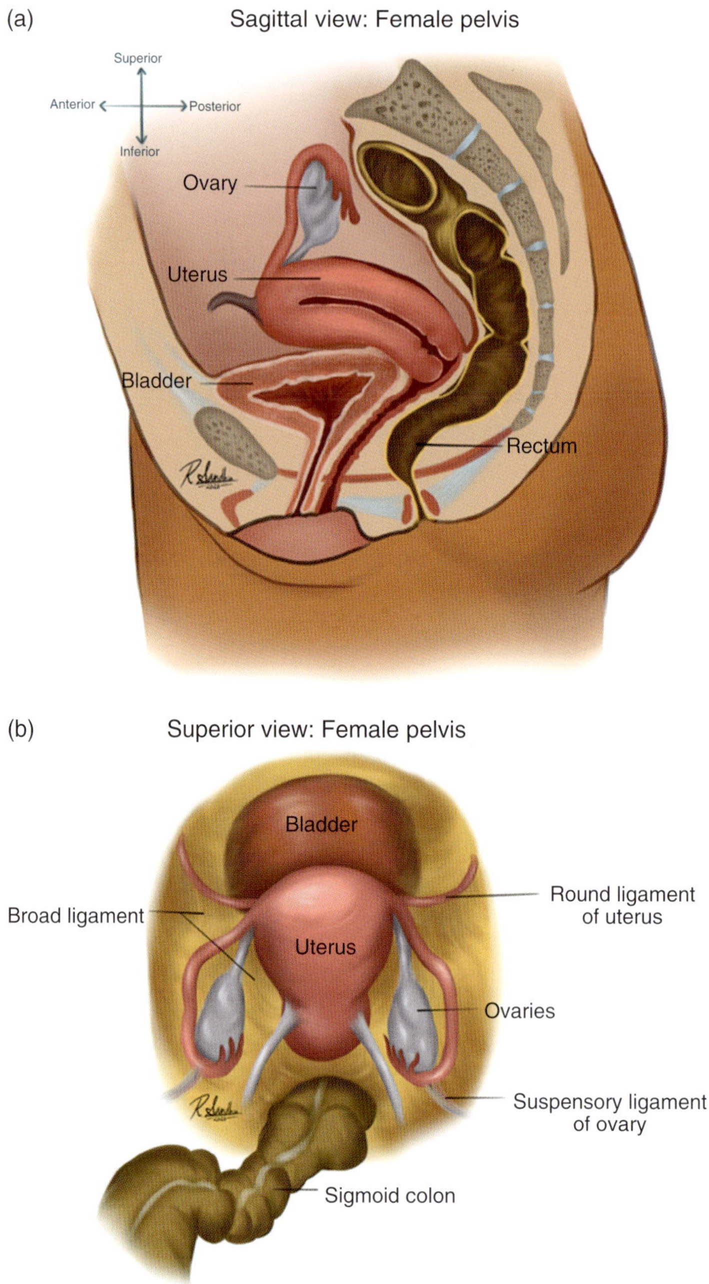

FIGURE 6.1 (a, b) Female pelvic anatomy in sagittal plane (a) and superior coronal plane (b).

The uterus can be found posterior to the bladder and anterior to the rectum. The uterine corpus is referred to as the body, which has a triangular shape, while the superior portion is called the fundus, and the inferior portion is the isthmus [3, 4]. The uterus has three layers. The innermost layer is the endometrium, which lines the uterine cavity and thickens during the menstrual cycle. The middle layer is the myometrium, which is the thickest portion and contains smooth muscle fibers. The outermost layer is a series, which envelopes the uterus and is made of visceral peritoneum [4]. This portion of the uterus can be found in several different positions: anteflexed or retroflexed, midline, or slightly lateral to midline. The uterine cervix is the structure that serves as the canal between the uterine cavity and the vagina, with the superior portion continuous with the uterus. The inferior portion is found protruding into the vagina. The cervix opening has two portions, the internal os, which opens into the endometrial cavity, and the external os, which opens into the vagina [4].

The adnexa consist of the ovaries and the fallopian tubes. The ovary is a fundamental organ in reproduction and is responsible for the production of many hormones. This is where the follicle matures during proliferation and is expelled when the Luteinizing hormone peaks. The ovaries can be found suspended laterally and possibly posterior to the uterus. There are many ligaments that support the ovary, including the utero-ovarian ligament, the suspensory ligament of the ovary (which contains the ovarian vessels), and the broad ligament [5]. The ovary has an outer cortex that contains the ova and follicles, and a medulla, which contains blood vessels and connective tissues forming the fibrous lunar tissue layer [4]. The fallopian tubes are supported by the broad ligament and are located posterior to the uterine corpus and superior to the round ligaments. There is a lumen that communicates with the uterine cavity and the intra-abdominal cavity. The fallopian tubes consist of two layers: an outer muscularis layer composed of longitudinal smooth muscle fibers and an inner layer that consists of circular smooth muscle fibers. There are four divisions to the fallopian tube: the interstitial portion, the isthmus, the ampulla, and the fimbria [5].

Pelvic organs have a blood supply and drainage via iliac vessels. The internal iliac artery, a branch from the common iliac artery, provides blood supply to the uterus and ovaries. The left common iliac vein can be found anterior to the sacrum and medial to the aortic bifurcation, where it will join the right common iliac vein to form the inferior vena cava [4].

The bladder is a midline structure found posterior to the pubic bone, separated by a potential space called the retropubic space (also known as the space of Retzius). In females, it is closely related to the anterior wall of the vagina [6]. When the bladder is empty, it is pyramidal in shape, with the apex pointed out toward the pubic bone. When full, it is spherical in shape and can hold approximately 400–500 mL of fluid. During this time, it has the ability to distend and expand above the pubic bone into the abdominal cavity [6].

The pouch of Douglas, also referred to as the posterior cul-de-sac or the recto-uterine pouch, is the space between the uterus and the rectum, the site where fluid is likely to collect. The pouch is formed by the rectouterine fold extending lower than the anterior fold and having peritoneum reflected from the posterior part of the vaginal fornix onto the anterior surface of the rectum. It is bound by the uterus and supravaginal part of the cervix anteriorly, by the rectum posteriorly, and by the uterosacral ligaments laterally [5].

Indications for Obstetric and Gynecological Ultrasound

Indications for performing obstetric ultrasound in pregnancy include, but are not limited to, the confirmation of intrauterine pregnancy, the number of fetuses, determination of gestational age, demonstration of cardiac activity, and assessment of the cause of abnormal bleeding in the first, second, and third trimesters [7].

Indications for performing gynecologic ultrasound include pelvic pain, pelvic mass (benign and malignant lesions), abnormal vaginal bleeding in premenopausal or postmenopausal patients, and the location of an intrauterine device (IUD) [7, 8].

Although the risks are low in ultrasound, potential risks and benefits should always be considered with any imaging modality. The as low as reasonably achievable (ALARA) principle is one that should be considered when checking on ultrasound machine settings, along with overall scanning time. In order to follow ALARA, a scanner must be sure to apply the correct examination presets (such as OB–First Trimester), based on the specific ultrasound machine being used. Adjusting the power to the lowest available setting that still allows a diagnostic-quality image will help to reduce the patient's exposure to ultrasound bioeffects. Monitor the mechanical and thermal indexes (MI and TI, respectively) and understand the upper limits of these based on the time of scanning (Chapter 1) [9].

Ultrasound Techniques

There are several ways in which a pelvic sonogram can be performed transabdominally, transvaginally, or both [8]. In relation to patient preparation, it is important that when performing a transabdominal sonogram, optimally the patient's bladder is full, but not overdistended. When performing a transvaginal ultrasound, the patients' bladder is to be empty in order to avoid obscuring pelvic structures and causing patient discomfort throughout the procedure. Having an understanding of optimal timing to evaluate the pelvis in relation to menstruation and the ultrasound appearance of the endometrium is also important. It is important to evaluate the endometrium and ovaries based on the menstrual cycle of the patient, because the variation in the thickness of the endometrium and the size of the ovarian follicles are strongly associated with the level of estrogen, progesterone, and corpus luteum. While a transvaginal ultrasound is preferred in the first trimester, a transabdominal ultrasound can also be performed.

A curvilinear array transducer (3–5 MHz) and transvaginal probe (5–10 MHz) are commonly used in obstetrics and gynecology (OB/GYN) ultrasound. When choosing scanning frequency, a balance between imaging penetration and resolution will depend on the clinical application. Curvilinear transducers are wide with a narrow convex surface with a narrow curve, allowing for excellent visualization of the abdomen. However, there are two major limitations in transabdominal ultrasound. The first is the need to use lower scanning frequencies (lower image resolution), and the other is the ultrasound attenuation degrading effect of the anterior abdominal wall for imaging the organs in the deep pelvis, especially in patients living with obesity. The application of transvaginal ultrasound can overcome these limitations. Ultrasound is the first-line imaging choice for assessing the female pelvis. Transabdominal and transvaginal are complementary. Transabdominal gives you a global view for assessing large ovarian cysts, multiple fibroids, as well as measuring the size of the uterus accurately. Transvaginal gives you a higher level of resolution because of the higher frequency probe (Fig. 6.2) but is limited by image depth and penetration.

The B-mode grayscale image is most commonly used in OB/GYN ultrasound. Color flow and spectral Doppler are supplemental to assess vascularity of the organ

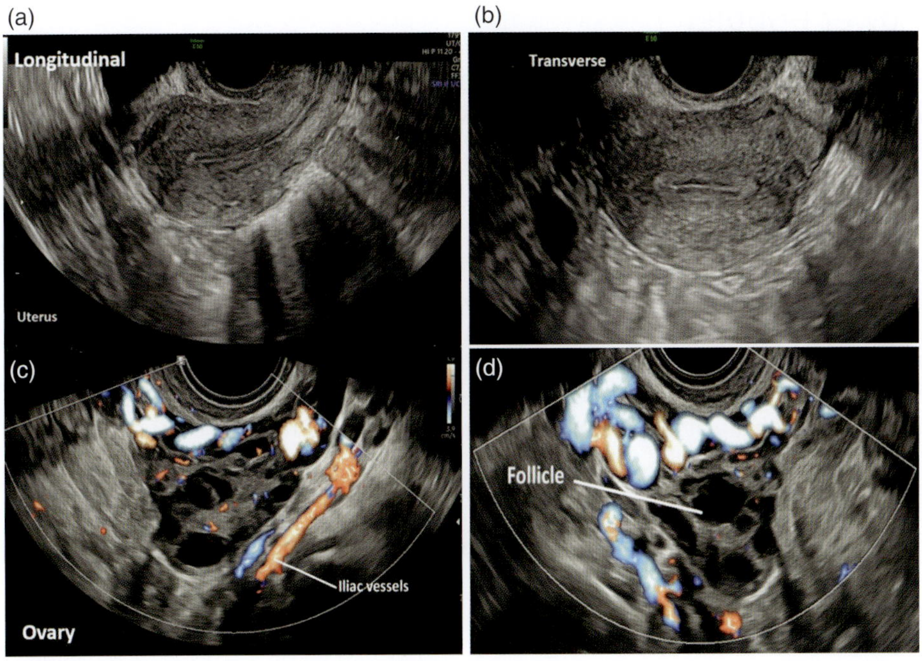

FIGURE 6.2 (a–d) Longitudinal (a) and transverse (b) planes of normal uterus in transvaginal ultrasound. Color flow imaging is useful to assess vascularity in the ovary and vessels adjacent to the ovary (c). The size and number of ovarian follicles can be evaluated via transvaginal ultrasound (d).

and hemodynamic status (such as patency and blood flow velocity) of vessels [7]. In the primary care clinical setting, these images will be seen as two-dimensional.

B-Mode Image

This form of imaging depends on the relative intensity of backscatters. These backscatters, as echoes return to the transducer, are dependent on the reflection of the various interfaces encountered. The brighter and more echogenic the display, the stronger the degree of the returning echoes. B-mode imaging displays varying degrees of brightness that allow the operator to evaluate the morphology of the pelvic organs and determine any possible pathological findings. Real-time B-mode image is important to demonstrate cardiac activity and movement of the fetus.

Color Flow Imaging

This method allows for visual detection of the mean velocity of blood flow utilizing a color map over grayscale image. By convention, the areas colored blue represent blood flowing away from the transducer, and the red areas represent blood flowing toward the transducer, vice versa. This technique is used in assessing vascularity of the organ and fetal cardiac activity, along with monitoring blood flow in the umbilical cord and placenta during pregnancy [7].

Power Doppler

This technique is more sensitive than conventional color flow imaging for depicting blood flow in the pelvic organs. It is especially useful when blood flow is very slow in smaller vessels [7].

Spectral Doppler

This approach is also known as pulsed wave Doppler mode. The pulsed wave Doppler is used to select the exact vascular location for scanning using the Doppler gate (Chapter 1). It provides quantitative hemodynamic information of the organ (such as ovary) and is useful in investigating the major vessels of the fetus. This mode can be used to evaluate blood flow velocity and resistance of the umbilical arteries [8].

Ultrasound in Normal Pregnancy

First-Trimester

Transvaginal ultrasound is commonly used in the first trimester to determine the location of a pregnancy. If ultrasound is performed very early during the gestational period, the intrauterine pregnancy will appear as a small, eccentric intrauterine collection of fluid in relation to the opposing walls of the uterine cavity, with an echogenic rim [8]. This can lead to what is known as pregnancy of uncertain location (PUL) or an intrauterine pregnancy of uncertain viability. If a viable embryo is detected at this time, a standard obstetric ultrasound examination should be performed, which includes assessment of gestational age, yolk sac, fetal number, and fetal cardiac activity [8]. The measurement of the crown-rump length (CRL) is the most accurate way to determine the gestational age of a fetus in the first trimester (Fig. 6.3). The CRL is the longest straight line of the embryo, measured from the

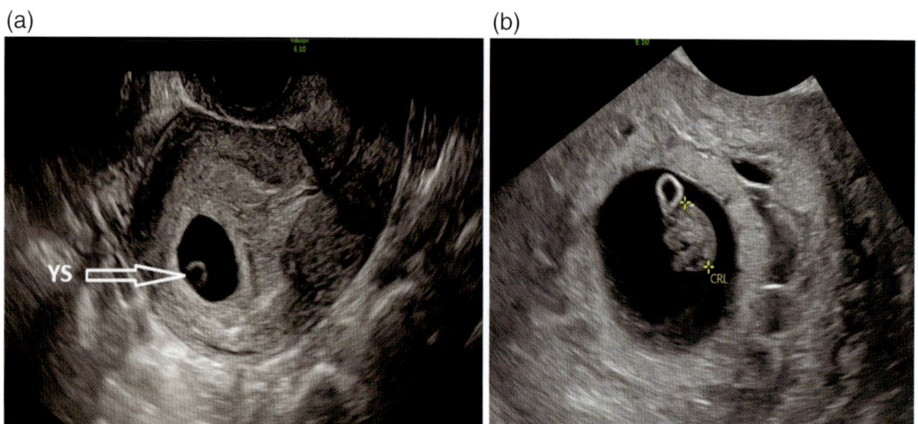

FIGURE 6.3 (a, b) Transvaginal ultrasound of the first-trimester pregnancy. Yolk sac (YS, arrow) is seen in the gestational sac (a) and measurement of crown-rump length (CRL, b).

outer margin of the cephalic pole to the rump of the embryo or fetus. Along with examining the fetus, certain maternal pelvic anatomy, including the uterus, cervix, adnexa, and cul-de-sac region, should be visualized [10].

When it comes to documenting fetal cardiac activity with the use of ultrasound, the AIUM recommends that M-mode or B-mode be used for scanning, keeping the machine thermal index (TI) as low as possible. A TI of 0.7 or less is preferable, and the operator should not scan for longer than needed to adequately assess the pregnancy. The use of spectral Doppler should not be routinely used in early pregnancy (first trimester) [9].

Second and Third Trimester

In the second and third trimesters, ultrasound can be used to answer specific clinical questions that one may have throughout the pregnancy. It is also done to evaluate fetal growth, cardiac activity, presentation, placental location in respect to the internal cervical os, and amniotic fluid volume [10].

Even after the first trimester, it is important to continue to monitor if the fetus is growing properly [11]. This can be accomplished through the measurement of the femur length (FL), biparietal diameter (BPD), and finally abdominal circumference (AC) (Fig. 6.4). The transducer should be aligned along the long axis of the femoral bone, and length should only include the span of ossified bone [10]. Biparietal diameter is taken at the level of the thalami and the cavum septi pellucidi (CSP) and is considered a standardized method of measurement. The image is obtained by placing the transducer perpendicular to the fetal parietal bones. The cursors should be placed on the outer edge of the proximal skull and the outer edge of the distal skull. An abdominal circumference (AC) is commonly used to estimate fetal weight. The AC is measured on the anatomic plane by visualizing the stomach and portal vein, also known as the portal sinus [12]. It is common to conduct an anatomic survey of the fetus in the second trimester. Approximately 3–5% of fetuses will have structural malformations that will require more routine ultrasounds to monitor progression throughout the second trimester as recommended by the American College of Obstetrics and Gynecology (ACOG) [13].

Being that the presentation of the fetus changes throughout the second trimester, scanning fetal presentation in the third trimester is more accurate. Having an understanding of fetal presentation during the third trimester can help better prepare for delivery, with the two most common late-stage presentations being breech and cephalic. The information of the placental location with respect to the internal cervical os, to exclude placenta previa, is critical when planning the approach for delivery as well [8].

Amniotic fluid volume (AFV) is considered a marker of fetal health. There are several factors affecting AFV, ranging from ruptured membranes to structural and chromosomal anomalies [14]. AFV can be measured by identifying and measuring the deepest vertical pocket (DVP) or the amniotic fluid index (AFI) as the operator places the transducer perpendicular to the skin. The single deepest pocket method consists of measuring the largest vertical pocket in the region with the greatest amount of amniotic fluid without the presence of fetal extremities or the umbilical cord. Oligohydramnios is defined as a single deepest pocket area of less than 2 cm (normal is between 2 and 8 cm), and polyhydramnios is greater than 8 cm [11, 14]. AFI is calculated by summing measurements of maximal amniotic fluid pocket

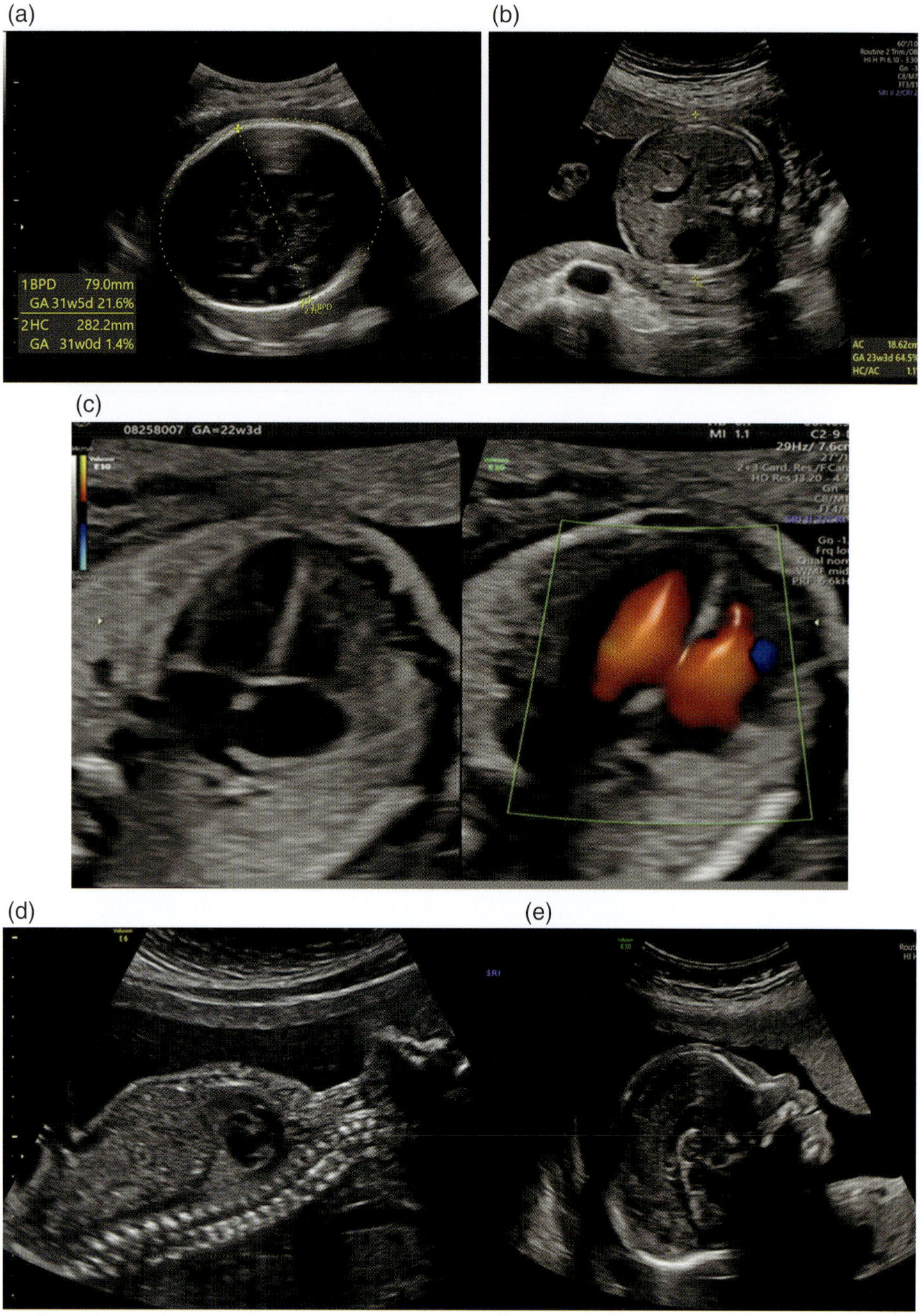

FIGURE 6.4 (a–e) Ultrasound of a normal second-trimester pregnancy is used to assess the anatomy of the fetus. Fetal anatomic surveys in the second semester include fetal head (a), abdomen (b), heart on B-mode (c, left) and color flow imaging (c, right), chest and abdomen (d), and profile (e) on B-mode images.

diameter in four quadrants (one from each quadrant of the uterus). Oligohydramnios is considered when AFI is less than 5 cm (normal 5–25 cm), and polyhydramnios is diagnosed when AFI is greater than 25 cm [14].

Ultrasound of Common Pathologies During Pregnancy

First-Trimester Bleeding

Miscarriage First-trimester bleeding prompts immediate evaluation to determine pregnancy viability. Pelvic ultrasound, along with serum human chorionic gonadotropin (HCG) concentration measurements, plays an essential role in the diagnosis and subsequent management of early-pregnancy problems. Criteria for diagnosing early-pregnancy loss (EPL) include (1) a gestational sac measuring around 25 mm without identification of an embryo; (2) an embryo with a CRL of about 7 mm without cardiac activity; and (3) absence of cardiac activity 2 weeks after an initial ultrasound demonstrating a gestational sac without a yolk sac [15].

Findings that are suspicious for, but are not diagnostic of EPL, include an embryo with a CRL less than 7 mm with no cardiac activity; a mean sac diameter between 16 and 24 mm with no embryo; absence of an embryo with cardiac activity 7–13 days after an ultrasound that demonstrated a gestational sac without a yolk sac; absence of an embryo with cardiac activity 7–10 days after an ultrasound that demonstrated a gestational sac with a yolk sac; absence of an embryo 6 weeks or more after the last menstrual period; an empty amnion; an enlarged yolk sac, greater than 7 mm; or a gestational sac that is small relative to the size of the embryo (less than 5 mm difference between the CRL and the mean sac diameter) (Fig. 6.5). Findings suspicious for, but not diagnostic of EPL,

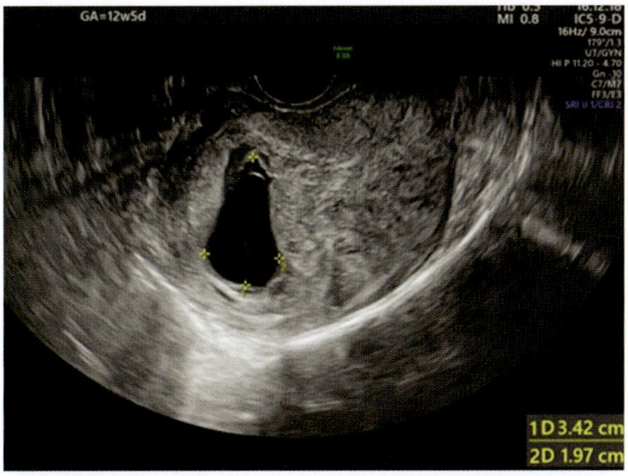

FIGURE 6.5 Emergency transvaginal ultrasound was performed on a 27-year-old woman with vaginal bleeding and 12 weeks and 5 days pregnancy based on her last menstrual period. There is a large empty gestational sac in the uterus. No fetal pole or yolk sac is identified in the gestational sac.

(a) (b)

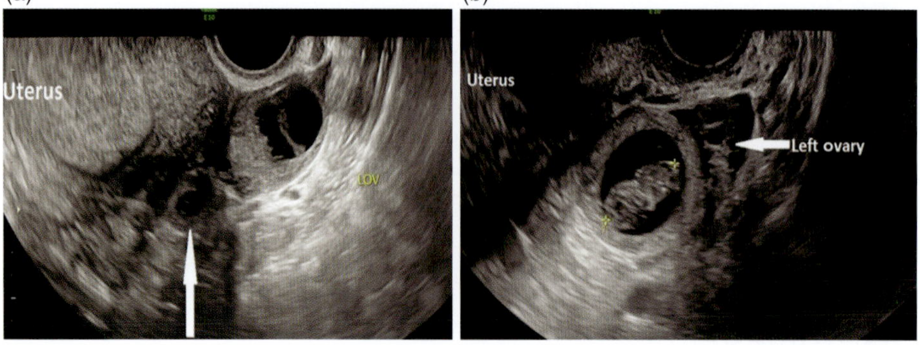

FIGURE 6.6 (a, b) Transvaginal ultrasound identified 6.5 weeks (a) and 9 weeks (b) ectopic pregnancies. B-mode images show a gestational sac located between the uterus and the left ovary. A yolk sac (long white arrow) is visualized on the image from a patient with 6.5 weeks of ectopic pregnancy (a). CRL of the fetus can be measured in the image (b) from the patient with 9 weeks of ectopic pregnancy.

follow-up transvaginal ultrasonography at 7–10 days after the initial ultrasound scan is requested to further assess pregnancy viability [15].

Ectopic Pregnancy An ectopic pregnancy is a pregnancy that occurs outside of the uterus, with 96% of ectopic pregnancies occurring in the fallopian tubes [16]. The most common presentation of an ectopic pregnancy is abdominal pain and/or first-trimester bleeding beginning 6–8 weeks after the last menstrual period. Ectopic pregnancy remains a significant cause of pregnancy-related morbidity and mortality. For that reason, all women of reproductive age presenting with acute abdominal pain and/or vaginal bleeding should be evaluated for ectopic pregnancy.

Transvaginal ultrasound, along with serum quantitative HCG levels, is the primary test used to diagnose ectopic pregnancies. The presence of a gestational sac with an embryo or yolk sac, with or without fetal cardiac activity, in an ectopic site confirms the diagnosis (Fig. 6.6) [17]. Inconclusive findings indicative of an ectopic pregnancy include an empty uterus, an inhomogeneous adnexal mass, known as a "blob" sign, and an adnexal mass composed of an empty gestational sac, also known as a "bagel sign" [18].

Expectant management of a confirmed ectopic pregnancy strongly depends on the clinical conditions of the patient. Medical management through the use of methotrexate can be considered for hemodynamically stable patients if they can comply with follow-up surveillance, ectopic pregnancy has not ruptured, they are not experiencing severe or persistent abdominal pain, and their liver and kidney function tests are within normal limits. Relative contraindications due to decreased probability of success when utilizing methotrexate in hemodynamically stable patients include, but are not limited to, HCG levels >5000 mIU/ml, the presence of embryonic cardiac activity in an ectopic pregnancy, and the size of the gestational sac >3.5 cm. During medical management, HCG levels should continue to be monitored regularly until levels reach about <5 mIU/mL [18].

However, surgical management is necessary in situations involving hemodynamic instability, signs of intraperitoneal bleeding (free fluid in the abdomen or pelvis), and symptoms of ectopic pregnancy rupture.

Second- and Third-Trimester Bleeding

Placenta Previa Placenta previa refers to the placenta being attached to the lower uterine segment, with its lower edge positioned below the presenting part of the fetus, reaching or covering the internal cervical os [19, 20]. Placenta previa occurs after 28 weeks of gestation, and it is the primary cause of bleeding during pregnancy [21]. Its etiology is associated with previous endometrial injury. Advanced maternal age, history of prior cesarean section or abortion, delayed development of the trophoblast layer of the fertilized ovum, and the use of assisted reproductive technology (ART) are all high-risk factors for placenta previa. As reported, the incidence of placenta previa in the third trimester is 0.5–1.2% among all pregnancies [21].

Based on the relationship between the lower edge of the placenta and the internal cervical os, placenta previa is classified into four types:

1. **Complete placenta previa or central placenta previa**:
   The placenta completely covers the internal cervical os (Fig. 5.7a,b).
2. **Partial placenta previa**:
   The lower edge of the placenta partially covers the internal cervical os.
3. **Marginal placenta previa**:
   The placenta is attached to the lower segment of the uterus and reaches the internal cervical os but does not cover the os (Fig. 6.7c).
4. **Low-lying placenta**:
   The placenta is attached to the lower uterine segment, with its edge located less than 2 cm from the internal cervical os (Fig. 6.7d).

The classification of placenta previa can change with the progression of pregnancy and labor. Classification may vary depending on the timing of diagnosis and should be determined based on the last examination prior to clinical management.

Complications of placenta previa include antepartum, intrapartum, and postpartum hemorrhage in the mother, increased risk of placenta accreta spectrum, increased risk of puerperal infection, and amniotic fluid embolism. Significant fetal blood loss can lead to fetal distress or even death. The rate of iatrogenic preterm delivery increases, along with perinatal morbidity and mortality [22–24].

To clearly define the relationship between the placenta and the internal cervical os, scanning can be performed transabdominal, transvaginal, or transperineal. Transvaginal ultrasound provides better visualization of the relationship between the internal cervical os and the lower placental edge, offering superior diagnostic accuracy for placenta previa compared to transabdominal ultrasound. For diagnostically challenging cases, a combination of transvaginal and transabdominal scans is recommended [25]. Evaluation of the relationship between the placenta and the internal os is standard practice during any second or third semester ultrasound, any patient presenting beyond 20 weeks of gestation with vaginal bleeding should be reexamined for possible placenta previa in the third trimester, as it is an obstetric emergency that can lead to continued severe bleeding, preterm birth, and/or cesarean delivery [26, 27].

Placental Abruption Placental abruption, also known as abruptio placentae, is placental detachment from the uterine wall prior to delivery of the fetus, occurring after 20 weeks of gestation or during labor. The main classic manifestations of

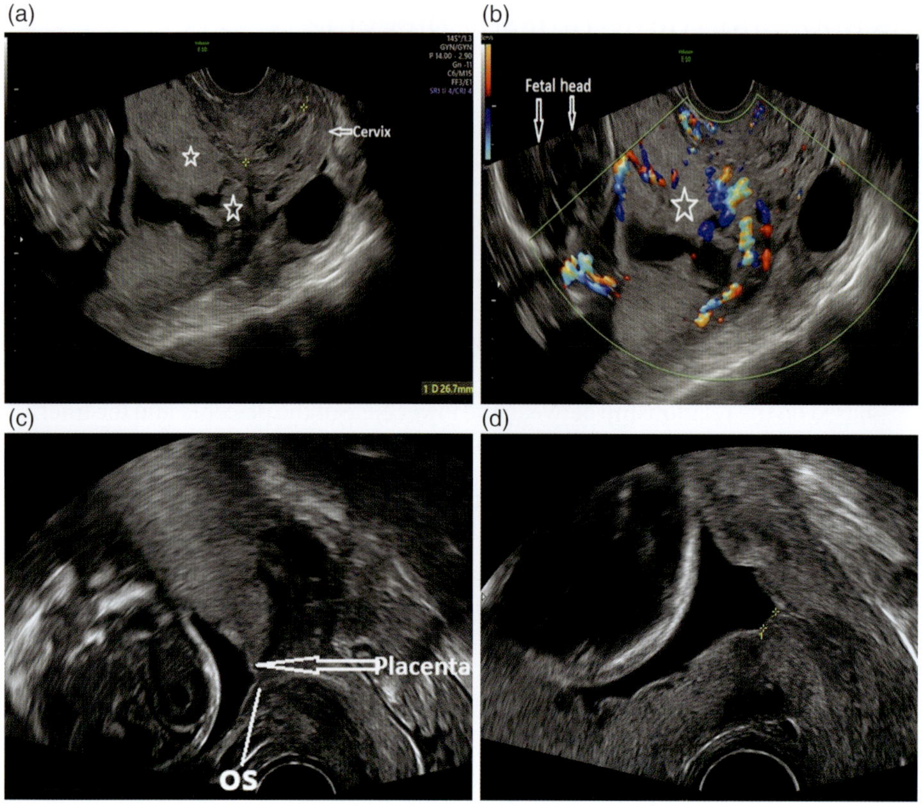

FIGURE 6.7 (a–d) Transvaginal B-mode (a) and color flow (b) images show a patient with complete placenta (*placenta tissue) previa. Marginal placenta previa (c) and low-lying placenta (d) can be observed in the second and third trimester pregnancy.

placental abruption include vaginal bleeding, uterine contractions, abdominal pain, often accompanied by uterine hypertonicity, uterine tenderness, and abnormal fetal heart rate [28–30]. Its occurrence is associated with factors such as maternal hypertension, severe preeclampsia, abdominal trauma, external cephalic version, polyhydramnios, and uterine malformations. However, placental abruption can also occur without any identifiable high-risk factors. The main consequence of placenta abruption is hemorrhage in the decidual layer. Based on the pattern of bleeding, placenta abruption can be classified into three types: revealed abruption, concealed abruption, and mixed abruption [29]. It is important to scan the entire placenta to observe placental thickness, parenchymal echogenicity, and the retroplacental space via transabdominal approach. On B-mode ultrasound, a revealed abruption shows thickened, heterogeneous placenta measuring more than 5 cm in a perpendicular plane, no significant change in placental morphology or fluid accumulation behind the placenta (Fig. 6.8a). In concealed abruption, retroplacental hematoma is present as a separate area between the uterus and placenta. The placenta appears thickened with disorganized variable echogenicity and absent blood flow on color flow imaging (Fig. 6.8b) [22, 29, 30]. Suspicion of placental abruption requires emergent evaluation in a labor and delivery unit and continued assessment of maternal and fetal status, as abruption can be deadly for both the mother and the fetus [30].

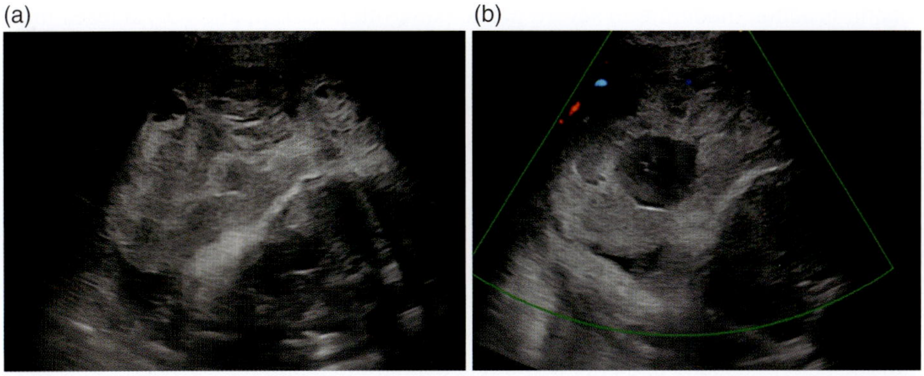

FIGURE 6.8 (a, b) A patient with intrauterine fetal demise in the gestational age of 36 weeks. The placenta appears markedly thickened with disorganized internal echogenicity (a), and no Doppler signals are displayed on color flow imaging (b). Placental abruption is the cause of fetal demise in this patient.

Ultrasound of Common Non-obstetric Pathologies

Ruptured Ovarian Cyst

Rupture of an ovarian cyst is a common cause of acute pelvic pain in women of reproductive age. The classic presentation of a ruptured ovarian cyst is acute onset of moderate to severe unilateral lower abdominal pain, often arising in association with strenuous physical activity, such as sexual intercourse or exercise [31]. This pain is thought to arise because of peritoneal irritation stemming from the material released from the ruptured cyst or hemorrhage.

Pelvic ultrasound is the imaging study of choice for the evaluation of a female patient with pelvic pain [1]. Sonographic imaging of a ruptured ovarian cyst may demonstrate the presence of an ovarian cyst and/or the presence of free peritoneal fluid. However, these findings often occur physiologically and therefore must be interpreted in the context of the entire clinical presentation. Sonographic features of hemorrhagic cysts may vary but can include an enlarged ovary containing a reticular pattern of echoes, indicating the presence of fibrin. Additionally, pressure with a transvaginal probe may induce a "jelly-like" wobble of the blood clot within a hemorrhagic cyst. Hemorrhage occurring within a physiologic cyst containing a corpus luteum may contain circumferential color flow, known as the "ring of fire." Once again, these images must be taken into the context of the clinical picture, as physiologic cysts, with minor hemorrhaging, are not uncommon in women of reproductive age [31].

Ovarian Torsion

Ovarian torsion describes the partial or complete rotation of the ovary on its ligamentous connections. Ovarian torsion is a common surgical emergency, accounting for around 2.7% of emergency surgical procedures. The classic presentation of ovarian torsion is acute, moderate to severe pelvic pain, often accompanied by nausea and/or vomiting, typically in a female with an adnexal mass. Ovarian torsion can result in significant sequelae, including but not limited to loss of the ovary, so early diagnosis is important [32–34].

Ultrasound is the study of choice for suspected ovarian torsion. Transabdominal and transvaginal ultrasound should be obtained in most patients. Sonographic features associated with this include a unilaterally enlarged, hyperechogenic ovary with heterogeneous stromal enhancement, often accompanied by an ovarian mass [33]. Multiple small peripheral follicles, commonly referred to as a "string of pearls," are present due to edematous displacement. While this can also be seen in polycystic ovarian syndrome, polycystic ovaries are often centrally echogenic and lack edema, and the patient usually presents without acute pain [34, 35].

Doppler ultrasound can be used to assist in diagnosis by demonstrating diminished or absent ovarian blood flow, which may indicate ovarian torsion (Fig. 6.9). However, this is controversial because some patients can have torsion and have essentially normal blood flow within the ovary because of the redundant blood supply [34]. Additionally, a "whirlpool sign," described as a rounded, hyperechoic structure with concentric hypoechoic lines or a tubular entity with circumscribed heterogeneous echoes, can be seen when moving the probe along the axis of suspected torsion. The whirlpool sign, indicative of a twisted pedicle, may be visualized on B-mode and color flow imaging depending on the level of blood flow interruption. Patients with confirmed diagnoses of ovarian torsion should be sent for surgical detorsion immediately to preserve the function of the ovary and prevent detrimental sequelae [32–34]. However, blood flow in the ovary cannot completely exclude ovarian torsion, and clinical information should be taken into consideration [34].

Adnexal masses, defined as masses originating from the ovary, fallopian tube, or adjacent connective tissue, are common gynecologic issues. Differentiation between benign masses and potential malignancies is of pivotal importance in the evaluation of adnexal masses, as clinical management varies greatly depending on this classification. Pelvic sonography, consisting of transabdominal and transvaginal imaging, is commonly used for assessing the size and sonographic characteristics of cystic or solid, and benign versus malignant potential [35, 36].

(a) (b)

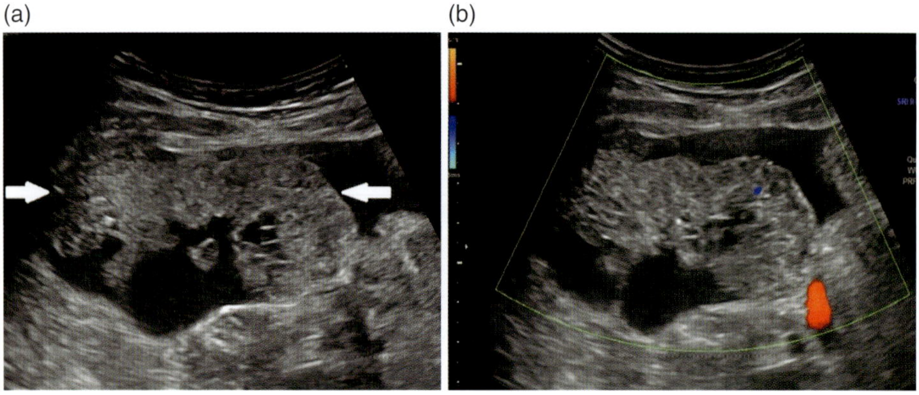

FIGURE 6.9 (a, b) B-mode (a) and color Doppler (b) images of ovarian torsion. The enlarged ovary (between two arrows) is heterogeneous (a), and absence of vascularity and normal follicles (b). Free fluid appears around the ovary.

Endometrioma

An endometrioma is an adnexal mass most commonly occurring in premenopausal women with endometriosis. Symptoms of an endometrioma vary widely, but can include pelvic pain, pelvic pressure, or dysmenorrhea. While endometriomas are benign, clear cell carcinoma or endometrioid adenocarcinoma may develop in endometriomas. Additionally, an association exists between endometriomas/endometriosis and infertility. For these reasons, it is important to differentiate between endometriomas and other pelvic masses. Transvaginal ultrasound is often utilized for this purpose [37, 38].

Upon sonographic examination, a typical endometrioma commonly presents as a tumor with one to four locules, ground glass echogenicity of cyst fluid, and no solid components. In premenopausal women exhibiting typical features of an endometrioma less than 10 cm in size, annual follow-up should be considered if it is not removed surgically. Enlargement, development of vascularity, or changing morphology should prompt referral to a specialist [37].

Traditionally, pathologies of the uterus and ovaries are assessed during a routine pelvic ultrasound. An extended ultrasound scan beyond the uterus and ovaries into the posterior and anterior pelvic compartments is helpful to look for deep infiltrating endometriotic nodules [38].

Dermoid Cyst

Dermoid cysts, also known as mature cystic teratomas, are germ cell tumors composed of sebaceous fluid and tissue arising from three germ cell layers: ectodermal, mesodermal, and endodermal tissue. They comprise nearly 30% of all ovarian tumors, making them the most common benign ovarian germ cell tumors [39]. The unique composition of dermoid cysts results in characteristic sonographic features, including a fat-fluid level, hyperechoic dots and lines, a shadowing known as the "tip of the iceberg" sign, and one or more hyperechoic regions within a hypoechoic mass, also known as the "dermoid plug" sign (Fig. 6.10). While definitive diagnosis is made upon histologic examination following surgical resection [39].

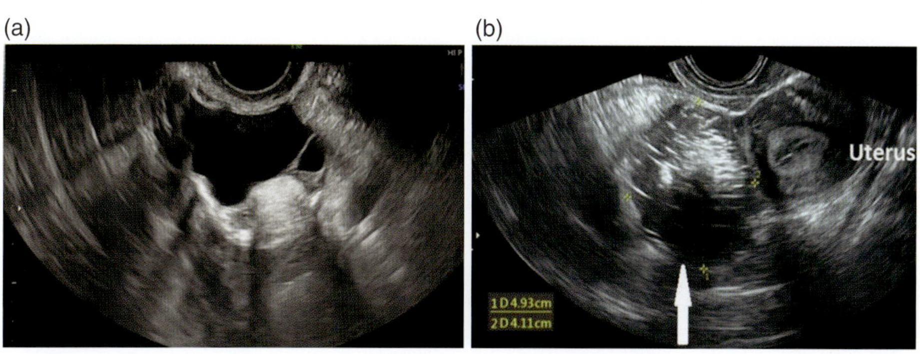

FIGURE 6.10 (a, b) B-mode images of dermoid cysts show fat-fluid level (a) in a 25-year-old female. There are hyperechoic lines, shadowing, and "tip of iceberg sign" (white arrow) appeared in the right adnexa region in another young female patient (b).

Ovarian Cancer

Ovarian cancer is the second most common gynecologic malignancy in the United States, with roughly 22,000 new cases each year, and accounts for roughly 14,000 deaths per year [40]. This is because nearly 60% of women with ovarian cancer developed metastasis by the time of diagnosis, as early-stage disease is often asymptomatic. Common symptoms of late-stage ovarian cancer are nonspecific, including back pain, fatigue, abdominal pain, bloating, constipation, and urinary symptoms [41]. These symptoms may be accompanied by paraneoplastic syndromes, such as Leser-Trelat sign, Trousseau syndrome, or subacute cerebellar degeneration, as well as symptoms of regional metastasis, including ureteral or bowel obstruction and shortness of breath [42]. A noteworthy exception to the late presentation of ovarian cancer symptoms is sex-cord stromal tumors, which are often detected in stage I. Diagnosis is determined by symptoms related to excessive hormone production, including precocious puberty, virilization, and abnormal uterine bleeding (AUB). Patients presenting with adnexal masses or clinical symptoms of ovarian cancer should undergo transvaginal ultrasound to assess ovarian morphology, further characterize masses, and determine the need for gynecologic oncology referral [43].

Ultrasound characteristics for predicting a benign mass include unilocular morphology, presence of solid components with the largest solid component measuring less than 7 mm in diameter, presence of acoustic shadowing, presence of a smooth, multilocular tumor measuring less than 100 mm at the largest diameter, and absence of blood flow. Ultrasound characteristics for predicting a malignant tumor include the presence of an irregular solid tumor, ascites, four or more papillary structures, and an irregular multilocular solid tumor measuring 100 mm or greater at its largest diameter with vascularity (Fig. 6.11) on color flow imaging [44]. A large meta-analysis performed to assess the ability of various models to correctly predict benign versus malignant adnexal masses found that the Simple Rules demonstrated a sensitivity and specificity of 93% and 81%, respectively, when classifying inconclusive masses as malignant, thereby providing an evidence-based framework for the sonographic interpretation of adnexal masses [44].

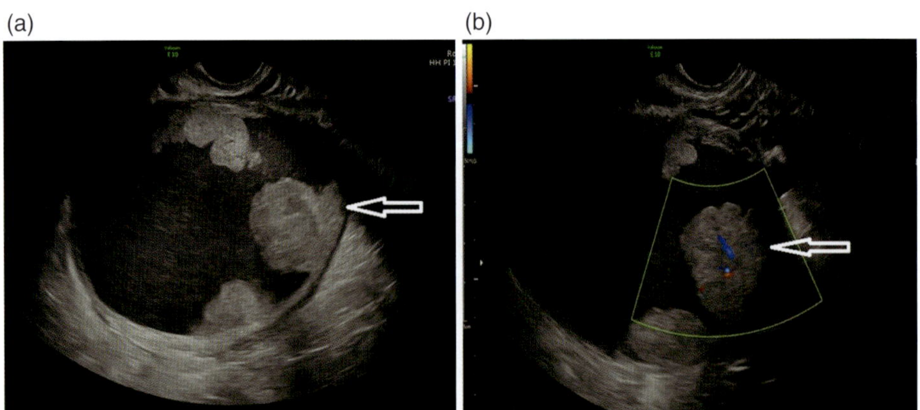

FIGURE 6.11 (a, b) Transvaginal B-mode image (a) and color flow imaging (b) of the ovary show a large complex cyst with solid nodules on the cystic wall. Ovarian carcinoma was confirmed by surgical pathology.

Abnormal Uterine Bleeding

AUB is a broad term utilized to describe any symptomatic deviation from normal menstruation in terms of frequency, duration, volume, or regularity. Due to the broad nature of this categorization, abnormal vaginal bleeding can be attributed to a multitude of causes. To simplify communication between researchers, clinicians, and patients, the International Federation of Gynecology and Obstetrics Menstrual Disorders Committee (FIGO MDC) created a classification system for potential etiologies of AUB consisting of nine basic categories arranged into the mnemonic PALM-COEIN: polyp, adenomyosis, leiomyoma, malignancy/hyperplasia, coagulopathy, ovulatory dysfunction, endometrial dysfunction, iatrogenic, and not otherwise specified [45]. Transvaginal ultrasound is the imaging study of choice for the detection of causes underlying AUB. Common ultrasound findings associated with several of these conditions will be listed below.

Uterine Polyps

Polyps are benign localized epithelial tumors that may be found throughout the endometrial cavity or cervical canal. Sonographic features of endometrial polyps include an echogenic lesion with a singular feeding vessel and/or an "interrupted mucosa sign." While a singular feeding vessel is considered a characteristic finding, it is not necessary for diagnosis. The interrupted mucosa sign describes the area in which the extremely echogenic linear interface between opposing mucosal surfaces of the endometrium is focally interrupted by a polyp. Although this sign may be visible during the second half of the menstrual cycle, polyp borders often appear indistinct and isoechoic to the endometrium [46]. This sign is often most apparent on transvaginal ultrasound images of the uterus in the transverse or longitudinal planes during the first half of the menstrual cycle, when the endometrium is at its thinnest. Around up to 25% of patients with endometrial polyps also have endocervical polyps [47].

Endocervical polyps can also be diagnosed with the use of a transvaginal ultrasound. Endocervical polyps demonstrate a reported incidence close to 4% in gynecologic patients, most commonly in multiparous women in their 3rd or 4th decade [46, 47]. On ultrasound, polyps typically present as slightly hyperechoic masses within the endocervical canal. Color Doppler may also demonstrate a singular vascular stalk entering the mass and originating from the endocervical mucosa (Fig. 6.12), further supporting the diagnosis.

Dislocated Intrauterine Device (IUD)

Ultrasound can be used in the localization and placement of IUDs. While ultrasound guidance is not required for IUD placement, it is currently used to overcome the challenges of difficult IUD insertions [48]. This is generally utilized in patients who have a history of difficult IUD insertions, cervical stenosis, or tortuous cervical canals. Ultrasound is also a first-line imaging tool for the evaluation of IUD positioning after placement in patients when the strings exiting the cervix cannot be visualized, or for patients experiencing pelvic pain or abnormal bleeding after IUD placement [47]. When visualized on ultrasound, the IUD has a very distinctive shape (Fig. 6.13) that can be visualized within the bottom portion of the uterus extending through the cervical canal [48].

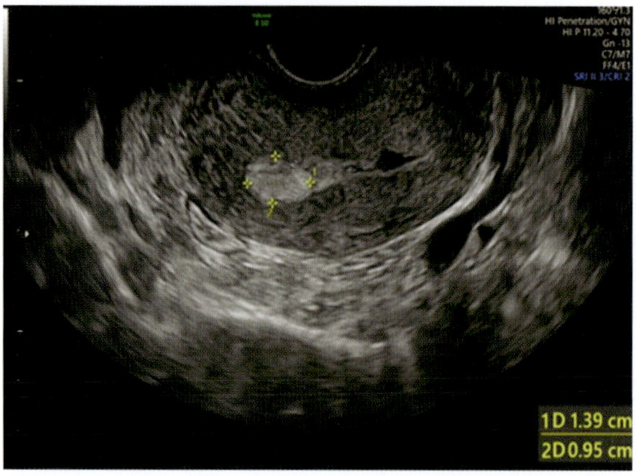

FIGURE 6.12 Transvaginal ultrasound of uterine polyps measures 1.39 × 0.95 cm.

(a) (b)

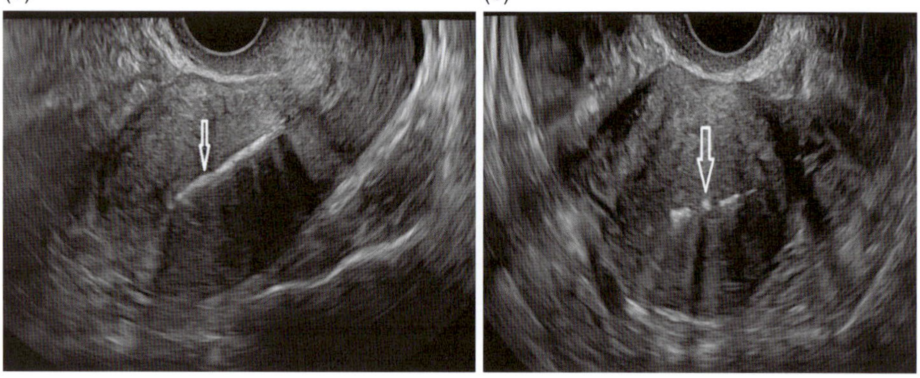

FIGURE 6.13 (a, b) Transvaginal ultrasound images show an IUD (arrow) in longitudinal (a) and transverse planes (b).

Endometrial Carcinoma

Endometrial carcinoma is a common cause of postmenopausal bleeding (PMB) that refers to any uterine bleeding in a postmenopausal woman. PMB is a common condition, accounting for roughly 5% of gynecologic visits [49]. The most common cause of PMB is atrophy of the endometrium or vaginal mucosa [50]. However, all postmenopausal women with unanticipated uterine bleeding should be assessed for endometrial carcinoma, a potentially lethal condition that accounts for roughly 10% of PMB [51].

Uterine cancer is the most common gynecological cancer in the United States.

More than 90% of uterine cancers originate from the uterine epithelium, also known as the endometrium, with the remainder arising from the myometrial muscle or, less commonly, the endometrial stroma. Endometrial carcinoma most commonly presents as PMB in women between the ages of 60 and 70 years old [52]. Diagnosis of endometrial carcinoma is based on histology. However, the

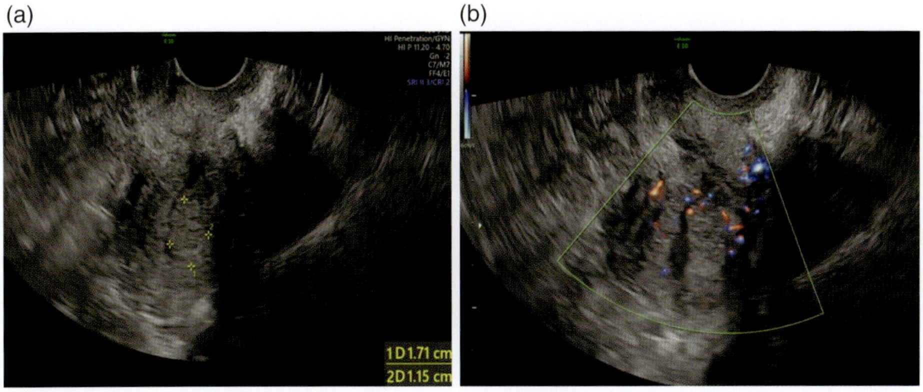

FIGURE 6.14 (a, b) Transvaginal ultrasound was performed to search for the cause of postmenopausal bleeding. Longitudinal B-mode image of the uterus measures an endometrial lesion (a) with hypervascularity on color flow imaging (b), which suggests possible malignancy. Endometrial biopsy confirmed endometrial carcinoma.

measurement of endometrial thickness via transvaginal ultrasound can assist in the diagnosis of both endometrial hyperplasia and endometrial carcinoma when the endometrium is homogenous. In postmenopausal women, an endometrial thickness of 4–5 mm or less is associated with a low risk for endometrial carcinoma [49]. The rate of carcinoma increases in likelihood as endometrial thickness increases. Endometrial thickness is measured by scanning the uterus in a sagittal plane, with results reported as the thickness of the endometrium from basalis layer to basalis layer in the anterior-posterior direction (Fig. 6.14), excluding fluid within the cavity [49, 52].

Currently, the American College of Obstetricians and Gynecologists, as well as the Society of Radiologists in Ultrasound, recommends the use of transvaginal ultrasound or endometrial sampling as the first diagnostic measures in women presenting with PMB. Women with an endometrial thickness of 4 mm or less can thereby avoid the use of more invasive procedures, such as endometrial biopsy or dilation and curettage, to further assess their risk of endometrial carcinoma [52]. Uterine polyps are another cause of PMB, especially in patients with hormone replacement, in addition to endometrial carcinoma.

Uterine Fibroids/Leiomyomas

Uterine leiomyomas, more commonly known as uterine fibroids, originate from the smooth muscle cells of the uterus [53]. They are the most common benign tumors in women, with an estimated cumulative incidence of 70% in Caucasian women and over 80% in black women before the age of 50 years old [54]. Leiomyomas typically appear as round, well-defined, solid, hypoechoic masses with or without calcification/acoustic shadowing (Fig. 6.15). However, factors, including calcification and necrosis, can result in different levels of echogenicity. Generally, transvaginal ultrasound is useful to define small fibroids and transabdominal ultrasound is required to assess multiple fibroids in an enlarged uterus [53, 54].

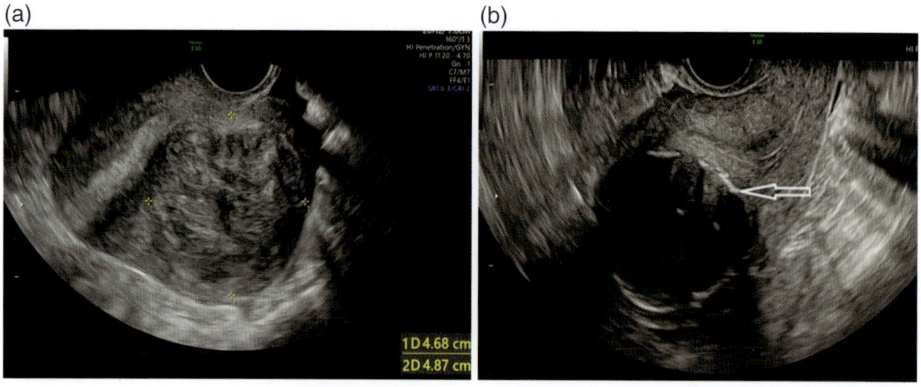

FIGURE 6.15 (a, b) B-mode image of uterine fibroid without (a) and with (b) calcification (arrow).

Summary

Ultrasound is a tool that is fundamental in the field of obstetrics and gynecology. It allows for the monitoring of pregnancy, along with the visualization of various pathologic conditions. It is critical to follow pregnancy with the use of ultrasound, providing information on gestation age, fetal weight, and evaluation of amniotic fluid volume. The ability to use transvaginal and transabdominal ultrasound to evaluate pathologies such as ectopic pregnancies, placental abruptions, and identification of pelvic masses allows for quicker diagnosis and treatment of these potentially life-threatening conditions. The basic understanding of concepts discussed in this chapter will be helpful in the proper use of ultrasound in OB/GYN.

Review Questions

1. What is the most accurate sonographic method to determine gestational age in the first trimester?
   - **a.** Amniotic fluid volume
   - **b.** Crown-rump length
   - **c.** Biparietal diameter
   - **d.** Fetal weight
2. At what point is a miscarriage confirmed with ultrasound?
   - **a.** Gestational sac has passed
   - **b.** Loss of previously visualized heartbeat
   - **c.** CRL measures 7 mm or greater without cardiac activity
   - **d.** All of the above
3. What are some of the characteristics associated with ALARA?
   - **a.** Grain adjustment
   - **b.** Different ultrasound techniques
   - **c.** Mechanical and thermal indexes
   - **d.** Prolonged transducer use

4. A 25-year-old woman presents with abdominal pain, vaginal bleeding, and a positive UPT in the emergency room. What is the possible diagnosis?
   a. Ovarian cyst
   b. Dermoid cyst
   c. Ectopic pregnancy
   d. Adenoma
5. What is the most common leading cause of third-trimester bleeding?
   a. Placental abruption
   b. Ruptured ovarian cysts
   c. Ovarian torsion
   d. Placenta previa
6. What material causes the pain in ovarian cyst rupture?
   a. Materials being excreted are irritating the peritoneal cavity
   b. Corpus leuteum follicles irritating the Adnexa
   c. Enzymes irritating the peritoneal cavity
   d. Pain receptors on the ovary stimulate the pain pathway
7. What is a possible consequence if an ovarian torsion is not diagnosed and managed in a timely manner?
   a. Can lead to blood clot
   b. Can lead to loss of fertility
   c. Can cause loss of the ovary
   d. It is not a medical emergency
8. What are sonographic features of dermoid cysts?
   a. Fat-fluid level
   b. Hyperechoic dots and lines
   c. "Tip of iceberg"
   d. "Dermoid plug"
   e. All of the above
9. What is the most common cause of benign postmenopausal bleeding?
   a. Uterine polys
   b. Cervical cancer
   c. Atrophy of the endometrium or vaginal mucosa
   d. Atrophy of the adnexa
10. What are possible causes for a patient with postmenopausal bleeding when the endometrial thickness measures 10 mm on transvaginal ultrasound image?
    a. Endometrial cancer
    b. Endometrial hyperplasia
    c. Normal postmenopausal changes
    d. Both a and b
    e. Both b and c

Correct answers: 1. b; 2. d; 3. c; 4. c; 5. d; 6. a; 7. c; 8. e; 9. c; 10. d.

References

1. Benacerraf BR, Abuhamad AZ, Bromley B, et al. Consider ultrasound first for imaging the female pelvis. *Am J Obstet Gynecol* 2015; 212: 450–455. https://doi.org/10.1016/j.ajog.2015.02.015.
2. Vrachnis N, Papageorghiou AT, Bilardo CM, et al. International society of ultrasound in obstetrics and gynecology (ISUOG) – the propagation of knowledge in ultrasound for the improvement of OB/GYN care worldwide: experience of basic ultrasound training in Oman. *BMC Med Educ* 2019; 19: 434. https://doi.org/10.1186/s12909-019-1866-6.
3. Dietrich CS 3rd, Gehrich A, Bakaya S. Surgical exposure and anatomy of the female pelvis. *Surg Clin North Am* 2008; 88: 223–243.
4. Balgobin S, Jeppson PC, Wheeler T 2nd, et al. Standardized terminology of apical structures in the female pelvis based on a structured medical literature review. *Am J Obstet Gynecol* 2020; 222: 204–218.
5. Barber MD. Contemporary views on female pelvic anatomy. *Cleve Clin J Med* 2005; 72(Suppl 4): S3–S11. https://doi.org/10.3949/ccjm.72.suppl_4.s3.
6. Moore KL, Agur AMR, Dalley AF II, Moore KL. Moore's essential clinical anatomy. 6, Chapter 6 ed. Pelvis and Perineum, 2019; 609–624 Wolters Kluwer.
7. Torloni MR, Vedmedovska N, Merialdi M, et al. Safety of ultrasonography in pregnancy: WHO systematic review of the literature and meta-analysis. *Ultrasound Obstet Gynecol* 2009; 33(5): 599–608.
8. Abinader R, Warsof SL. Benefits and pitfalls of ultrasound in obstetrics and gynecology. *Obstet Gynecil Clin North Am* 2019; 46: 367–378.
9. AIUM official statement for recommended maximum scanning times for displayed thermal index values. *J Ultrasound Med* 2023; 42(12): E74–E75. https://doi.org/10.1002/jum.16322.
10. AIUM practice parameter for the performance of limited obstetric ultrasound examinations by advanced clinical providers. *J Ultrasound Med* 2018; 37: 1587–1596. https://doi.org/10.1002/jum.14677.
11. Abuhamad A, Minton KK, Benson CB, et al. Obstetric and gynecologic ultrasound curriculum and competency assessment in residency training programs: consensus report. *Am J Obstet Gynecol* 2018; 218: 29–67. https://doi.org/10.1016/j.ajog.2017.10.016.
12. Bushman ET, Thompson N, Gray M, et al. Influence of estimated fetal weight on labor management. *Am J Perinatol* 2020; 37: 252–257.
13. Mai CT, Isenburg JL, Canfield MA, et al. National population-based estimates for major birth defects, 2010–2014. *Birth Defects Res* 2019; 111: 1420–1435. https://doi.org/10.1002/bdr2.1589.
14. Magann E, Whittington JR, Morrison JC, Chauhan SP. Amniotic fluid volume assessment: eight lessons learned. *Int J Women's Health* 2021; 14: 773–779.
15. Doubilet PM, Benson CB, Bourne T, et al. Diagnostic criteria for nonviable pregnancy early in the first trimester. *N Engl J Med* 2013; 369: 1443–1451.
16. Bouyer J, Coste J, Fernandez H, et al. Sites of ectopic pregnancy: a 10-year population-based study of 1800 cases. *Hum Reprod* 2002; 17: 3224–3230.
17. Webster K, Eadon H, Fishburn S, et al. Ectopic pregnancy and miscarriage: diagnosis and initial management: summary of updated NICE guidance. *BMJ* 2019; 367: l6283.
18. Sivalingam VN, Duncan WC, Kirk E, et al. Diagnosis and management of ectopic pregnancy. *J Fam Plann Reprod Health Care* 2011; 37: 231–240.
19. Faiz AS, Ananth CV. Etiology and risk factors for placenta previa: an overview and meta-analysis of observational studies. *J Matern Fetal Neonatal Med* 2013; 13: 175–190.
20. Vimercati A, Galante A, Fanelli M, et al. PAS or Not PAS? The sonographic assessment of placenta accreta spectrum disorders and the clinical validation of a new diagnostic and prognostic scoring system. *J Imaging* 2024; 10(12): 315.
21. Oyelese Y, Shainker SA. Placenta previa. *Clin Obstet Gynecol* 2025; 68: 86–92.

22. Melamud K, Wahab SA, Smereka PN, et al. Imaging of antepartum and postpartum hemorrhage. *Radiographics* 2024; 44(4): e230164.
23. Smith DD, Adesomo AA, Gonzalez-Brown VM, et al. Sonographic predictors of antepartum bleeding in placenta previa. *Am J Perinatol* 2024; 41: 961–968.
24. Otake Y, Ugajin A, Takahashi H, et al. Prediction of antenatal bleeding and preterm deliveries using placental magnetic resonance imaging in patients with placenta previa. *Jpn J Radiol* 2024; 42: 630–638.
25. Aryananda RA, Duvekot JJ, Van Beekhuizen HJ, et al. Transabdominal and transvaginal ultrasound findings help to guide the clinical management of placenta accreta spectrum cases. *Acta Obstet Gynecol Scand* 2024; 103: 93–102.
26. Fadl S, Moshiri M, Fligner CL, et al. Placental imaging: normal appearance with review of pathologic findings. *Radiographics* 2017; 37: 979–998.
27. Olive EC, Roberts CL, Nassar N, Algert CS. Test characteristics of placental location screening by transabdominal ultrasound at 18–20 weeks. *Ultrasound Obstet Gynecol* 2006; 28: 944–949.
28. Joo EH, Kim N, Ryu HM, et al. Clinical factors associated with developmental delay in placental abruption. *Front Med (Lausanne)* 2025; 12: 1544679.
29. Schneider E, Kinzler WL. Placental abruption: pathophysiology, diagnosis, and management. *Clin Obstet Gynecol* 2025; 68: 98–104.
30. Oyelese Y, Ananth CV. Placental abruption. *Obstet Gynecol* 2006; 108: 1005–1016.
31. Bottomly C, Bourne T. Diagnosis and management of ovarian cyst accidents. *Best Pract Res Clin Obstet Gynaecol* 2009; 23: 711–724. https://doi.org/10.1016/j.bpobgyn.2009.02.001.
32. Valsky DV, Esh-Broder E, Cohen SM, et al. Added value of the gray-scale whirlpool sign in the diagnosis of adnexal torsion. *Ultrasound Obstet Gynecol* 2010; 36: 630–634. https://doi.org/10.1002/uog.7732.
33. Anthony EY, Caserta MP, Singh J, Chen MYM. Adnexal masses in female pediatric patients. *AJR* 2012; 195(5): W426–W431.
34. Moro F, Bolomini G, Sibal M, et al. Imaging in gynecological disease: clinical and ultrasound characteristics of adnexal torsion. *Ultrasound Obstet Gynecol* 2020; 56: 934–943. https://doi.org/10.1002/uog.21981.
35. Van Nagell JRJ, Miller RW. Evaluation and management of ultrasonographically detected ovarian tumors in asymptomatic women. *Obstet Gynecol* 2016; 127: 848–858.
36. Testa AC, Bourne TH. Characterising pelvic masses using ultrasound. *Best Pract Res Clin Obstet Gynaecol* 2009; 23: 725–738.
37. Guerriero S, Condous G, van den Bosch T, et al. Systematic approach to sonographic evaluation of the pelvis in women with suspected endometriosis, including terms, definitions, and measurements: a consensus opinion from international deep endometriosis analysis (IDEA) group. *Ultrasound Obstet Gynecol* 2016; 48: 318–332.
38. Piessens S, Edwards A. Sonographic evaluation for endometriosis in routine pelvic ultrasound. *J Minim Invasive Gynecol* 2020; 27: 265–266. https://doi.org/10.1016/j.jmig.2019.08.27.
39. Ayhan A, Bukulmez O, Genc C, Karamursel BS. Mature cystic teratomas of the ovary: case series from one institution over 34 years. *Eur J Obstet Gynaecol Reprod Biol* 2000; 88: 153–157.
40. Siegel RL, Miller KD, Jemal A. Cancer statistics, 2020. *CA A Cancer J Clin* 2020; 70: 7–30. https://doi.org/10.3322/caac.21590.
41. Goff BA, Mandel LS, Melancon CH, Muntz HG. Frequency of symptoms of ovarian cancer in women presenting to primary care clinics. *JAMA* 2004; 291: 2705–2712.
42. Cannistra SA. Cancer of the ovary. *N Engl J Med* 2004; 351: 2519–2529.
43. Liu JH, Zanotti KM. Management of the adnexal mass. *Obstet Gynecol* 2011; 117: 1413–1428.
44. Timmerman D, Testa AC, Bourne T, et al. Simple ultrasound-based rules for the diagnosis of ovarian cancer. *Ultrasound Obstet Gynecol* 2008; 31: 681–690.

45. Munro MG, Critchley HO, Broder MS, Fraser IS. FIGO classification system (PALM-COEIN) for causes of abnormal uterine bleeding in nongravid women of reproductive age. *Int J Gynaecol Obstet* 2011; 113: 3–13.
46. Kamaya A, Yu PC, Lloyd CR, et al. Sonographic evaluation for endometrial polyps: the interrupted mucosa sign. *J Ultrasound Med* 2016; 35: 2381–2387.
47. Lentz GM, Lobo RA, Gershenson M, Katz VL (eds). Comprehensive gynecology. 6th ed. Philadelphia, Pa: Elsevier Mosby, 2012; 383–432.
48. Nowitzki KM, Hoimes ML, Chen B, et al. Ultrasound of intrauterine devices. *Ultrasonography* 2015; 34: 183–194.
49. Moodley M, Roberts C. Clinical pathway for the evaluation of postmenopausal bleeding with an emphasis on endometrial cancer detection. *J Obstet Gynaecol* 2004; 24: 736–741.
50. Smith PP, O'Connor S, Gupta J, Clark TJ. Recurrent postmenopausal bleeding: a prospective cohort study. *J Minim Invasive Gynecol* 2014; 21: 799–803.
51. Prendergast EN, Misch E, Chou YA, et al. Insufficient endometrial biopsy results in women with abnormal uterine bleeding. *Obstet Gynecol* 2014; 123(Suppl 1): 180S–181S.
52. American College of Obstetricians and Gynecologists. The role of transvaginal ultrasonography in the evaluation of postmenopausal bleeding. *Obstet Gynecol* 2009; 114: 409–411.
53. Baird DD, Dunson DB, Hill MC, et al. High cumulative incidence of uterine leiomyoma in black and white women: ultrasound evidence. *Am J Obstet Gynecol* 2003; 188: 100–107.
54. Woźniak A, Woźniak S. Ultrasonography of uterine leiomyomas. *Prz Menopauzalny* 2017; 16: 113–117. https://doi.org/10.5114/pm.2017.72754.

CHAPTER 7

Genitourinary System

Anton Pham[1], Qing Zhong[1], Ryan Geist[1], Stella Chan[1], and Johnson Chen[2]

[1] Rocky Vista University, College of Osteopathic Medicine, Ivins, Utah, USA

[2] Department of Radiology, Weill Cornell Medicine, Cornell University, New York, USA

Introduction

Renal ultrasound provides a fast, radiation-free, and inexpensive alternative to computed tomography (CT) and magnetic resonance imaging (MRI) for the initial workup of patients who present with acute symptoms ranging from abdominal pain, hematuria, renal failure, and uncontrolled hypertension [1, 2]. With ultrasound, one can directly visualize renal calculi, cysts, or solid masses without the use of radiation. When stone disease or renal pathology is clinically less likely, ultrasound can assist in evaluation for other pathologies, such as an abdominal aortic aneurysm, gallbladder disease, or ovarian torsion. These specific examples illustrate the central diagnostic role of renal ultrasound. By using ultrasound as the first imaging choice, results can be obtained faster and accurately [3]. This chapter will cover ultrasonography of the genitourinary system, including anatomy and characteristics of common pathologies.

General Anatomy

The kidneys are a pair of bean-shaped organs located along the posterior abdominal wall in the retroperitoneal space between the T12 and L3 vertebrae [4]. They are approximately 10 cm in length, with the right kidney positioned slightly lower than the left due to the location of the liver [4]. The diaphragm, the psoas major, and the quadratus lumborum muscles are directly adjacent to the kidneys [5]. The ureters descend along the posterior abdominal wall along the ventral surface of the psoas major muscle and cross the pelvic brim to enter the pelvic cavity [5].

The kidney itself is composed of three major regions: the hilum, cortex, and medulla. The hilum is the point of entrance and exit for the renal vessels and ureter [4]. The upper expanded portion of the ureter is called the renal pelvis and divides into two or three major calyces and several minor calyces [4, 6]. The cortex has several renal columns that penetrate the entire depth of the kidney, while the medulla forms a series of pyramids that direct the urinary stream into a minor calyx [6].

The urinary bladder is a muscular sac in the pelvis, positioned just above and behind the pubic bone when empty [4]. The muscular tissue layers of the bladder wall serve to stretch and accommodate urine with a normal capacity of 300–400 mL of fluid [7]. During urination, the bladder contracts along with internal and external sphincters, relaxing to allow urine to flow and exit through the urethra [8].

The prostate gland is typically about the size of a walnut, located just below the bladder and surrounding the prostatic urethra [4, 9]. The prostate is partly muscular and partly glandular, with ducts opening into the prostatic portion of the urethra [4]. It is made up of five zones: fibromuscular stroma, transition zone, central zone, periurethral zone, and peripheral zone [9].

The testes are paired ovoid structures contained within the scrotum and serve as the site of androgen and sperm production in males [10]. Each testis is covered by the tunica albuginea [4]. Immediately external to the tunica albuginea is the tunica vaginalis, which is derived from parietal peritoneum and aids in the frictionless motion of the testes within the scrotal sac [4]. The tunica vaginalis is comprised of a visceral layer and a parietal layer [11]. The visceral layer covers the entire surface of the testis, except where the efferent ductules connect the testis to the epididymis [11]. The parietal layer of the tunica vaginalis is located adjacent to and external to the visceral layer [4]. There is typically a small amount of fluid located in the space between the visceral layer and the parietal layer, which allows for the reduction in friction [10].

The spermatic cord passes through the inguinal canal from the abdomen into the scrotum and supplies the innervation, lymphatic drainage, and blood supply to the testes [10]. The artery responsible for supplying most of the blood to the testicle is the testicular artery that arises from the aorta bilaterally (Fig. 7.1) and travels within the spermatic cord to the testicle [4]. The principal venous drainage of the testicle is provided by the pampiniform venous plexus, which arises

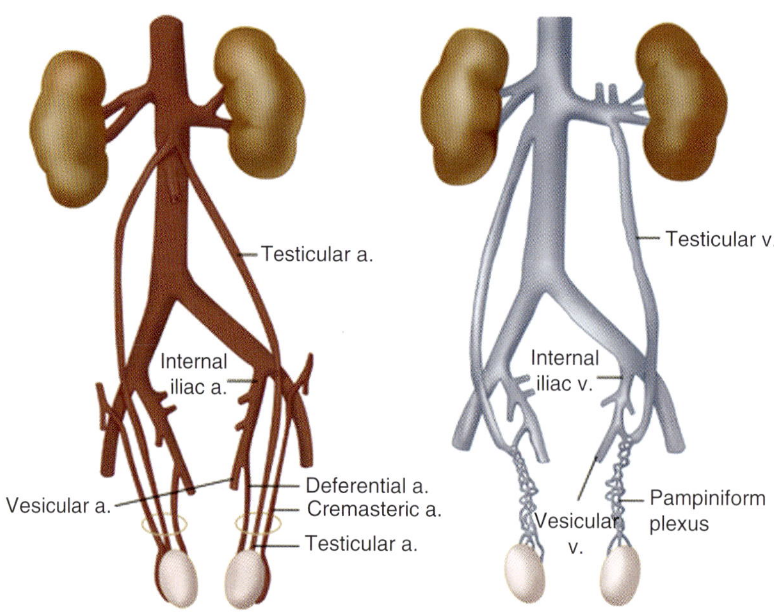

FIGURE 7.1 Arterial and venous systems of kidneys and testicles. a, artery; v, vein.

within the scrotum and ascends within the spermatic cord [4]. The plexus eventually coalesces within the inguinal canal to form the testicular veins [11]. A notable difference in the venous drainage of the left testicle as compared to the right testicle is the drainage of the left testicular vein into the left renal vein, whereas the right testicular vein drains directly into the inferior vena cava (Fig. 7.1) [10]. The lymphatic vessels draining the testes travel alongside the blood supply and drain to the lumbar lymph nodes [4].

Indications for Genitourinary Ultrasound

1. Flank pain/suspected renal colic with or without hydronephrosis
2. Acute or chronic renal failure
3. Acute infection/suspected acute pyelonephritis or renal abscess
4. Hematuria/suspected renal calculi or malignancy
5. New hypertension/uncontrolled hypertension
6. Urinary retention
7. Proteinuria
8. Trauma
9. Transplanted kidney
10. Testicular pain, enlarged testes, or testicular mass
11. Suspected prostate enlargement and/or abnormal digital rectal exam
12. Infertility

Ultrasound Techniques

Techniques for Imaging the Kidney

Patients are in the supine or lateral decubitus position, and a curvilinear transducer of 3–6 MHz will be used to image kidneys [3]. To view the right kidney, the transducer is placed on the right along the lateral subcostal edge between the 7th and 10th intercostal spaces at the anterior or middle axillary or posterior axillary line [1]. Due to its proximity to the liver, the right kidney will display using the liver as an acoustic window, making it easier to identify than the left [1]. The probe should be moved along the skin to obtain a longitudinal image of the right kidney, using a rocking technique once the kidney is visualized, and then it is rotated 90° to visualize transverse images of the kidney [1]. To locate the left kidney, the probe is placed at the posterior axillary line and scanned longitudinally first, as the kidney is easiest to identify in this view and is often obscured by intestinal air. The spleen can be used as an acoustic window to image the left kidney [3]. The normal kidney appears bean-shaped in long

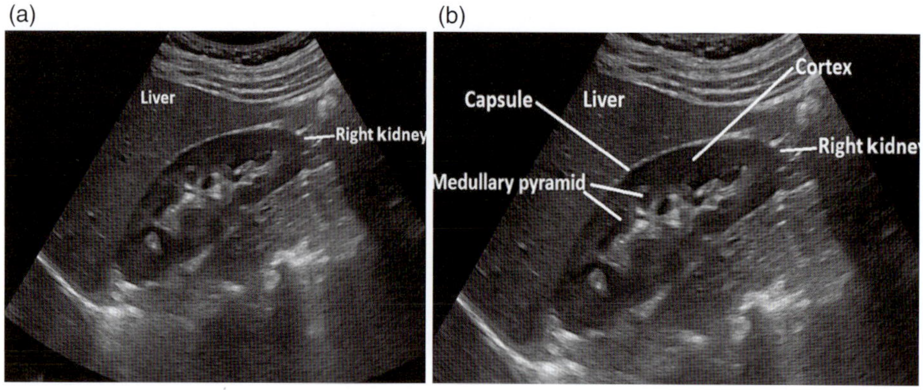

FIGURE 7.2 Longitudinal kidney without (a) and with labels (b) in B-mode ultrasound images.

axis and round-shaped in short axis on B-mode ultrasound imaging (Figure 7.2). The renal sinus is hyperechoic, and medullary pyramids are hypoechoic relative to the renal cortex [3]. Some technical considerations in performing a kidney ultrasound include re-scanning post-void to establish if hydronephrosis may be physiological in the setting of an extremely full bladder [12].

Ultrasound Techniques for Imaging the Bladder and Prostate

A curvilinear transducer of 3.5–5.5 MHz will be used to image the bladder and prostate [12, 13]. The transducer is placed above the pubic bone, and sound beam is directed toward the deep pelvis. It is important to scan all walls of the bladder carefully to detect any small bladder lesions [12].

Using a transabdominal approach, a full bladder is needed to act as an acoustic window to visualize the prostate [14]. A urinary bladder volume of 50–99 mL may be adequate for scanning the prostate gland and is likely to be tolerated much better by patients [13, 14].

Ultrasound Techniques for Imaging the Testis

A transducer with a high-frequency (7.5–15 MHz) is used to observe the internal structures of the testis [15]. The patient is placed in a supine position with a towel draped across the thighs to support the scrotum [16]. Using an adequate amount of warm gel to eliminate any gas trapped in the skin folds of the scrotum and to reduce the cremasteric reflex, begin with short-axis grayscale as well as a color flow imaging down the scrotum to compare the echogenicity and blood flow of both testes [11]. This is called the "buddy shot" or "sunglasses view." Each testicle is evaluated independently in both the long and transverse axes, noting the size and appearance of the testicle and epididymis. If a mass is found, an ultrasound can be used to determine if the mass is intratesticular or extratesticular. Low flow velocity color flow imaging and power Doppler can be used, in addition, to visualize the blood flow in the testes and nearby structures [17].

Common Pathologies in Genitourinary System

Kidney Cysts

Kidney cysts are classified by the Bosniak classification system: I. simple cyst; II. cyst with smooth and thin (≤2 mm) wall and septa; IIF. cyst with smooth and minimally thickened (3 mm) wall or septa; III. indeterminate cyst with thickened wall with more than three septa or irregular margin and is enhanced by contrast medium in CT; IV. likely malignant cystic masses [18].

Simple renal cysts are often unilateral and increasing in prevalence to 50% of people who are older than 50 [3]. These cysts are typically round in shape, containing anechoic fluid and demonstrating a smooth thin capsule [18]. Cystic fluid reduces attenuation of ultrasound waves and results in posterior enhancement (Fig. 7.3) [3]. Although possibly distorting adjacent renal parenchyma, simple renal cysts are benign and do not require treatment [3, 18].

Complex renal cysts can demonstrate multiple features, including septa, irregular thickened walls, calcification, or solid nodularity. Bosniak IV cystic masses have solid components and an 85–100% chance of developing malignancy [3, 18].

Autosomal-Dominant Polycystic Kidney Disease (ADPKD) Patients most at risk for ADPKD carry mutations in *PKD1* (85%) and *PKD2* (15%) [19, 20]. Age-dependent ultrasound diagnostic criteria for ADPKD have been established, where those at risk between 15 and 39 years of age will have a total of at least three renal cysts (either unilateral or bilateral) and between 40 and 59 years of age, at least 2 cysts seen in each kidney [20]. In adulthood, kidneys may be enlarged by hundreds to thousands of cysts bilaterally [1, 3]. Despite being the most common hereditary kidney disorder, only half of the patients with ADPKD are diagnosed during their lifetime [19]. Enlarged polycystic kidneys can be 4 times the normal size and 20 times

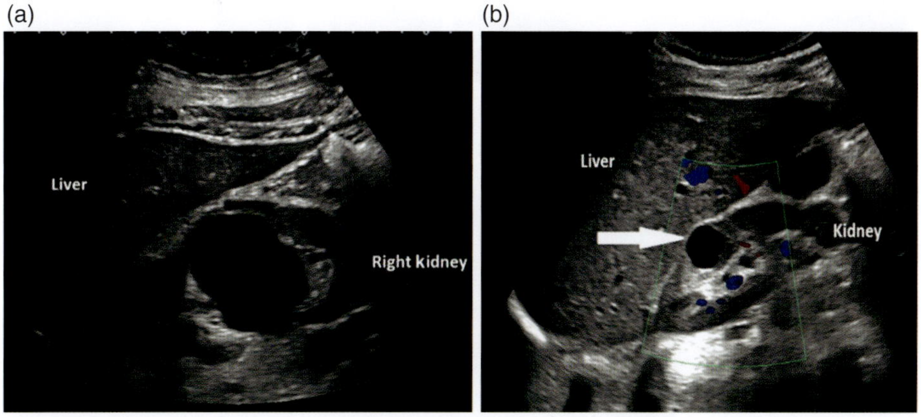

FIGURE 7.3 B-modeultrasound image of longitudinal plane of the right kidney with a cyst (a). A simple kidney cyst (arrow) is in the midpole of the right kidney. No Doppler signals appear in simple syst on color flow imaging (b).

the normal weight [21]. Patients may also present with liver cysts, pancreatic cysts, and cerebral aneurysms [19, 21]. Patients are usually asymptomatic until 40–50 years old, when back pain, hypertension, and chronic renal failure may manifest. ADPKD contributes to 10–15% of all kidney failure [21].

Solid Renal Masses

Benign Solid Mass An angiomyolipoma is composed of fat, smooth muscle tissue, and vessels. It is the most common benign tumor, especially in middle-aged women, and has no malignant potential. The lesion is often homogeneously hyperechoic; however, when its size is larger than 4 cm, bleeding within the mass may occur (Fig. 7.4) [3]. Smaller angiomyolipomas may be followed with imaging to monitor for growth, whereas intervention may be considered for larger ones. Renal oncocytomas are another benign solid renal mass, one which is difficult to differentiate from a malignant tumor on imaging, including by ultrasound.

Malignant Solid Mass Renal cell carcinoma (RCC) accounts for 86% of malignancy in the kidney and is the most common solid renal mass. RCCs occur more frequently in those who are older than 60, with a male-to-female ratio of 2:1 [3]. Because of the widespread use of ultrasound and CT scanning, renal tumors are

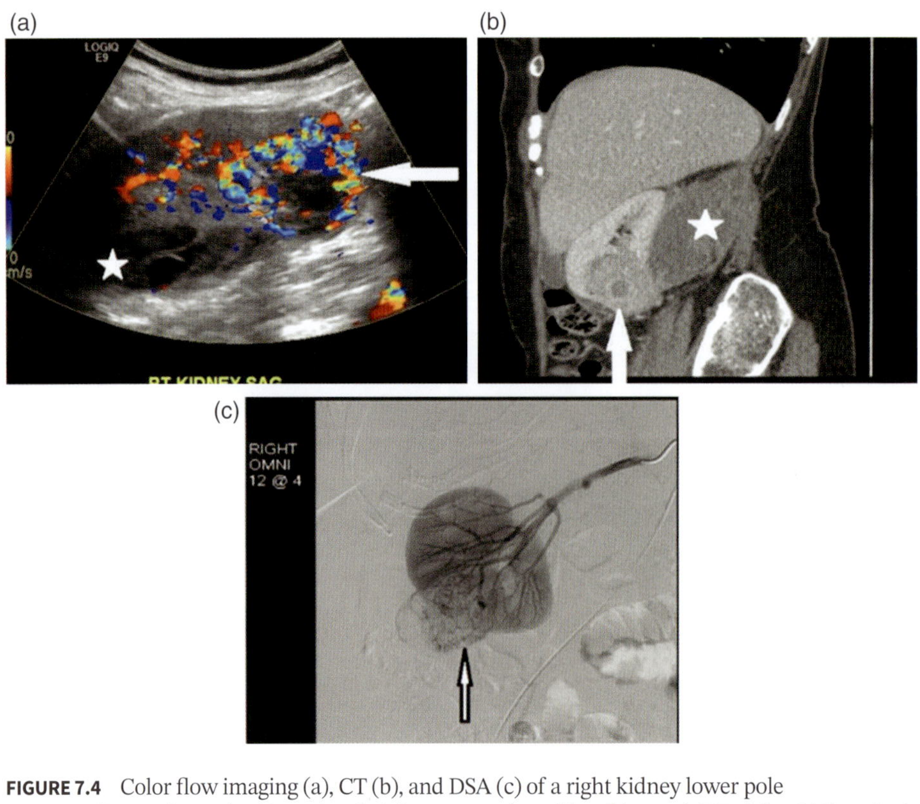

FIGURE 7.4 Color flow imaging (a), CT (b), and DSA (c) of a right kidney lower pole angiomyolipoma (arrow) with perinephric hematoma (a and b, white star). RT, right; SAG, sagittal.

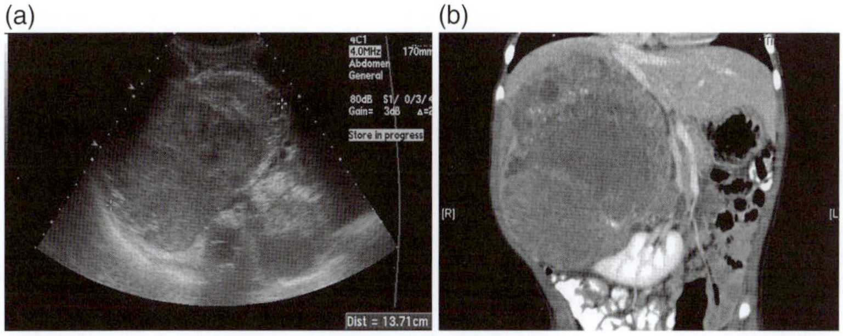

FIGURE 7.5 Wilms tumor on B-mode ultrasound (a) and contrast-enhanced CT (b).

frequently detected incidentally in individuals with no urologic symptoms. RCCs have a variety of sonographic appearances both in terms of a spectrum of solid to cystic composition and echogenicity [3]. CT and MRI are frequently utilized when renal cell cancer is suspected on ultrasound images to confirm the character of the mass and to further stage the lesion with respect to local involvement (i.e. renal vein) as well as metastatic disease.

Wilms Tumor In pediatric patients younger than age 15, Wilms tumors account for 95% of all renal malignancies [22]. In the United States, the most common age range affected by this malignancy is three to five years old, and it has the highest rate of occurrence in the African American population [23]. Wilms tumor often presents with abdominal pain and a firm abdominal mass in the right or left upper quadrant of a young child [22]. Typically, the first modality of imaging used for the evaluation of Wilms tumor is ultrasound, and then CT may be utilized for the assessment of the extent and nature of the tumor [24]. On B-mode ultrasound, Wilms tumor will present as an echogenic intrarenal mass with hyperechoic rings around the renal pyramids (Fig. 7.5). Color flow imaging can also be used to visualize increased vascularity within the tumor [25].

Hydronephrosis

Hydronephrosis is most often caused by urinary tract obstruction and can result from blockage at any location along the length of the urinary tract. Common causes include renal calculi, renal carcinoma, prostatic enlargement, urethral stricture, urinary tract infection, and retroperitoneal fibrosis. In adults, hydronephrosis occurs more commonly in men, as a complication of benign prostatic hypertrophy [26]. Overall, hydronephrosis is more commonly observed in children compared to adults secondary to congenital defects of the urinary tract [3]. The presentation is frequently asymptomatic when mild, but severe cases can manifest with flank pain, dysuria, hematuria, oliguria, and fever [27]. Ultrasound is typically the preferred imaging modality for diagnosing hydronephrosis [28]; however, a non-contrast CT scan may be appropriate if the suspected cause is a renal calculus. On ultrasound, hydronephrosis manifests as anechoic dilation of the renal pelvis and calyces [3]. In more severe cases, thinning of the cortex will occur and cortico-medullary differentiation may be lost (Fig. 7.6) [29].

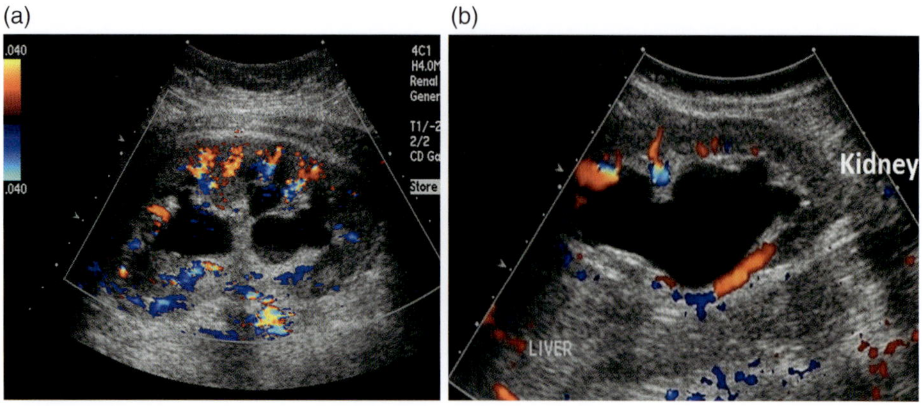

FIGURE 7.6 Moderate (a) and severe (b) hydronephrosis on color flow image of the longitudinal kidney.

Renal Calculi

Renal calculi, also known as kidney stones or nephrolithiasis, are deposits of minerals and salts that occur in 8.8% of the population [30]. Stones may contain calcium, such as calcium oxalate, which makes up the majority of kidney stones, or calcium phosphate. Other compositions include struvite (magnesium ammonium phosphate), uric acid, and, more rarely, cystine stones [31, 32]. Symptoms of renal calculi often include hematuria and pain in the abdomen, flank, and groin. The gold standard for imaging renal calculi is non-contrast CT, but US may be used on initial evaluation of the urinary tract, noting potential for some difficulty in identifying smaller stones and distal ureteral stones. On ultrasound, renal calculi may appear as echogenic foci with associated acoustic shadowing (Fig. 7.7). With color flow imaging, comet-tail artifacts appearing as twinkling may be present [33].

Acute Kidney Injury and Chronic Kidney Disease

Acute kidney injury: Prerenal renal failure is the most common form of acute renal injury; however, the mild changes that are associated with the pathology can be easily missed on ultrasound [34]. Acute tubular necrosis from poor renal perfusion could appear as an enlarged kidney with increased cortical echogenicity, indicating prerenal renal failure [3]. Postrenal renal failure is typically caused by urinary obstruction and would need further evaluation via renal sonography to assess for hydronephrosis or outlet obstruction [34].

Chronic kidney disease: Early diagnosis can be difficult, as the kidney appears normal on B-mode sonography in the early stages of chronic kidney disease. In late-stage kidney disease, the kidney becomes hyperechoic with a decreased longitudinal dimension and parenchymal thickness [2, 35]. Color flow imaging will often reveal decreased renal perfusion [35]. In end-stage chronic kidney disease, the kidney demonstrates homogenous echogenic architecture without visible differentiation between parenchyma and sinus as well as reduction in size (Fig. 7.8) [2].

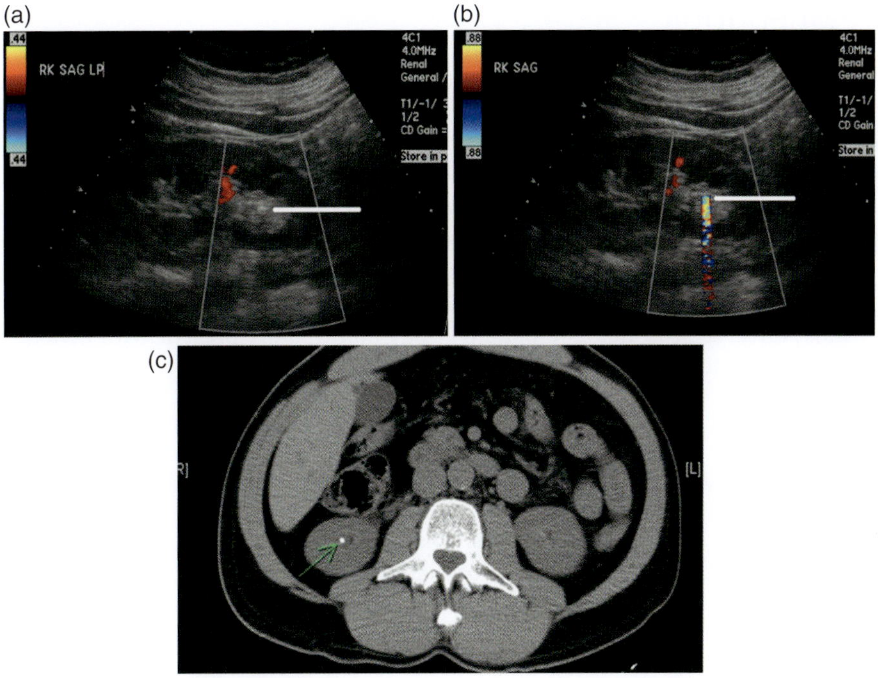

FIGURE 7.7 A small nonobstructive renal calculus (lower pole) appears as echogenic foci with acoustic shadowing on B-mode image (a, pointed by a white solid line). Twinkling artifact (pointed by a white line) appears deep to the calculus (b) on color flow imaging. Non-contrast CT (c) confirms the ultrasound result.

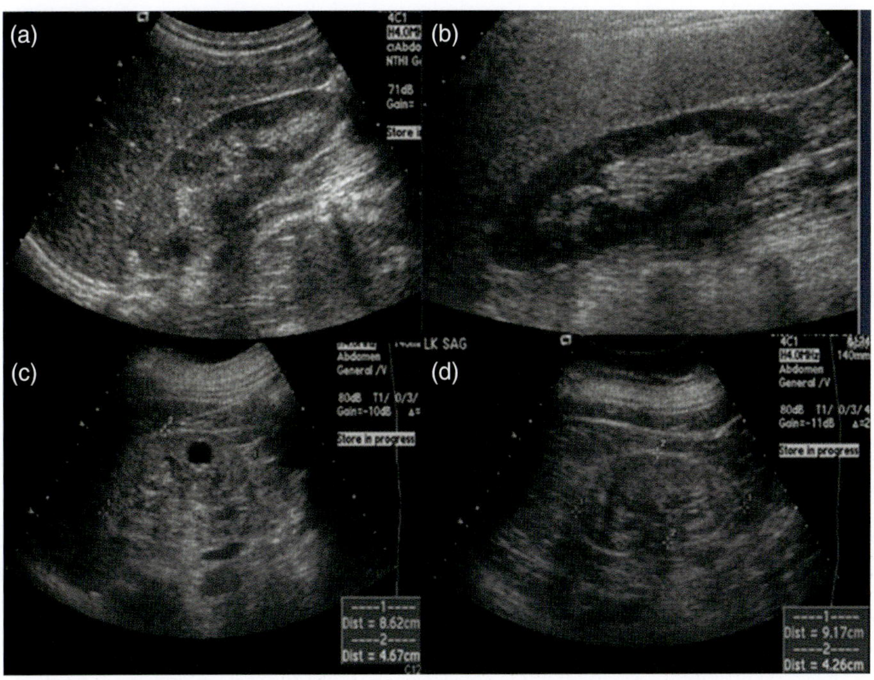

FIGURE 7.8 (a) Normal kidney; (b) a normal kidney in a patient with hepatic steatosis; (c) atrophic kidney measures 8.62 cm; (d) atrophic kidney in a patient with renal failure.

Pyelonephritis

Acute pyelonephritis is a renal tubulointerstitial inflammation caused by ascending or hematogenous infection. Patients may experience fever, flank pain, pyuria, and bacteriuria. On ultrasound, acute pyelonephritis may be presented as hyperechoic areas within the cortex [3]. In complicated cases, the kidney may be enlarged with focal cortical changes that are either hyperechoic or hypoechoic and may also show decreased vascularity in the region of a developing abscess [36]. Fluid can accumulate in the perirenal space with the development of abscesses that appear as well-defined hypoechoic masses on ultrasound exam [36]. Emphysematous pyelonephritis, rare and most often seen in diabetic patients, may additionally present with echogenic foci with associated ring-down artifact.

Renal Artery Stenosis

About 1–10% of Americans with hypertension suffer from renal artery stenosis, a pathology caused by atherosclerotic occlusive disease (90% of patients) or fibromuscular dysplasia (10% of patients, mostly <40 years) [37]. Symptoms of renal artery stenosis include hypertension and an abdominal bruit on the affected side [37]. On grayscale sonography, the affected kidney may become smaller and echogenic due to hypoperfusion and with atherosclerotic plaques that can be observed on grayscale imaging [38]. The diagnosis of renal artery stenosis on color duplex sonography includes direct criteria: peak systolic velocity (PSV) in main renal artery >2.0 m/sec (Fig. 7.9) and PSV ratio of renal artery/aorta >3.5; and indirect criteria: acceleration time >0.07 m/sec and parvus-tardus waveform in the intrarenal artery distal to the stenosis [38]. Stenosis can be confirmed by conventional angiography and/or MRA. Generally, a patient's blood pressure will normalize after correction of the stenosis either by angioplasty with stenting or surgery.

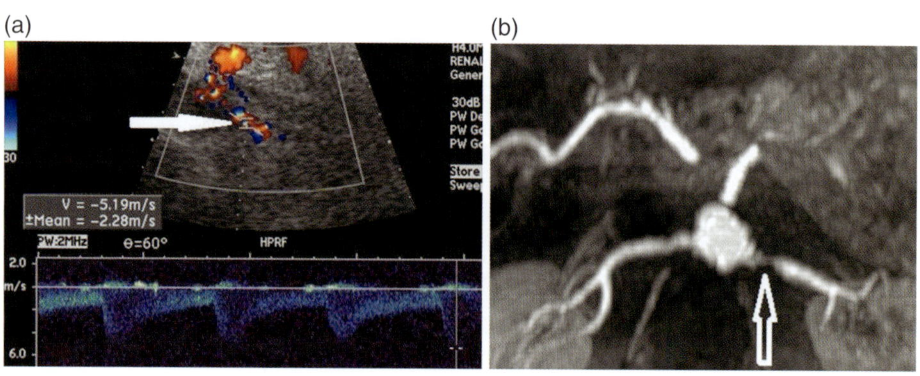

FIGURE 7.9 Renal artery stenosis: (a) Duplex ultrasound image shows a turbulent flow (white arrow) at the stenosis in color flow imaging and increase of peak systolic velocity (V 5.19 m/sec) at stenotic proximal left renal artery. (b) Left renal artery stenosis (arrow) is confirmed with digital subtraction angiography.

Congenital Abnormalities

Solitary Kidney A solitary kidney is determined when only one kidney is present or functional. This can be secondary to congenital defects or surgical removal of one kidney and is easily identified by sonography. Most people who have a solitary kidney experience no health consequences; however, solitary kidneys have been shown to have an association with an increased risk of chronic kidney disease and will need proper surveillance [39]. Patients with a solitary kidney need to monitor blood pressure, glomerular filtration rate, and urine protein content regularly [39, 40].

Horseshoe Kidney Horseshoe kidney occurs in about 1 in 500, where during renal development the two kidneys fuse across the midline into a U-shaped configuration, similar to a horseshoe [41]. Abnormal positioning of the umbilical artery may interfere with kidney migration, resulting in the fusion, most often of the lower poles [42]. More than 70% of people with horseshoe kidneys will have symptoms, including abdominal pain, nausea, kidney stone, and urinary tract infection [41]. Ultrasound exam is useful in diagnosing horseshoe kidney as this abnormality is easily visualized, with lower-than-normal kidney position extending below the inferior mesenteric artery with an isthmus joining the two kidneys [42].

Renal Transplantation

Surgical Anatomy

During kidney transplantation, the allograft kidney is placed in the left or right extraperitoneal iliac fossa. The donor kidney will have its own ureter, renal artery, and vein, so that the donor renal artery is commonly anastomosed to the external iliac artery of the recipient and the donor renal vein to the external iliac vein [43]. The donor ureter is attached to the recipient's bladder by ureteroneocystostomy with a new orifice above the native orifice [43].

Indications for ultrasound scan posttransplantation

1. Routine baseline ultrasound is performed 24–48 hours after operation
2. Renal failure
3. Uncontrolled hypertension
4. Hematuria
5. Abdominal pain at the location of transplanted kidney
6. Fever

Ultrasound Techniques

Renal transplant patients are in supine position for ultrasound assessment. The allograft kidney is easily located due to its superficial location as compared to the native kidney [43]. Curvilinear or sector transducers can be used with frequencies between 2 and 6 MHz for adults; however, children may require a higher frequency

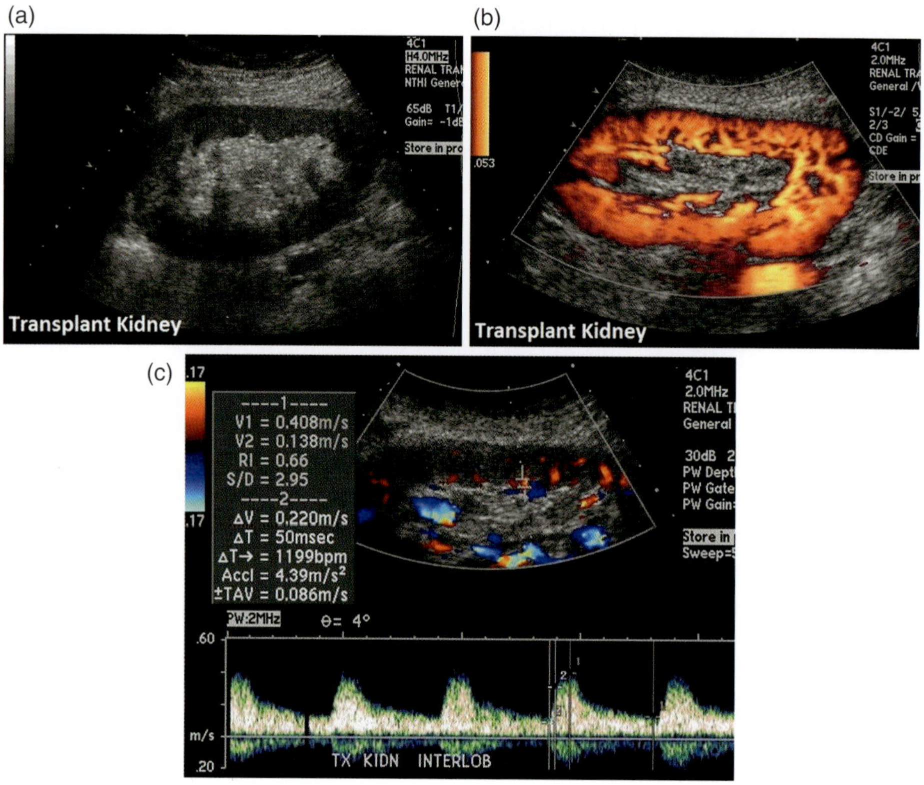

FIGURE 7.10 B-mode ultrasound (a), power Doppler (b), and spectral Doppler parameters of the intrarenal artery (c) in a normal transplanted kidney. TX, transplant; KIDN, kidney; INTERLOB, interlobar artery.

transducer [44]. Grayscale, color flow imaging (Fig. 7.10), and spectral Doppler ultrasound should be performed to assess for obstruction, hydronephrosis, and evaluation of transplant vasculature [44].

Acute Rejection

Acute rejection will usually occur within the first three months after kidney transplantation with a peak within the first 1–3 weeks. An episode of acute rejection adversely predicts long-term graft loss [43].

Although renal histology by biopsy is the gold standard to diagnose acute rejection, biopsy is invasive and can cause complications, such as intrarenal arteriovenous fistula, aneurysm, and hemorrhage. Ultrasound is convenient, noninvasive, and is routinely performed in the first 24–48 hours after transplantation as a baseline evaluation [45].

With acute rejection, ultrasound may find the kidney to be normal, enlarged, or having an obscured differentiation between the cortex and medulla [45]. Spectral Doppler ultrasound may show an elevated resistive index (RI) value (>0.8) and a reversal of diastolic flow in severe cases. These findings, however, are nonspecific and can also be an indication of acute proximal tubular necrosis (ATN) [43, 45].

Chronic Rejection

Chronic rejection occurs after the first three months posttransplantation with eventual failure of the donor kidney [43]. The main predictive factor is a previous attack of acute rejection. Like acute rejection, ultrasound findings for chronic rejection are nonspecific such as thinning of the cortex, increased echogenicity, or decreased vascularity [43, 46]. Diagnosis should be confirmed by histology with changes, including interstitial cellular infiltration and fibrosis, tubular atrophy, and glomerular sclerosis [46]. When chronic renal failure occurs, immunosuppressant toxicity should be considered. In particular, calcineurin inhibitors can cause acute and chronic renal injury, with afferent arteriole constriction, the cause of acute nephrotoxicity [43]. The blood level of calcineurin inhibitors should be monitored and switched to other immunosuppressants when warranted [43].

Vascular Complications

Renal Artery Stenosis Renal artery stenosis occurs in approximately 10% of patients after kidney transplantation [43, 47]. Stenosis most often happens at the anastomosis and is related to surgical technique [47]. The direct indicators on Doppler imaging include PSV at the stenotic site greater than 2–2.5 m/sec, and a PSV ratio of the renal artery at the stenosis to the external iliac artery greater than 3.5 [43, 48]. Indirect indicators are distal turbulent or distal parvus-tardus waveform [43, 47, 48]. Angiography remains the gold standard to confirm renal artery stenosis (Fig. 7.11); however, color duplex ultrasonography is the screening method of choice to assess for stenosis and monitor revascularization [48].

Renal Vein Thrombosis Renal vein thrombosis, while rarely a cause of transplant dysfunction, is a common result of early graft loss, occurring in 0.4–6% of patients early posttransplantation [47, 48]. Patients may experience pain over the graft, sudden swelling, and renal failure. The allograft may be enlarged and hypoechoic on grayscale ultrasound [47]. On spectral Doppler ultrasound, the absence of venous blood flow and a reversal of diastolic flow in the renal artery are diagnostic for renal vein thrombosis [43, 48]. This is different from the reversal of flow limited to early diastole in acute renal rejection and ATN [48]. Once a diagnosis of renal vein thrombosis is found, anticoagulant therapy and surgical intervention may be initiated as soon as possible.

Arteriovenous Fistula Intrarenal arteriovenous fistulas are a complication of graft kidney biopsy occurring when the needle penetrates both arterial and venous walls [43]. On color flow imaging, intrarenal arteriovenous fistulas will appear as a mosaic pattern, with turbulent flow, and will need to be confirmed with spectral Doppler sonography. Spectral Doppler will show high velocity, low resistance arterial flow, and severe turbulence as well as with the draining vein having an arterialized flow appearance [47, 48].

Most of the fistulas are small and asymptomatic and able to resolve spontaneously [43]. However, with large high-flow arteriovenous shunting, renal ischemia or bleeding into the collecting system may occur, resulting in hydronephrosis [47].

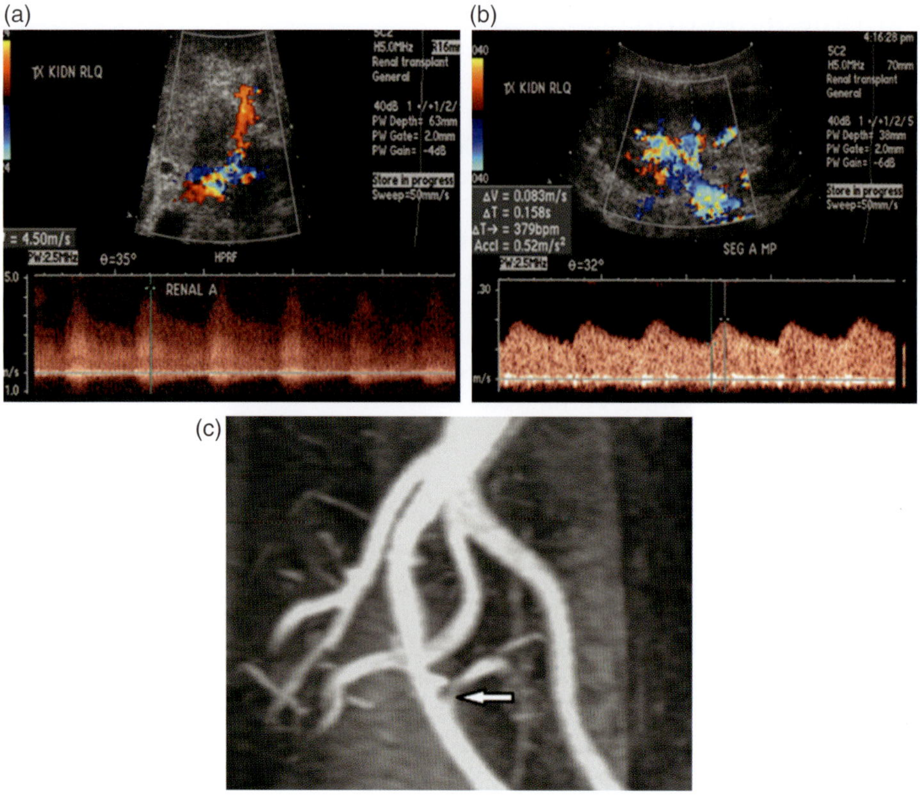

FIGURE 7.11 Peak systolic velocity measures 4.5 m/sec at the proximal main transplant renal artery (RENAL A, a), and parvus-tardus Doppler waveform appears in the intrarenal artery (b) indicate a transplant renal artery stenosis. DSA shows a stenosis at the renal/iliac arterial anastomosis (arrow, c). SEG A, segmental artery; MP, mid-pole.

Hematoma Hematomas most often occur shortly after transplantation in the intrarenal parenchyma or perirenal space but may also arise after trauma or biopsy [43]. Other perinephric fluid collections that should be considered include lymphocele, urinoma, or abscess [47]. On ultrasound, hematomas appear echogenic during their acute phase and will develop into a more cystic appearance with internal fibrinous septa and clot debris [43]. Hematomas are common after surgery and should be monitored for increasing size to determine if intervention is necessary [47].

Urinary Bladder

Transabdominal ultrasound imaging of the bladder is best performed with a distended bladder and should include an examination of the ureterovesical junction and surrounding structures and wall [8, 49]. The examination technique may use either a sector or curvilinear transducer with a frequency of 5 MHz or greater and should be viewed in both transverse and longitudinal scans [49]. Transrectal, transvaginal, or transrectal approaches can also be used to better visualize the bladder if necessary [8]. A normal bladder on ultrasound examination is anechoic with some degree of posterior enhancement behind the bladder. The bladder volume can be calculated using the vesicle volume formula: width × height × length × a correction factor between 0.52 and 0.7 that accounts for the varying shape of urinary bladders [8]. Wall thickness, presence of discrete lesions, and urinary retention are commonly assessed during bladder ultrasonography, aiding in the evaluation for cystitis, calculi, clots, tumors, or traumatic injury [8].

The normal prostate gland is hypoechoic and is located deep and inferior to the bladder. Due to its oval or apple-shaped appearance, the prostate size is calculated using an ellipsoid volume formula: width × height × length × 0.52 [13]. A normal prostate size is 20 g (or 20 cc) in a young male and 30 g in an older male, with a prostate larger than 30 g regarded as prostatomegaly [12].

Post-void Residual Volume

The primary application of the calculation of bladder volume by sonography is the assessment of post-void residual (PVR) volume. This volume may be elevated in a number of disease states, including outlet obstruction and neurogenic bladder. The assessment of bladder volume is usually via a transabdominal approach, based on maximum dimensions obtained from images in both the sagittal and transverse planes (Fig. 7.12). The volume is calculated using the vesicle volume formula: width x height x length x a correction factor, which is typically 0.52 (but may vary up to 0.7) [8]. When obtaining the PVR, the imaging should be performed immediately following voiding.

Bladder Calculi

Bladder calculi typically form primarily within the bladder in the setting of urinary stasis, though some may have originated as renal calculi that migrated into the bladder [50]. These calculi have a similar sonographic appearance to renal calculi,

(a) (b)

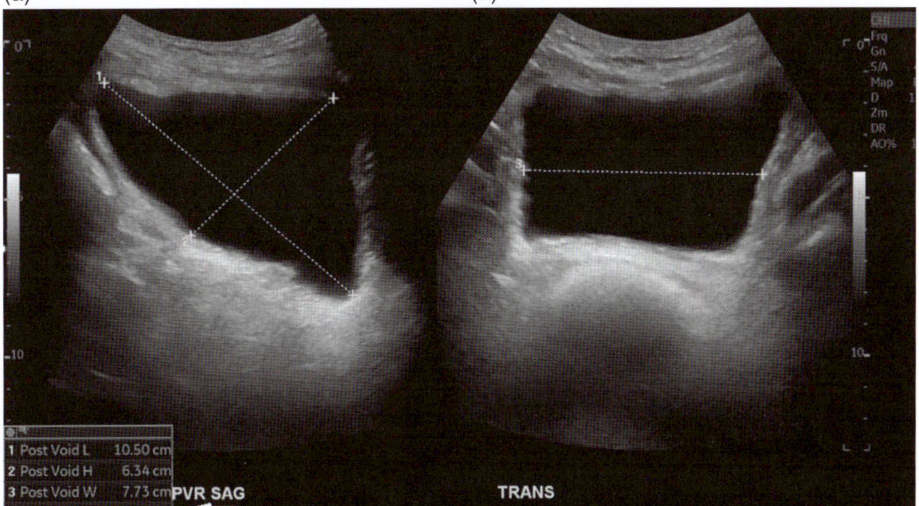

FIGURE 7.12 B-mode sagittal and transverse images of the urinary bladder following voiding, with measurements to estimate the post-void residual volume.

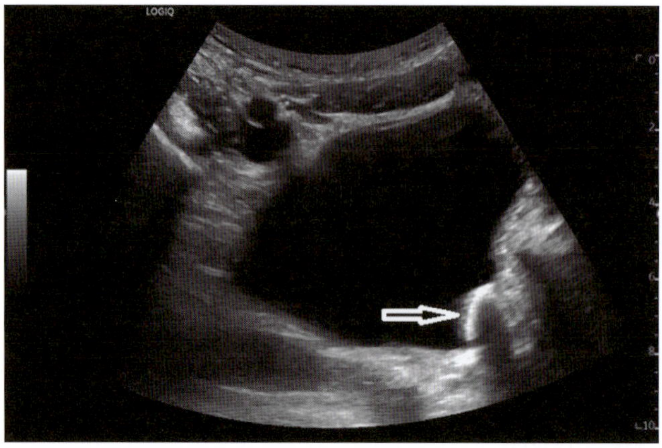

FIGURE 7.13 B-mode transverse image of the urinary bladder with an intraluminal echogenic structure (arrow) with posterior shadowing, which was mobile when the patient was imaged in the left decubitus position, compatible with a bladder calculus.

namely echogenic foci with associated posterior acoustic shadowing (Fig. 7.13). When color Doppler is employed, associated twinkle artifact may be seen. The calculi should be dependent in position, and thus patient rotation may be employed to demonstrate their mobility, such as imaging in a decubitus position following the initial supine position.

Tumors

Bladder tumors are usually malignant, with transitional cell carcinomas being the most common, accounting for about 90% [50]. They can largely be categorized as superficial or invasive, and of the superficial tumors, most demonstrate a papillary pattern. These sonographically appear as polypoid lesions projecting into the lumen, which may demonstrate vascularity on color flow imaging, and which are fixed upon changes in patient position (Fig. 7.14). An associated contour deformity of the bladder suggests invasion, noting that ultrasound does not have a significant role in tumor staging.

(a) (b)

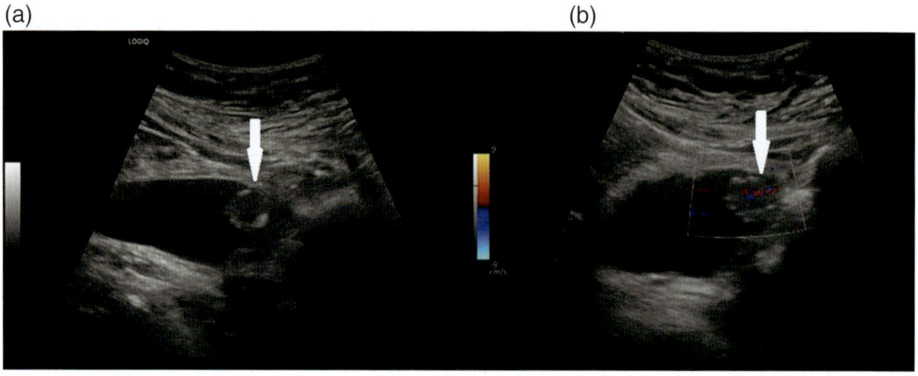

FIGURE 7.14 Rounded intraluminal lesion (arrows) along the bladder wall, predominantly hypoechoic (a), with internal vascularity (b).

Prostate Gland

The normal prostate gland is situated between the bladder neck and the urogenital diaphragm. From a transabdominal approach, it is thus located deep and inferior to the bladder. The prostate is positioned anterior to the rectum and is well-suited for imaging via a transrectal approach. The prostate can be divided into different zones: peripheral zone, transitional zone, central zone, and anterior fibromuscular stroma.

Prostatomegaly

The prostate gland can be enlarged secondary to different etiologies, including benign prostatic hyperplasia and prostate cancer. Prostate volume can be estimated based on transabdominal imaging via a suprapubic approach, with dimensions obtained from images in both the sagittal and transverse planes (Fig. 7.15). Due to its ovoid or apple-shaped configuration, the prostate size is calculated using an ellipsoid volume formula: width × height × length × 0.52 [13]. A normal prostate size is 20 mL in a young male and 30 mL in an older male, with a prostate larger than 30 mL regarded as prostatomegaly [12]. Benign prostatic hypertrophy may be evidenced by other sonographic findings besides prostatomegaly, including a heterogeneous central gland, calcifications, and median lobe hypertrophy with protrusion into the bladder.

Testes

Orchitis

Orchitis, inflammation of one or both testes, is most commonly seen in combination with epididymitis, called epididymo-orchitis [17]. When isolated orchitis occurs, it is most commonly caused by mumps viral infection in children and is rare in adults [14, 51]. Symptoms include sudden onset of fever, nausea, and vomiting with swelling and tenderness of the affected testis [51]. On ultrasound, orchitis can be present as focal or diffuse parenchymal hypoechogenicity [17]. Hypervascularity

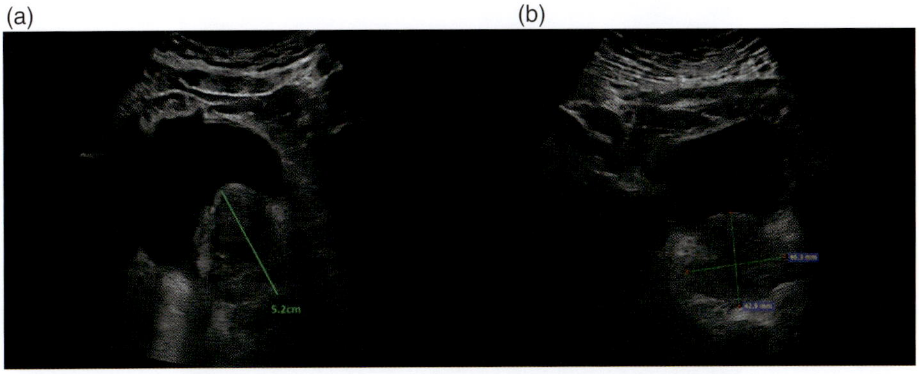

FIGURE 7.15 B-modesagittal and transverse images of enlarged prostate gland, with corresponding measurements for gland size in longitudinal (a) and transverse (b) planes.

and a thickened scrotal wall may also be present [52]. If not treated, orchitis can progress to ischemia, infarction, abscess, and infertility [17].

Hydrocele

A hydrocele can be classified as communicating or noncommunicating. Communicating hydroceles have a persistent connection to the fluid within the peritoneal cavity of the abdomen, whereas noncommunicating hydroceles have no connection to the peritoneal cavity [52]. The fluid accumulated in noncommunicating hydroceles results from fluid secreted by the lining of the tunica vaginalis [52, 53]. During embryological development, the testes form along the posterior body wall of the fetus and proceed to descend through the inguinal canal into the scrotal sac. Therefore, communication is initially present between the parietal and visceral layers of the tunica vaginalis and the peritoneal cavity, known as the processus vaginalis [54]. As a result, communicating hydroceles are particularly common in newborns due to the patent processus vaginalis and potentially affect up to 4.7% of all newborns; however, the majority resolve spontaneously within the first two years of life without intervention [52, 55]. Noncommunicating hydroceles are far more common among adolescents and adults and often caused by trauma, epididymo-orchitis, testicular torsion, or tumors [56].

Clinically, patients with a hydrocele will present with a scrotal mass that will transilluminate upon examination with a light source. The diagnosis can be confirmed with use of ultrasound imaging, where a hydrocele can appear as an anechoic collection about the testicle (Fig. 7.16). In some cases, the hydrocele may contain septa, calcifications, or even cholesterol deposits [54].

Cancer

While only accounting for 1% of all male cancers, testicular cancers are the most common solid malignancy in males from ages 15–35, with seminomas and nonseminomatous germ cell tumors accounting for the majority [52]. Fortunately, testicular cancer only accounts for 0.1% of all deaths of cancer in men within the United States, and the 5-year survival rate is well over 95% [52]. In the majority of cases, testicular cancer

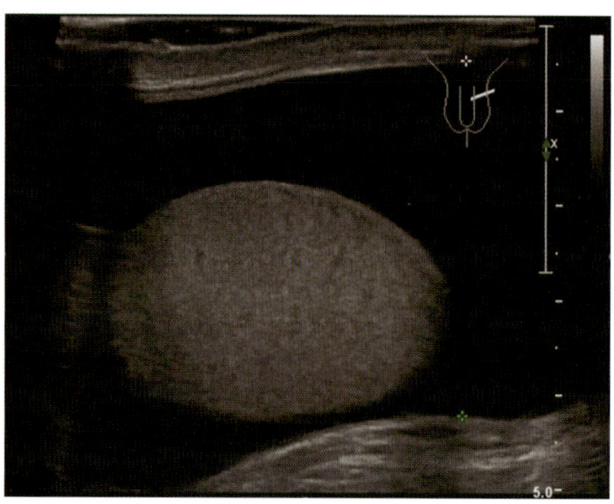

FIGURE 7.16 B-mode image of the left testis shows a large amount of fluid surrounding the testis, suggesting a hydrocele.

presents as a painless nodule or swelling of one testicle but can also present symptoms that overlap with other entities, such as orchitis [17, 52]. On ultrasound imaging, tumors will appear as hypoechoic lesions with hypervascularity and ill-defined borders that can be large enough to displace the normal testis [17]. Assessment of patients with suspected testicular cancer may include blood levels of alpha fetoprotein and beta-hCG, as well as potentially biopsy to confirm malignancy [52].

Testicular Torsion

Testicular torsion is considered a surgical emergency that is most often seen in neonates and postpubertal boys [57]. This occurs when there is either absent or faulty fixation of the testes to the tunica vaginalis, allowing for torsion about the spermatic cord. This may reduce or stop blood flow, subsequently producing ischemia and potentially irreversible damage within seven hours if no intervention is enacted. Testicular torsion often presents as an acute onset of testicular pain with a negative cremasteric reflex [52]. Although most cases of testicular torsion can be diagnosed using history and physical examination, ultrasound can be utilized. On ultrasound, the affected testis may be increased in size with altered or absent blood flow. Color flow imaging can assess the spermatic cord all the way up to the deep inguinal ring to evaluate for adequate blood flow (Fig. 7.17). In addition, high-resolution ultrasound of the spermatic cord may visualize the torsion, often appearing as an inhomogeneous

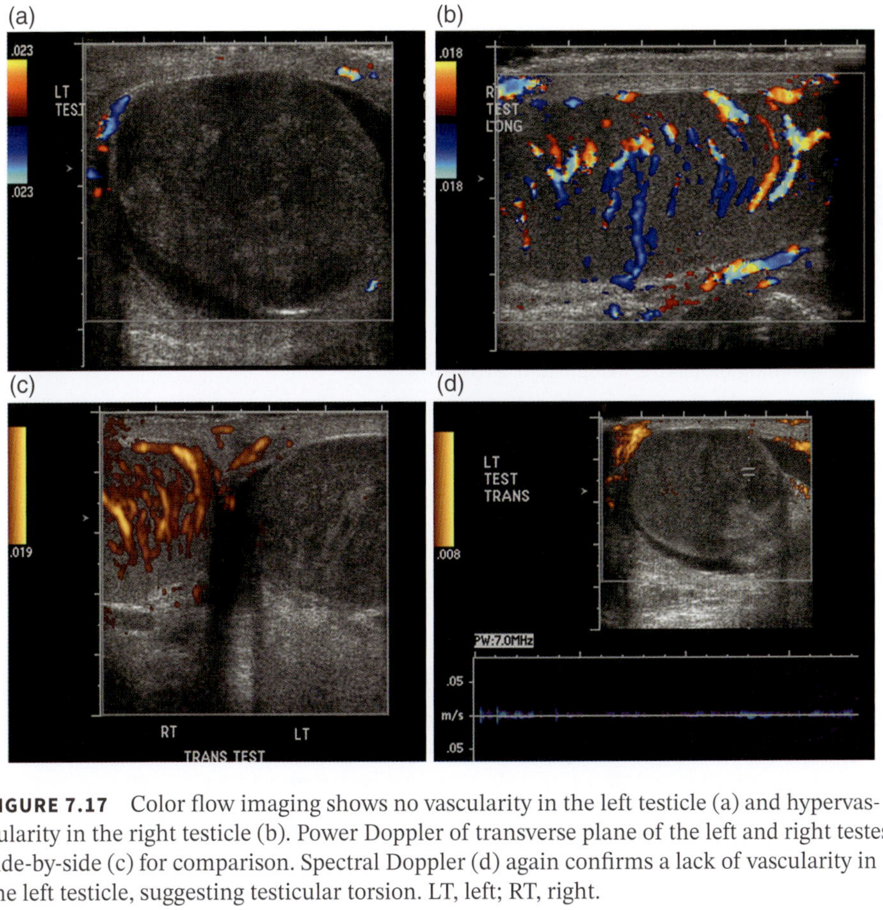

FIGURE 7.17 Color flow imaging shows no vascularity in the left testicle (a) and hypervascularity in the right testicle (b). Power Doppler of transverse plane of the left and right testes side-by-side (c) for comparison. Spectral Doppler (d) again confirms a lack of vascularity in the left testicle, suggesting testicular torsion. LT, left; RT, right.

mass in an inguinal or paratesticular position with so-called whirlpool sign [58]. Treatment of testicular torsion includes emergent surgical exploration with intraoperative detorsion and fixation of the testes to prevent irreversible damage.

Summary

Ultrasound is a valuable imaging technique in the assessment of pathologies in the genitourinary (GU) system. Morphology, hemodynamics, and functional conditions of the organs in the GU system can be evaluated using grayscale and Doppler techniques. With its high accuracy, repeatability, and low cost, ultrasound plays an important role in disease screening, diagnosis, and monitoring. Ultrasound-guided procedures in the GU system will be introduced in Chapter 13 of this book.

Review Questions

1. A 25 y/o man comes to the clinic because he has had vomiting and diarrhea for seven days and oliguria for two days. Past medical history is unremarkable. He is not allergic to any food or medication. Physical examination: BP 80/40 mmHg, T 37 °C, HR 100 /min, R 20 /min. He is dehydrated. There is no pallor in conjunctiva. No rales are heard in both lungs. No murmur is heard on the front chest. No extremity edema is observed.

Lab:

Urine:

Urine: gravity: 1.025, no protein, no RBC, no white blood cells

Urine FE_{Na}: <1%

Urine volume (24 hours): 300 mL

Serum:

Creatinine (Scr): 3 mg/dL (normal <1.3 mg/dL),

Blood urea nitrogen (BUN): 40 mg/dL (normal <20 mg/dL)

Hemoglobin: 15 g/dL (normal >13 g/dL).

Ultrasound of kidney shows that both kidneys measure 12x5x3 cm (normal), and no hydronephrosis.

What is the most likely diagnosis?

a. Prerenal acute renal failure

b. Acute renal tubular necrosis

c. Postrenal acute renal failure

d. Chronic renal disease

e. Minimal change glomerulonephritis

2. A 50 y/o woman comes to the clinic with complaints of anorexia and fatigue for four months. Physical examination finds conjunctival pallor. Her BP is 170/95 mmHg. Urine analysis is normal. Serum: creatinine 6 mg/dL, BUN 60 mg/dL, hemoglobin 6 g/dL. Longitudinal kidneys measure 8.5 × 3 × 2 cm (normal 9–12 cm long × 5–6 cm width × 2–3 cm thickness) on ultrasound. Which is the most likely diagnosis?

a. Prerenal acute renal failure

b. Acute tubular necrosis

c. Postrenal acute renal failure
d. Chronic renal disease (failure)
e. Minimal change glomerulonephritis

3. A 50 y/o woman comes to clinic with complaint of anorexia, fatigue, and ankle swelling for four months. Physical examination finds conjunctival pallor. Her BP is 170/95 mmHg, edema in both ankles. Urine analysis is normal. Serum: creatinine 6 mg/dL, BUN 60 mg/dL, hemoglobin 6 g/dL. Ultrasound on kidney shows size of both kidneys 8.5 × 3 × 2 cm (normal 9–12 cm long × 5–6 cm width × 2–3 cm thickness). Blood smears show normal morphology of red blood cells. What is the most likely reason that this patient has low hemoglobin level?
   a. Kidney releases less renin
   b. Kidney synthesizes less 1-alpha hydroxylase
   c. Kidney synthesizes less erythropoietin
   d. Kidney release less angiotensin II
   e. Kidney releases less aldosterone

4. A 14 y/o boy is brought to the clinic because his urine color has been dark for two days. He does not have any urinary urgency, frequency, or irritation of urination. He does not have joint pain or abdominal pain. He did not have any skin infection, sore throat, or cold in the last three months. His past medical history is unremarkable. Physical examination does not find anything abnormal, and he does not have fever, edema, hypertension, skin rash, petechiae, or purpura.

Laboratory test:

Urine: red blood cell 10/high power field (400×) (normal <3), protein (+) (normal [−]).

24 hour-urine protein: 500 mg (normal <150 mg)

Stool: occult blood test (−)

Serum: Hemoglobin: 14 g/dL (normal >12 g/dL),

Serum creatinine: 1.1 mg/dL (normal <1.3 mg/dL),

Blood urea nitrogen (BUN): 20 mg/dL (normal <20 mg/dL)

Red blood cells: 5 trillion cells/L (normal: 4.35–5.65 trillion cells/L)

White blood cells: 5 billion cells/L (3.4–9.6 billion cells/L)

Platelet: 300,000 cells/μL (150,000–350,000/μL)

Bleeding time: 5 minutes (normal with 1–9 minutes)

Prothrombin time: 10 seconds (normal 9.6–11.8 seconds)

Activated partial thromboplastin time: 25 seconds (normal 20–36 seconds)

Ultrasound of kidney: normal sonography of kidney, size of both kidneys 12 × 5 × 3 cm (normal 9–12 cm long × 5–6 cm width × 2–3 cm thickness), no kidney stone, no hydronephrosis.

Plain abdominal X-ray: no stone in urinary tract and kidney

What is the most likely cause of his hematuria?
   a. Kidney stone
   b. Urinary tract infection
   c. Thrombocytopenia
   d. Henoch-Schonlein purpura
   e. Glomerulonephritis

5. A 70 y/o healthy man comes to the clinic for a checkup. He has no complaints. He does not have any chronic disease, diabetes, or hypertension. Sonography of his right kidney shows a hypervascular solid lesion in the kidney. His urinalysis: red blood cells 10/high power

field (400×), protein (+). Blood tests show normal hemoglobin, and normal liver and renal function. Which disorder is most likely needed to exclude or confirm?

a. Simple kidney cyst

b. Autosomal-dominant polycystic kidney disease

c. Kidney stone

d. Hydronephrosis

e. Renal cell cancer

6. A 40 y/o man is found to have hypertension recently. Bruits can be heard on his mid abdomen bilaterally. Ultrasound of the kidney has not found an abnormality. Angiogram shows bilateral renal artery stenosis. Which drug is contraindicated for use to reduce his blood pressure?

a. Angiotensin II receptor blocker (ARB)

b. Calcium channel blocker

c. Beta blocker

d. Loop Diuretic

e. Corticosteroid

7. A 50 y/o diabetic male comes to clinic for a checkup. He has uncontrolled hypertension and hyperlipidemia for 20 years. He has also smoked for 30 years. B-mode, color flow imaging, and spectral Doppler are requested to assess renal arteries to rule out which of the following:

a. Renal artery stenosis

b. Nephrolithiasis

c. Hydronephrosis

d. Renal benign tumor

e. Renal malignant tumor

8. A 45 y/o hypertensive man complains of abdominal pain and red-colored urine for one day. Physical examination finds abdominal masses bilaterally with irregular surface. Urinalysis shows hematuria and mild proteinuria. Ultrasound of kidneys show numerous anechoic rounded of anechoic circular structures in bilateral kidney regions.

What is the ultrasound result?

a. Nephrolithiasis

b. Pyelonephritis

c. Polycystic kidney disease

d. Hydronephrosis

e. Kidney solid tumor

9. A 33 y/o pregnant woman presents to the ER with left flank pain radiating down to her left groin that began last night. The patient also states she saw blood in her urine this morning and has nausea as well. You suspect nephrolithiasis, which imaging option is best to use on this pregnant woman?

a. CT scan without contrast

b. MRI

c. Ultrasound

d. X-ray

e. Nuclear imaging

Correct answers: 1. a; 2. d; 3. c; 4. e; 5. e; 6. a; 7. a; 8. c; 9. c.

References

1. Noble VE, Brown DFM. Renal ultrasound. *Emerg Med Clin North Am* 2004; 22: 641–659.
2. Gao J, Perlman A, Kalache S, et al. Multiparametric quantitative ultrasound imaging in assessment of chronic kidney disease. *J Ultrasound Med* 2017; 36: 2245–2256.
3. Hansen KL, Nielsen MB, Ewertsen C. Ultrasonography of the kidney: a pictorial review. *Diagnostics (Basel)* 2015; 6(1): 2. https://doi.org/10.3390/diagnostics6010002.
4. Moore KL, Dalley AF, Agur AMR. Clinically oriented anatomy. 7th ed. Philadelphia, PA: Lippincott Williams & Wilkins, 2014.
5. Fröber R. Surgical anatomy of the ureter. *BJU Int* 2007; 100(4): 949–965.
6. Soriano RM, Penfold D, Leslie SW. Anatomy, abdomen and pelvis, kidneys. In: StatPearls [Internet]. New York, New York: McGraw Hill Publishing, 2020.
7. Lukacz ES, Sampselle C, Gray M, et al. A healthy bladder: a consensus statement. *Int J Clin Pract* 2011; 65: 1026–1036.
8. Pavlica P, Gaudiano C, Barozzi L. Sonography of the bladder. *World J Urol* 2004; 22: 328–334.
9. Mitterberger M, Horninger W, Aigner F, et al. Ultrasound of the prostate. *Cancer Imaging* 2010; 10: 40–48.
10. SEER Training Modules. Testicular cancer. U.S. National Institutes of Health, National Cancer Institute, 2026. https://training.seer.cancer.gov.
11. Rebik K, Wagner JM, William M. Scrotal ultrasound. *Radiol Clin North Am* 2019; 57: 635–648.
12. Nuraj P, Hysenj N. The diagnosis of obstructive hydronephrosis with color Doppler ultrasound. *Acta Inform Med* 2017; 25: 178–181.
13. Brakohiapa EK, Botwe BO, Sarkodie BD. Prostatic volume determination by transabdominal ultrasonography: does accuracy vary significantly with urinary bladder volumes between 50 to 400 mL. *J Med Radiat Sci* 2019; 66: 81–90.
14. Correas JM, Halpern EJ, Barr RG, et al. Advanced ultrasound in the diagnosis of prostate cancer. *World J Urol* 2020.
15. Rafailidis V, Apostolou D, Charsoula A, Rafailidis D. Sonography of the scrotum. *J Ultrasound Med* 2015; 34: 507–518.
16. Dogra VS, Gottlieb RH, Oka M, Rubens DJ. Sonography of the scrotum. *Radiology* 2003; 227: 18–36.
17. Sommers D, Winter T. Ultrasonography evaluation of scrotal masses. *Radiol Clin North Am* 2014; 52: 1265–1281.
18. Silverman SG, Pedrosa I, Ellis JH, et al. Bosniak classification of cystic renal masses, version 2019: an update proposal and needs assessment. *Radiology* 2019; 292: 475–488.
19. Pei Y, Obaji J, Dupuis A, et al. Unified criteria for ultrasonographic diagnosis of ADPKD. *J Am Soc Nephrol* 2009; 20: 205–212.
20. Chapman AB, Devuyst O, Eckardt KU, et al. Autosomal-dominant polycystic kidney disease (ADPKD): executive summary from a kidney disease: improving global outcomes (KDIGO) controversies conference. *Kidney Int* 2015; 88: 17–27.
21. Rumack CM, Wilson SR, Charboneau JW, Levine D. Diagnostic ultrasound. 4th ed. Philadelphia, PA: Elsevier, 2011; 371.
22. Fernandez C, Geilla JI, Ehrlich PF, et al. Renal tumors. In: Pizzo PA, Poplack DG (eds). Principles and practice of pediatric oncology. 6th ed, 2011; 861.
23. Grimsby GM, Ritchey ML. Pediatric urologic oncology. *Pediatr Clin N Am* 2012; 59: 947–959. https://doi.org/10.1016/j.pcl.2012.05.018.
24. McDonald K, Duffy P, Chowdhury T, McHugh K. Added value of abdominal cross-sectional imaging (CT or MRI) in staging of Wilms' tumor. *Clin Radiol* 2013; 68: 16–20.
25. Kosiak M, Stefanowicz J, Adamkiewicz-Drożyńska E, et al. Sonographic image of solitary kidney in Wilms tumour survivors. *Kidney Blood Press Res* 2018; 43: 1363–1374. https://doi.org/10.1159/000492951.

26. Meldrum KK. Pathophysiology of urinary tract obstruction. In: Campbell-W urology. Vol 2. 11th ed. Philadelphia, PA: Elsevier, 2016; 1109–1103.
27. O'Neill WC. Atlas of renal ultrasonography. 1st ed. Philadelphia, PA: Elsevier Inc., 2000.
28. Leo M, Langlois B, Pare J, et al. Ultrasound vs. computed tomography for severity of hydronephrosis and its importance in renal colic. *West J Emerg Med* 2017; 18: 559–568.
29. Springer DA, Allen M, Hoffman V, et al. Investigation and identification of etiologies involved in the development of acquired hydronephrosis in aged laboratory mice with the use of high-frequency ultrasound imaging. *Pathobiol Aging Age Relat Dis* 2014; 4: 24932.
30. Curhan G. Nephrolithiasis. In: National kidney foundation primer on kidney diseases. Philadelphia, PA: Elsevier, 2014; 405–411.
31. Singh P, Enders FT, Vaughan LE, et al. Stone composition among first-time symptomatic kidney stone formers in the community. *Mayo Clin Proc* 2015; 90: 1356.
32. Lieske JC, Rule AD, Krambeck AE, et al. Stone composition as a function of age and sex. *Clin J Am Soc Nephrol* 2014; 9: 2141–2146.
33. Sorensen MD, Harper JD, His RS, et al. B-mode ultrasound verses color Doppler twinkling artifact in detecting kidney stones. *J Endourol* 2013; 27: 149–153.
34. Rahman M, Shad F, Smith MC. Acute kidney injury: a guide to diagnosis and management. *Am Fam Physician* 2012; 86: 631–639.
35. Petrucci I, Clementi A, Sessa C, et al. Ultrasound and color Doppler applications in chronic kidney disease. *J Nephrol* 2018; 31: 863–879.
36. Fontanilla T, Minaya J, Cortes C, et al. Acute complicated pyelonephritis: contrast-enhanced ultrasound. *Abdom Imaging* 2012; 37: 639–646.
37. Safian RD. Renal artery stenosis. *Prog Cardiovasc Dis* 2021; 65: 60–70.
38. Gao J, Shih G, Auh YH, et al. Pitfall and sources of error of color duplex sonography in screening for renovascular hypertension. *Int J Nephrol Urol* 2010; 2: 212–223.
39. Kim S, Chang Y, Rae Lee Y, et al. Solitary kidney and risk of chronic kidney disease. *Eur J Epidemiol* 2019; 34: 879–888.
40. Solitary Kidney. NIH NIDDK web. 2020. https://www.niddk.nih.gov/health-information/kidney-disease/solitary-kidney.
41. Taghavi K, Kirkpatrick J, Mirjalili SA. The horseshoe kidney: Surgical anatomy and embryology. *J Pediatr Urol* 2016; 12(5): 275–280.
42. Sakala MD, Dyer RB. The horseshoe kidney. *Abdom Imaging* 2015; 40: 2910–2911.
43. Kolofousi C, Stefanidis K, Cokkinos D, et al. Ultrasonographic features of kidney transplants and their complications: an imaging review. *ISRN Radiol* 2013; 2013: 480–862.
44. AIUM. AIUM practice guideline for the performance of an ultrasound examination of solid-organ transplants. *J Ultrasound Med* 2014; 33(7): 1309–1320.
45. Piyasena RV, Hamper UM. Doppler ultrasound evaluation of renal transplants. *Appl Radiol* 2010; 39(9): 24–32.
46. Gao J, Rubin J, Xiang DY, et al. Doppler parameters in renal transplant dysfunction. *J Ultrasound Med* 2011; 30: 169–175.
47. Brown ED, Chen MYM, Wolfman NT, et al. Complications of renal transplantation: evaluation with US and radionuclide imaging. *Radiographics* 2000; 20: 607–622.
48. Gao J, Ng A, Shih G, et al. Intrarenal color duplex ultrasonography: a window to vascular complications of renal transplants. *J Ultrasound Med* 2007; 26: 1403–1418.
49. American Institute of Ultrasound in Medicine; American Urological Association. AIUM practice guideline for the performance of an ultrasound examination in the practice of urology. *J Ultrasound Med* 2012; 31(1): 133–144.
50. Kim SE, Cho JY, Lee HK, et al. Ultrasound of the urinary bladder, revisited. *J Med Ultrasound* 2007; 15: 77–90.
51. Başekim CC, Kizilkaya E, Pekkafali Z, et al. Mumps epididymo-orchitis: sonography and color Doppler sonographic findings. *Abdom Imaging* 2000; 25: 322–325.
52. Wampler SM, Llanes M. Common scrotal and testicular problems. *Prim Care* 2010; 37: 613–626.
53. Hall NJ, Ron O, Eaton S, Pierro A. Surgery for hydrocele in children—an avoidable excess? *J Pediatr Surg* 2011; 46: 2401–2405.

54. Garriga V, Serrano A, Marin A, et-al. US of the tunica vaginalis testis: anatomic relationships and pathologic conditions. *Radiographics* 2009; 29: 2017–2032.
55. Acer-Demir T, Ekenci BY, Özer D, et al. Natural history and conservative treatment outcomes for hydroceles: a retrospective review of one center's experience. *Urology* 2018; 112: 155–160.
56. Hoang VT, Van HAT, Hoang TH, et al. A Review of Classification, Diagnosis, and Management of Hydrocele. *J Ultrasound Med.* 2024; 43(3): 599–607.
57. Molokwu CN, Somani BK, Goodman CM. Outcomes of scrotal exploration for acute scrotal pain suspicious of testicular torsion: a consecutive case series of 173 patients. *BJU Int* 2011; 107: 990–993.
58. Vijayaraghavan SB. Sonographic differential diagnosis of acute scrotum: real-time whirlpool sign, a key sign of torsion. *J Ultrasound Med* 2006; 25: 563–574.

CHAPTER 8

Peripheral Vascular Ultrasound

Andy Thai[1], Giovanni Montesano[1], and Jing Gao[2]

[1] Rocky Vista University, College of Osteopathic Medicine, Ivins, Utah, USA

[2] Rocky Vista University, Montana College of Osteopathic Medicine, Billings, Montana, USA

Introduction

Ultrasound has been an important diagnostic tool in the assessment of vascular morphology and function. Compared to conventional plethysmography, venography, and digital subtraction angiography (DSA), ultrasound has numerous advantages in screening and diagnosing vascular diseases [1–3]. Ultrasound provides clinical physicians with observations of two-dimensional and three-dimensional vessel texture, real-time blood flow in the vessels, and quantitative parameters of arterial and venous hemodynamics. Ultrasound has high accuracy, acceptability, portability, low cost, and has no radiation exposure [4]. Following the development of new ultrasound transducers, hardware, and image processing software, vascular ultrasound advanced to evaluate microvasculature, vessel wall mechanical properties, and complicated pathologies in vessels [5, 6]. Contrast-enhanced computed tomography (CT), magnetic resonance angiography (MRA), and DSA are able to display the large arterial and venous systems in their entirety. However, the requirement of contrast agent administration, contraindications, availability, and high costs limit the use of CT, DSA, and MRA as routine imaging techniques in screening for peripheral vascular disease or as a common tool in rural medicine [7]. Along with all the benefits, there are also some limitations to vascular ultrasound. Microvasculature can be more difficult to visualize and evaluate than its larger counterparts. It is often difficult to optimize vessels in a deep location or behind intestines and bones, compared to superficial vessels. Other imaging tests (CT, MRA) may be required if clinically indicated [4].

In this chapter, we discuss the clinical applications of ultrasound for assessing common peripheral arterial diseases (PADs) and detecting deep vein thrombosis (DVT). Ultrasound of the carotid artery and the abdominal aorta is introduced in this book separately (Chapter 10).

General Anatomy

Extremity Arteries

Upper Extremity Arteries The major blood supply to the upper extremity arises from the axillary artery, a continuation of the subclavian artery. The subclavian artery becomes the axillary artery at the lateral border of the first rib, and then becomes the brachial artery at the inferior border of the teres major muscle. The axillary artery has several branches to supply the muscles of the anterior chest, shoulder, and scapula when passing posterior to the pectoralis minor muscle [8].

The brachial artery, a continuation of the axillary artery, provides the major blood supply to the arm. It courses down the medial aspect of the humerus, giving off numerous unnamed muscular branches, the humeral nutrient artery, the profunda brachii artery, and the superior and inferior ulnar collateral arteries. These arteries descend along the humerus and contribute to the periarticular arterial anastomosis of the elbow region. As the brachial artery approaches the distal humerus, it courses anterior to the medial supraepicondylar ridge and trochlea of the humerus, and then ends at the cubital fossa, where it divides into the radial and ulnar arteries. The radial, ulnar, and interosseous arteries run laterally, anteriorly, and medially in the forearm. Radial and ulnar arteries form palmar arches that branch into common and then proper palmar digital arteries to supply blood flow to hands and fingers [9].

Lower Extremity Arteries The primary arterial supply of the lower extremity is the femoral artery. This is a continuation of the external iliac artery, which passes posterior to the inguinal ligament. It then courses through the femoral triangle with the femoral vein and nerve. This is where the profunda femoris artery branches off. One branch is the medial circumflex artery that supplies the head and neck of the femur, adductor and hamstrings muscles, and the sciatic nerve [9]. The femoral artery continues through the adductor canal and into the popliteal fossa. After the adductor hiatus, the femoral artery becomes the popliteal artery. In the popliteal fossa, the popliteal artery then branches into the anterior tibial, posterior tibial, and fibular (peroneal) arteries [8]. The anterior tibial artery courses anterior to the interosseous membrane within the anterior compartment and becomes the dorsalis pedis artery over the superior aspect of the foot. The posterior tibial artery courses posterior to the interosseous membrane and enters the posterior compartment of the leg and then branches into the medial and lateral plantar arteries at the level of the medial malleolus (Fig. 8.1). The fibular artery descends into the posterior compartment [10].

Extremity Veins

Upper Extremity Veins Venous drainage of the upper limb is comprised of superficial and deep components, which are connected via perforating veins. The cephalic and basilic veins are the main superficial veins of the upper limb and originate in the subcutaneous tissue of the dorsum of the hand. The cephalic vein travels from the dorsal venous network of the hand up the lateral border of the wrist and anterolateral forearm (Fig. 8.2). At the cubital fossa, the cephalic vein communicates

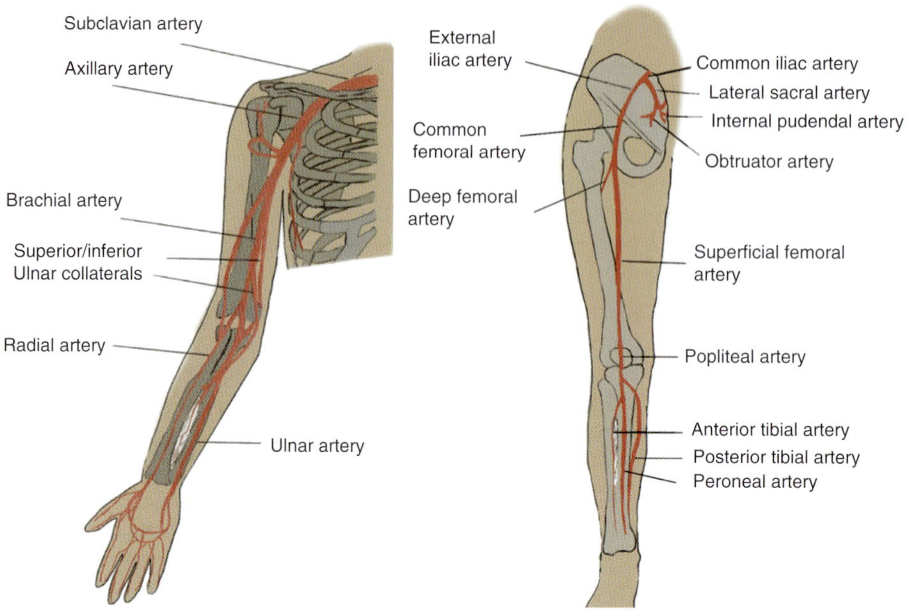

FIGURE 8.1 Anatomy of upper and lower extremity arteries.

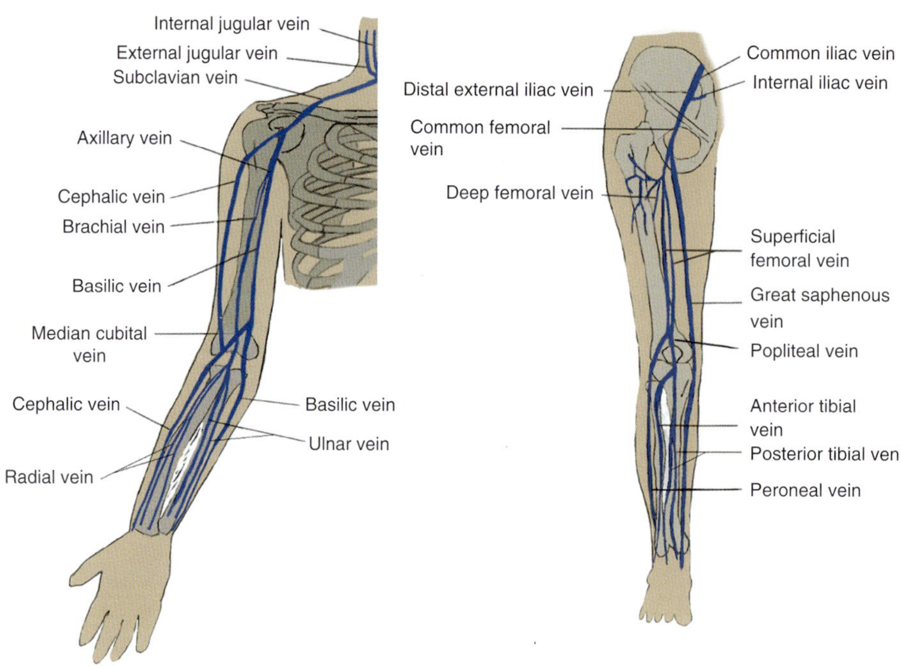

FIGURE 8.2 Anatomy of upper and lower extremity veins.

with the median cubital vein. It then continues its course superiorly up the arm, travels between the deltoid and pectoralis major muscles, and enters the clavipectoral triangle to terminate in the axillary vein [8]. The axillary vein further drains into the subclavian vein, then the superior vena cava [8].

The basilic vein ascends from the medial end of the dorsal venous network along the medial side of the forearm and inferior arm. About halfway up the arm, it pierces the brachial fascia and runs in parallel with the brachial artery to the axilla. It then merges with accompanying veins running in parallel with the axillary artery to form the axillary vein. The median vein of the forearm, while highly variable, begins at the base of the thumb and ascends the middle and anterior aspect of the forearm between the cephalic and basilic veins. In general, deep veins lie under the deep fascia and travel as pairs while parallel to the major arterial supply. Paired veins consist of radial (lateral) and ulnar (medial) veins in the forearm, and brachial veins in the upper arm, traveling along with arteries [9].

The bilateral internal jugular veins (IJVs) are the major vessels that drain the cranium and face. Each sigmoid sinus drains into the IJV, which courses through the jugular foramen. After exiting the skull, it descends through the carotid sheath along with the internal carotid artery and vagus nerve into the thorax, where it merges with the subclavian vein to form the brachiocephalic vein. Ultrasound of the IJV is commonly included in the upper extremity venous Doppler study to assess the presence of venous thrombosis [9, 10].

Lower Extremity Veins The venous drainage of the lower extremity consists of both the superficial and deep drainage. The superficial drainage goes into the great saphenous vein in the medial leg and drains into the common femoral vein near the femoral head in the femoral triangle. The small saphenous vein drains into the popliteal vein in the popliteal fossa. The deep venous drainage, consisting of anterior tibial, posterior tibial, peroneal in the lower leg, popliteal in the popliteal fossa, and superficial femoral in the upper leg accompanies the main arteries of the limb (Fig. 8.2). The popliteal vein becomes the femoral vein as it passes through the adductor hiatus, then becomes the external iliac vein in the pelvis [10].

Ultrasound Techniques and Normal Ultrasound Images

Patient Position

An ultrasound exam requires the patient to be in a prone, supine, or lateral position based on the anatomic location of the vessel being scanned. When scanning the axilla, have the patient lie supine with the ipsilateral arm outstretched and behind the patient's head. To scan the popliteal region, the patient is placed prone or on their side ipsilateral to the operator. Ensure the patient is lying comfortably. The exam times can vary depending on the complexity of the exam but are often completed within approximately 30 minutes.

Scanning Protocol

Vascular ultrasound is commonly performed with a linear array transducer (6–12 MHz). Application of a clear water-based gel to the site of scanning helps the transducer firmly contact the skin and eliminates air bubbles between the skin and transducer

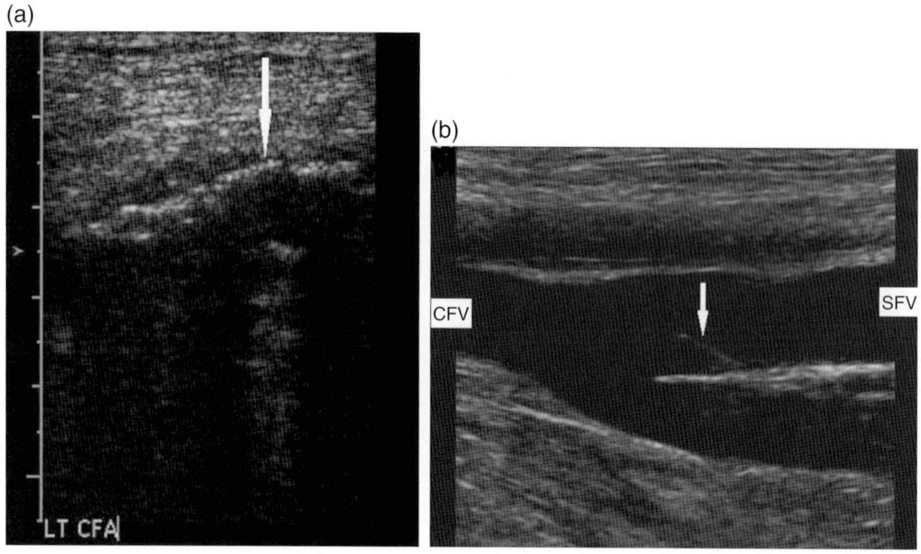

FIGURE 8.3 Longitudinal B-mode image of the left common femoral artery (LT CFA) shows diffuse atherosclerotic plaque (white arrow) on the anterior arterial wall with acoustic shadowing in B-mode ultrasound image (a). B-mode image is also useful in observing the activity of venous valves (white arrow, b) in normal superficial femoral veins (SFV). CFV, common femoral vein.

surface that can affect the sound waves transmitting into the body. The transducer can be placed anteriorly, posteriorly, or laterally to improve the image of the vessels investigated based on their anatomic locations [11].

To evaluate arterial and venous structures and blood flow hemodynamics, grayscale image, color flow, and spectral Doppler are all important [11]. B-mode grayscale image displays the wall and lumen of the vessels to observe the presence of arterial plaques along the arterial wall (Fig. 8.3) and a thrombus in the venous lumen. The free movement of the venous valve can be demonstrated in real time grayscale image (Fig. 8.3b). Compression on the transverse section of the vein in a grayscale image and color flow imaging using the scanning transducer is important to confirm the presence of thrombosis in venous lumen (Fig. 8.4).

Color flow imaging assesses the mean velocity and direction of the blood flow through tracking and measuring red blood cells traveling throughout the sampled site. When red blood cells move interacting with an ultrasound beam, they produce Doppler effects (Chapter 1) that can be calculated with software and processed to create both color-coded images (color flow imaging) and a graphical representation (spectral Doppler, Fig. 8.5) of blood flow at the site of investigation. Color flow imaging displays the patency of the vessels. It is also useful to guide spectral Doppler to sample the range of velocities at the site with arterial pathology. The waveform of the spectrum changes following the alteration of the flow velocity, pattern, and resistance in the artery and vein. This spectrum change can be seen in individuals with stenosis, abnormal communication between the artery and vein (arteriovenous fistula, AVF), and venous obstruction [4].

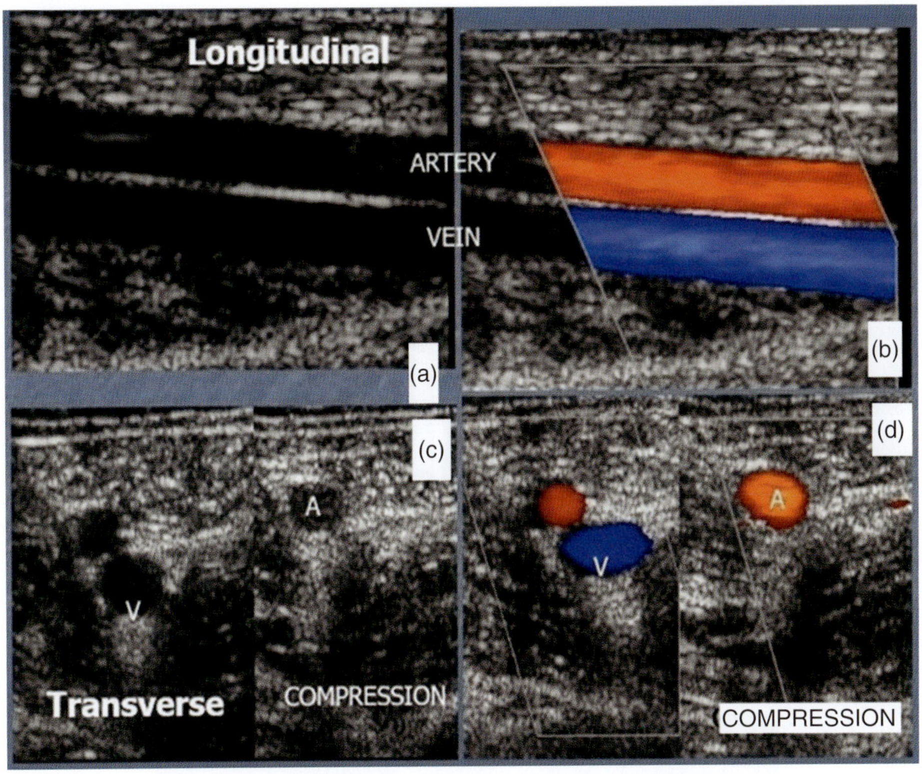

FIGURE 8.4 B-mode (a) and color flow imaging (b) of the normal superficial femoral artery and vein demonstrate that no internal echoes (free of thrombus) appear in venous lumen (a) and complete color fills in the vein (b). An adequate compressibility in the transverse plane of the vein in B-mode image (c) and color flow imaging (d) demonstrates no evidence of venous thrombosis. A, artery; V, vein.

Common Clinical Indications for Vascular Ultrasound

Circulatory status of arterial and venous systems can be assessed using vascular ultrasound. Common applications for vascular ultrasound include, but are not limited to, assessing arterial atherosclerosis, stenosis, aneurysm, and venous embolism, mapping normal anatomy to guide vascular interventions, as well as monitoring complications (such as AFV) of interventional procedures [12]. A focal narrowing of the artery as a result of atherosclerosis is a common pathology. A severe consequence of occlusive atherosclerosis is limb ischemia that typically presents with pain, numbness, coldness, weak pulse, and myalgias in the extremity distal to the stenosis. In addition, atherosclerosis is a general process that may affect the entire arterial system in the body, major arteries, as well as small arteries in the distal extremities. Therefore, the change in extremity arteries may indicate the disease involving other arteries, such as the coronary arteries with atherosclerosis [4, 11].

DVT is a common indication for venous ultrasound of the extremities. Patients at high risk of developing DVT (long time bed rest, major abdominal and orthopedic surgery, pregnancy, chemotherapy, venous catheter placement, etc.) and with

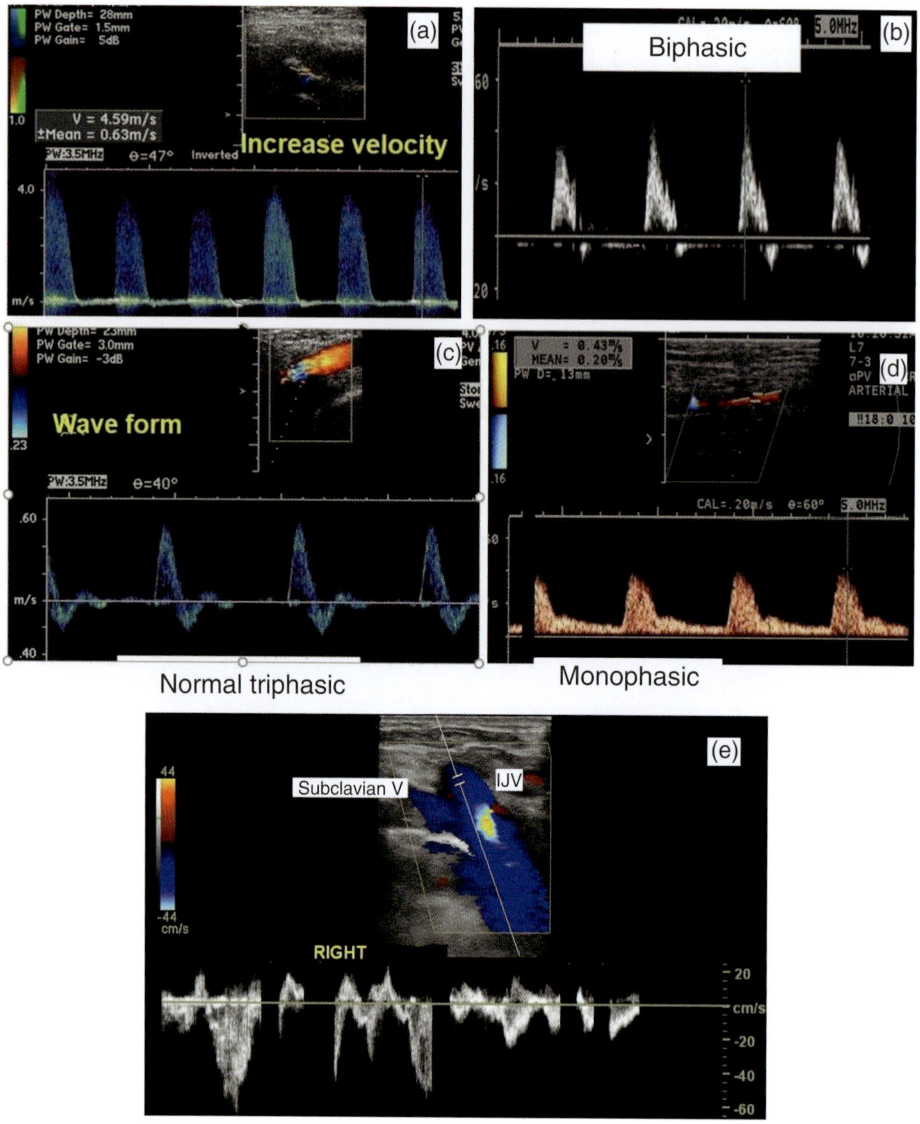

FIGURE 8.5 Both flow velocity (a) and spectral waveform are important in vascular ultrasound. In arterial ultrasound, spectral waveform changes from triphasic (c, normal), biphasic (b, mild stenosis or stiff arterial wall), to monophasic (d, distal to severe stenosis or occlusion) based on the severity of arterial flow obstruction and/or arterial compliance. In venous ultrasound (e), duplex Doppler (color flow and spectral Doppler) image can demonstrate the patency of the junction (brachiocephalic vein) of IJV and the subclavian vein (V) in color flow and spectral pattern of respiratory variation in spectral Doppler.

suspicion of DVT may present symptoms of pulmonary embolism (chest pain, shortness of breath) (Fig. 8.6), localized extremity pain, swelling, erythema, and/or warmth. Ultrasound is considered to be the first imaging study for screening and diagnosing DVT. A dislodged thrombi can travel to the lung and cause pulmonary embolism [13]. Clinically, the result of a vascular ultrasound can provide important information to physicians for determining the next step in patient management.

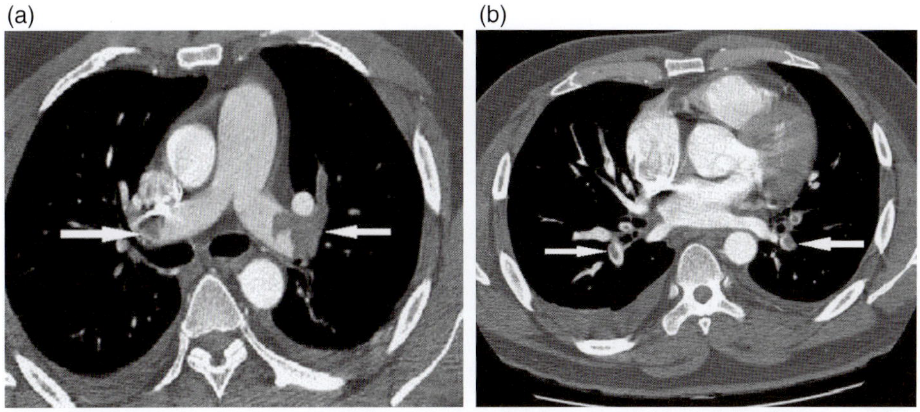

FIGURE 8.6 Images of contrast computed tomography show embolism (defect of contrast enhancement, white arrows) in the right and left main pulmonary arteries (a) and in small branches of the pulmonary artery (b).

Common Arterial Pathology of the Extremities

Peripheral Arterial Disease

The common cause of PAD is a result of fat, cholesterol, and other substances depositing on the arterial intima-media (atherosclerosis). PAD is a circulatory issue in which stenotic (narrowed) arteries reduce blood flow to the extremities distal to the stenosis. Patients present with intermittent pain in the extremities due to compromised flow and may be at risk for arterial occlusion. A common complaint of patients with PAD is leg pain when walking (claudication). An acute arterial embolism and occlusion may require emergency surgical intervention [12, 14].

The superficial femoral artery (SFA) is one of the most common vessels in the lower extremity to develop PAD [14]. It is reported that patients with atherosclerotic plaques in the SFA will likely be present with plaques in the coronary arteries and associate with a higher patient susceptibility to coronary death. The progress of atherosclerotic plaque formation in arteries of the lower extremities appears slower than that in the coronary system [12]. Therefore, ultrasound examination of the peripheral vasculature, most notably of the SFA, is important in designing a medical, surgical, or endovascular plan or to suggest further workup for suspected cardiovascular disease. Similar to the SFA, the popliteal artery is another common site for atherosclerosis and PAD, sharing the same indications for ultrasound examination, particularly if symptoms occur more distally in the feet [14]. Tests such as the ankle brachial index (ABI) are used to determine whether a patient with distal lower extremity symptoms needs further imaging assessment and are usually complementary to sonographic examination in determining the severity of PAD [15].

Doppler ultrasound is the definitive screening tool for arterial stenosis, with the use of peak systolic velocity (PSV) value and waveform morphology. When scanning regional arterial segments, deviation from triphasic, more pulsatile arterial morphology to a monophasic waveform is indicative of a proximal stenosis [11]. The area in question

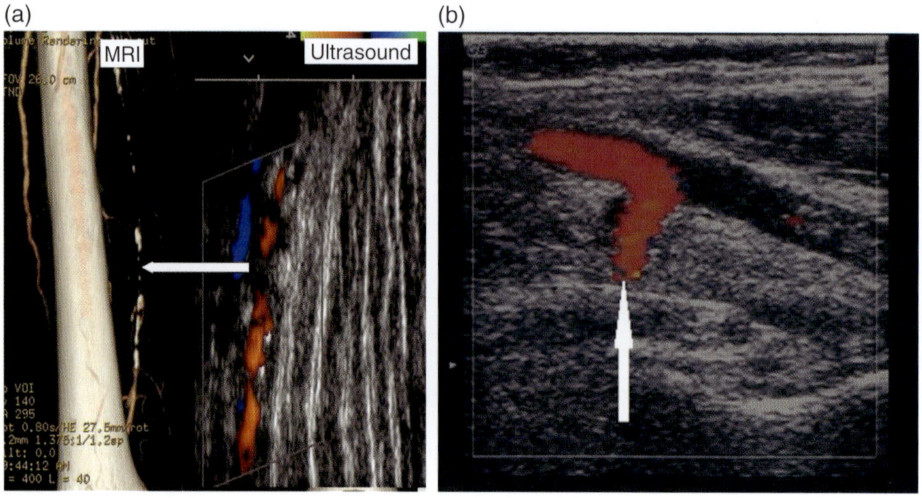

FIGURE 8.7 Color flow imaging and MRA demonstrate the occlusion of the superficial femoral artery (a, white arrow). Arterial occlusion with collateral vessel formation can be optimized using color flow imaging (b, white arrow).

on grayscale images should be evaluated further using color flow and spectral Doppler to identify any focal velocity elevation associated with visible arterial lumen reduction. An increase of PSV will occur at the site of hemodynamically significant stenosis (>70% lumen reduction), with lower flow proximal and distal to the stenosis. Waveforms are also useful in characterizing stenosis. An abnormal waveform, such as monophasic waveform (Fig. 8.5), is associated with flow in the artery distal to a hemodynamically significant stenosis or occlusion in addition to decrease in blood flow. Increases of PSV greater than 200 cm/sec and a PSV ratio (PSV at stenosis/PSV proximal to the stenosis) of 2:1 are associated with arterial lumen reduction of greater than 70% [16]. At the site of the occlusion, arterial lumen typically fills with medium-echogenicity thrombus in grayscale image and no flow on color flow imaging (Fig. 8.7).

Arteriovenous Fistula

Arteriovenous fistulas (AVFs) are acquired (post traumatic injuries, invasive procedures, or surgeries), congenital, or spontaneous, and are characterized by abnormal connections between arterial and venous circulations. Disruptions are present throughout all layers of the arterial and venous structures due to high pressures. Most small AVFs are asymptomatic and resolve spontaneously. However, symptomatic AVF that cannot spontaneously resolve requires interventions (surgery or embolization) [17].

AVFs can be identified through noninvasive color flow imaging. The presence of tissue vibration artifacts suggests AVF because of the blood flow turbulence and high-pressure within the artery and vein. Often, spectral Doppler waveforms may demonstrate arterialized waveforms and increased velocity in the venous side of the fistula and decreased arterial resistance on the arterial side of the fistula (Fig. 8.8). This is due to the fistulas bypassing the capillary bed and communication between the artery and vein [4, 11].

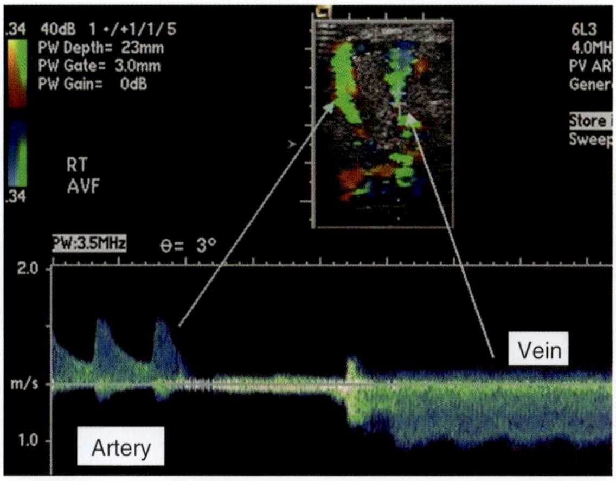

FIGURE 8.8 An AVF between the right common femoral artery (CFA) and common femoral vein developed after angiography of coronal artery via puncturing the right CFA. The resistance of CFA decreases, and flow velocity in CFV increases due to the communication between CFA and CFV. RT, right.

Aneurysm

An aneurysm is a result of a weakened arterial wall, leading to localized bulging or focal enlargement of 20% of the initial vessel diameter [18]. Aneurysms may occur unilaterally or bilaterally, commonly in the popliteal region. Risk factors for the development of a popliteal artery aneurysm include tobacco use, hypertension, clotting, embolism, ischemia, infarction, and abdominal aortic aneurysms [18].

Aneurysms can appear with a fusiform anechoic or hypoechoic mass along the course of an artery in a grayscale image. They can be saccular and develop at branching points of the arterial circulation. Calcification of the aneurysm walls may occur, which can inadvertently provide protection against ruptures [11]. Color flow imaging is effective to confirm blood flow in the aneurysm, differing from nonvascular fluid collection. If detected, spectral Doppler is used to differentiate between arterial and venous flows, as well as exclude superimposed AVF. Flow velocity in the aneurysm depends on the amount of thrombus, the size of the aneurysm, and the presence of wall calcification. Additionally, the use of pre- and post-operative ultrasound can improve the success of surgical intervention for popliteal artery aneurysms and monitor the patency of the arterial stent and graft if applicable [19].

Pseudoaneurysm

Approximately one-third of pseudoaneurysms require repair, making ultrasound evaluation a valuable tool in patient management [11]. A pseudoaneurysm, known as a false aneurysm, is caused by damage to the arterial wall by way of trauma or inflammatory erosion. At least one layer of the arterial wall is breached, differentiating this from a true aneurysm. The pseudoaneurysm sac is contained by outer arterial layers, perivascular tissue, clots, or reactive fibrosis [20]. Adjacent to the injured artery, a hematoma develops, and eventual lysis of the clot forms the pseudoaneurysm (Fig. 8.9).

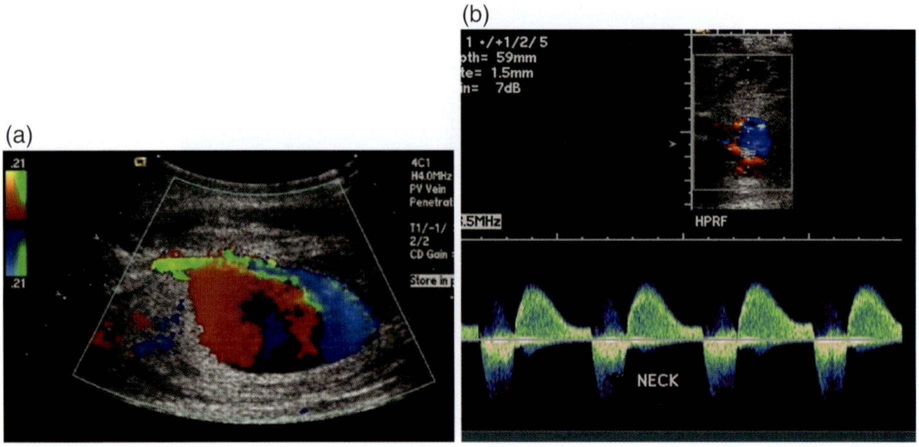

FIGURE 8.9 The sac (a) and the neck (b) of the pseudoaneurysm can be demonstrated in color flow imaging (a) and spectral Doppler (b). NECK, the neck is the connection between the wall of the injured artery and the sac of the pseudoaneurysm with a typical to-and-fro spectral Doppler pattern.

A pseudoaneurysm appears as a round or oval anechoic structure in grayscale ultrasound. A pseudoaneurysm sac less than 1.8 cm in diameter has a good prognosis with spontaneous closure [21]. The thrombus may or may not develop in the sac of the pseudoaneurysm. Thrombus may appear isoechoic or hypoechoic and can be located along the pseudoaneurysm lumen. In the patent area of a pseudoaneurysm, turbulent flow following a *Yin-Yang* pattern appears in color flow imaging (Fig. 8.9a). The pseudoaneurysm sac and its injured artery communicate through a neck, which is characterized as a "to-and-fro" biphasic flow pattern on spectral Doppler (Fig. 8.9b) [22].

Thoracic Outlet Syndrome

Another form of arterial stenosis caused by external pressure, elicited by specific positioning of the arm, is called thoracic outlet syndrome (TOS). Due to compression of the artery by adjacent musculature during movement of the arm, patients can experience pain anywhere in the upper extremity. If embolic events occur, these emboli can travel distally and cause pain in the hands and fingers. It is important to note that compression of upper extremity arteries can also be caused by bone or rib anomalies [23].

Ultrasound is useful in the evaluation of TOS by scanning patients in a neutral or adducted position and comparing the velocities in the artery to those when the arm is abducted [11]. Tests such as Adson's maneuver are used to test for TOS by way of inspiration, breath holding, neck extension, and turning the neck to the affected side. This maneuver can be used in combination with Doppler scanning to establish a baseline and observe for any abnormal or disrupted waveform morphology changes downstream of the upper extremity artery [24]. Furthermore, the artery can become injured over time, increasing the risk for occlusion or formation of emboli, adding to the importance of vascular ultrasound for timely evaluation and intervention [23, 24].

Common Venous Pathology of the Extremities

Acute Deep Vein Thrombosis

Acute DVT is the most common pathology of the subclavian vein and femoropopliteal vein [25]. An upper extremity DVT commonly develops in patients with a venous line, such as peripherally inserted central catheter (PICC) (Fig. 8.10a). Patients with DVT usually present with unilateral extremity pain, swelling, erythema, and/or warmth [26]. Ultrasound examination is the gold standard for diagnosing DVT, with compression ultrasound shown to have 95% of accuracy with 98% of specificity [27].

The main ultrasound finding in acute DVT is the presence of intraluminal thrombus (hypoechoic). A free tail floating proximally from the attachment site of

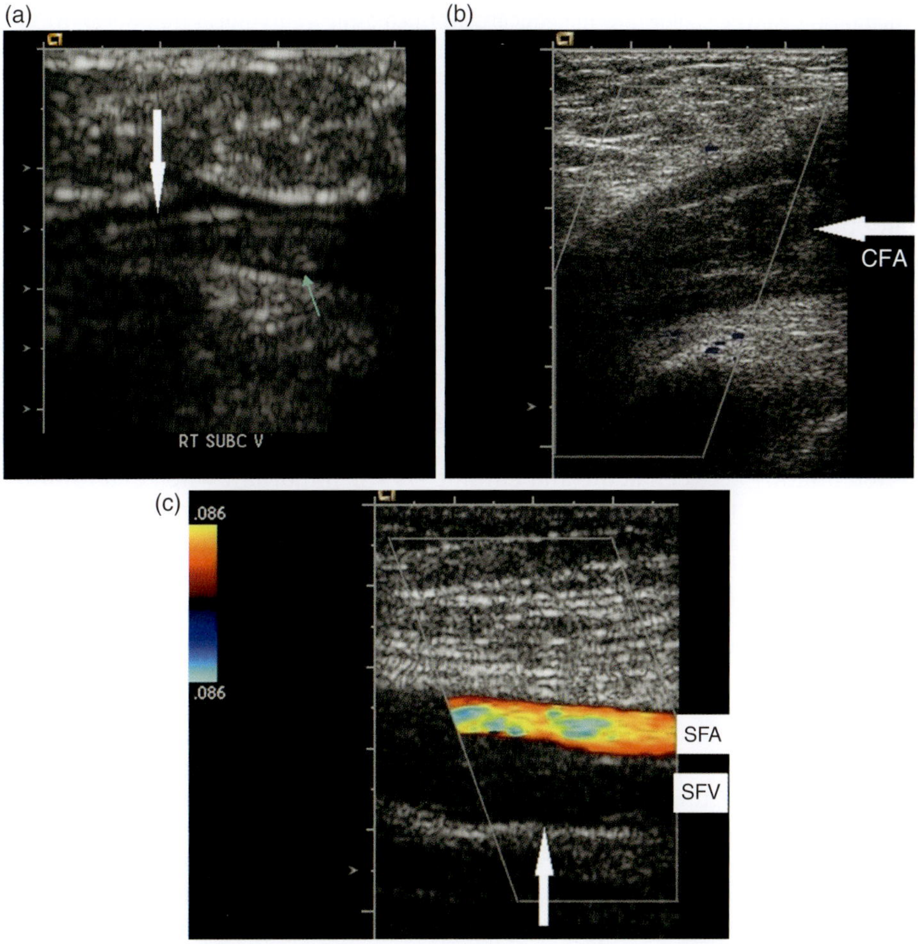

FIGURE 8.10 A thrombus (small green arrow) attaches to the catheter of venous line (white arrow) in the right subclavian vein (RT SUBC V) (a). The thrombus (white arrow) appears echogenic in subacute deep vein thrombosis in the common femoral vein in B-mode image (CFV, b). Color flow imaging (c) can demonstrate no color filling, indicating no venous flow when an occlusive DVT develops in the superficial femoral vein (SFV). SFA, superficial femoral artery.

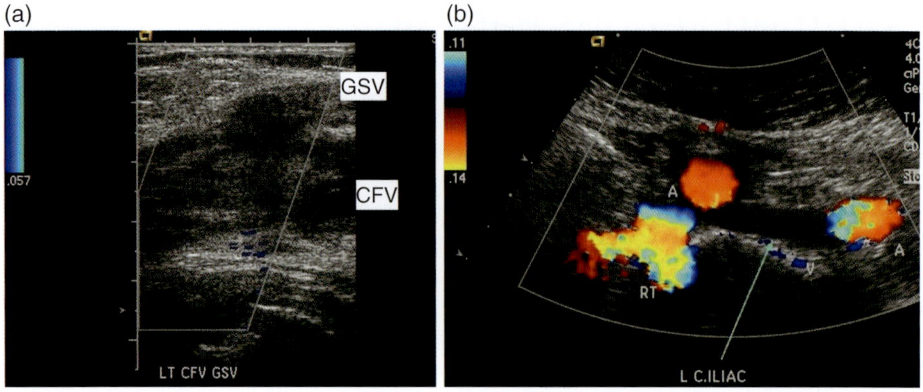

FIGURE 8.11 No venous flow (no color signals) in venous lumen is observed even when power Doppler setting is very sensitive (power Doppler scale 0.057). The thrombosis is located at the junction of the left common femoral vein (CFV) and great saphenous vein (GSV) (a). The extension of the thrombosis up to the left common iliac vein (green arrow) is demonstrated when color flow imaging is performed using a curvilinear transducer (b). The right common iliac vein (RT) and bilateral iliac arteries (A) are patent in this color flow imaging. A, artery; LT or L, left; C, common.

the clot on the vein may appear [28]. In grayscale image, the vein with direct visualization of the thrombus in the lumen will be incompressible (Fig. 8.10) [11]. Thrombi may or may not occlude the lumen. It is important to investigate the extension of the thrombus (Fig. 8.11) to determine medical management and if an inferior vena cava (IVC) filter is needed to prevent the development or recurrence of pulmonary embolism if the thrombus is visualized in the femoral veins [29].

Chronic Deep Vein Thrombosis

Differentiating between acute and chronic DVT is important when determining the appropriate therapeutic approach. With compression ultrasound, acute and chronic DVT may look the same, but there are some subtleties to help differentiate between the two. In chronic DVT's, the residual thrombus may become hyperechoic and decrease in size, while the vessel may appear normal (or smaller) in size [11]. This is thought to occur due to the fibrotic component of the residual thrombus and therefore adheres to the vein wall. Thickened venous walls may appear in grayscale images (Fig. 8.12). Additionally, there may be echogenic, web-like structures associated with chronic DVT seen within the vein or collateral vessels. Thrombus echogenicity is not a definitive method to differentiate between acute and chronic DVT; however, calcifications in the thrombus may be indicative of a chronic element [28].

Venous Insufficiency

Venous insufficiency affects the lower extremities and is caused by venous valvular damage, commonly due to damage after a DVT. Patients with venous insufficiency can have lower extremity swelling, induration, chronic skin changes, and venous

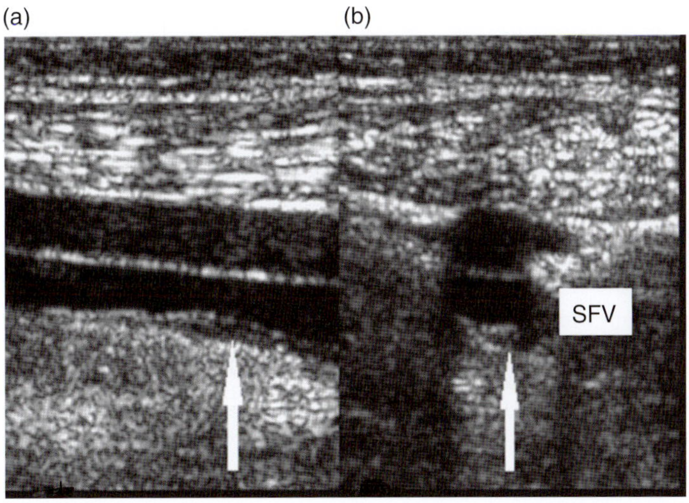

FIGURE 8.12 In longitudinal (a) and transverse (b) - B-mode images, venous wall thickening (white arrow) is noted in the vein with previous thrombosis. SFV, superficial femoral vein.

stasis ulcers. There can be superficial and deep venous insufficiency. Superficial insufficiency has a better prognosis, as deep venous insufficiency is associated with varicosities [30].

Ultrasound is useful in assessing a patient with venous insufficiency and is best observed with the patient in an upright position. The patient should support their body weight on the contralateral lower extremity in order to cause hydrostatic pressure significant enough to reproduce venous insufficiency. Provocative maneuvers, such as the Valsalva maneuver, are commonly used in conjunction with spectral analysis to scan at different levels of the venous system, including the common femoral vein, proximal great saphenous vein, popliteal vein, and saphenopopliteal junction. Venous insufficiency will show a greater degree of reversed flow for a longer duration compared to normal veins, which show antegrade flow for a very brief period [11, 13]. Distal augmentation of the extremity is performed by an examiner during spectral waveform examinations. A normal vein distally augmented will show antegrade flow with a short period of flow reversal, whereas insufficient veins will show increased and prolonged reversed flow [11].

Summary

Vascular ultrasound plays an important role in assessing arterial pathology and detecting DVT. Acute ischemic changes of the artery in the extremities may require urgent intervention, and the treatment for DVT is important in managing pulmonary embolism. The enhancement of knowledge in anatomy and ultrasound techniques, along with scan skill training, can provide patients with high quality of peripheral vascular ultrasound exams and accurate interpretations in clinical patient care.

Review Questions

1. When examining the superficial femoral artery, how should the patient be positioned?
   a. Sitting upright against the examination table with legs adducted
   b. Supine with hips externally rotated
   c. Supine with legs adducted
   d. Sitting upright against the examination table with one leg externally rotated
   e. Sitting upright with legs crossed
2. Which transducer is commonly used for lower extremity vascular ultrasound?
   a. Linear array
   b. Curvilinear
   c. Phased-array
   d. Convex
   e. Biplanar
3. If there is an obstruction to arterial blood flow in a low extremity and a patient is immobile, which examination would be preferred first?
   a. Sonohysterography
   b. Doppler ultrasound
   c. M-mode ultrasound
   d. Saline infusion sonography
   e. EMG
4. What is the main artery for supplying blood to the entire lower extremity?
   a. Anterior tibial artery
   b. Femoral artery
   c. Tibial artery
   d. Dorsalis pedis artery
   e. Popliteal vein
5. Which of the following will improve observing venous waveform variation?
   a. Valsalva maneuver
   b. Lay the patient supine
   c. Ask patient to hold their breath for 3–5 seconds
   d. Lay the patient on the ipsilateral lateral decubitus
   e. Using an ice bag
6. What is preferred as the first-line study when screening for extremity artery aneurysms?
   a. Color Doppler
   b. B-mode ultrasound
   c. MRI
   d. CT
   e. Digital subtractive angiography
7. How do you treat a small (diameter <2 cm) AV fistula?
   a. Spontaneously reduces itself and compression
   b. Surgical excision

c. Antibiotics
d. Radiographic ablation therapy
e. Heparin

8. Which spectral waveform in distal artery is most indicative of severe or occlusive arterial stenosis?
   a. Monophasic
   b. Biphasic
   c. Triphasic
   d. Multiphasic
   e. Variant
9. Subclavian steal syndrome "steals" blood from which artery?
   a. Subclavian artery
   b. Vertebral artery
   c. Radial artery
   d. Basilar artery
   e. Ulnar artery
10. Pulmonary embolism is a critical consequence of:
   a. Deep vein thrombosis
   b. AV fistula
   c. Arterial emboli
   d. Anastomosis stenosis
   e. Intima-media thickness

Correct answers: 1. b; 2. a; 3. b; 4. b; 5. a; 6. a; 7. a; 8. a; 9. d; 10. a.

References

1. Pellerito J, Taylor K. Peripheral arteries. *Clin Diagn Ultrasound* 1992; 27: 97–112.
2. Lee DK, Ahn KS, Kang CH, Cho SB. Ultrasonography of the lower extremity veins: anatomy and basic approach. *Ultrasonography* 2017; 36: 120–130.
3. Gerhard-Herman M, Gardin JM, Jaff M, et al. Guidelines for noninvasive vascular laboratory testing: a report from American society of echocardiography and the society of vascular medicine and biology. *J Am Soc Echocardiogr* 2006; 19: 955–972.
4. Mennitt K, Deol M, Gao J. Emergency color Doppler sonography of the extremity artery: a pictorial essay. *Clin Imaging* 2017; 42: 240–248.
5. Rafalidis V, Sidhu PS. Vascular ultrasound, the potential of integration of multiparametric ultrasound into routine clinical practice. *Ultrasound* 2018; 26: 136–144.
6. Hoskins PR, Kenwright DA. Recent development in vascular ultrasound technology. *Ultrasound* 2015; 23: 158–165.
7. Sibley RC, Teis SP, MacFarlane JJ, et al. Noninvasive physiologic vascular studies: a guide to diagnosing peripheral arterial disease. *Radiographics* 2017; 37: 346–357.
8. Netter FH. Atlas of human anatomy. 6th ed. Philadelphia, PA: Saunders/Elsevier, 2014.
9. Gilroy AM, MacPherson BR, Ross LM. Atlas of anatomy. 3rd ed. Stuttgart: Thieme, 2016.
10. Drake RL, Vogl A, Tibbits M, Richardson R. Gray's atlas of anatomy. 2nd ed. Philadelphia, PA: Churchill Livingstone, 2015.

11. Hwang JY. Doppler ultrasonography of the lower extremity arteries: anatomy and scanning guidelines. *Ultrasonography* 2017; 36: 111–119.
12. Dalager S, Falk E, Kristensen IB, et al. Plaque in superficial femoral arteries indicates generalized atherosclerosis and vulnerability to coronary death: an autopsy study. *J Vasc Surg* 2008; 47(2): 296–302.
13. Sadick M, Overhoff D, Baessler B, et al. Peripheral vascular anomalies - essentials in periinterventional imaging. *RöFo* 2020; 192: 150–162.
14. Kasapis C, Gurm HS. Current approach to the diagnosis and treatment of femoral-popliteal arterial disease: a systematic review. *Curr Cardiol Rev* 2009; 5: 296–311. https://doi.org/10.2174/157340309789317823.
15. American Institute of Ultrasound in Medicine. AIUM practice guideline for the performance of peripheral arterial ultrasound examinations using color and spectral Doppler imaging. *J Ultrasound Med* 2014; 33: 1111–1121.
16. Khan M, Panigrahi S. Frontmatter. In: Principles of engineering physics 1. Cambridge: Cambridge University Press, 2016; I–IV.
17. Kelm M, Perings SM, Jax T, et al. Incidence and clinical outcome of iatrogenic femoral arteriovenous fistulas: implications for risk stratification and treatment. *J Am Coll Cardiol* 2002; 40: 291–297. https://doi.org/10.1016/s0735-1097(02)01966-6.
18. Warren DJ, Craven I, Romanowski CA, Coley SC. Spontaneous closure of a type 2a dural arteriovenous fistula following late recanalization of the occluded sinus. *Interv Neuroradiol* 2010; 16: 282–285.
19. Wei YH, Xu JW, Shen HP, et al. Laparoscopic ligation of proximal splenic artery aneurysm with splenic function preservation. *World J Gastroenterol* 2014; 20: 4835–4838.
20. Schoen FJ. Blood vessels. In: Kumar V, Abbas AK, Fausto N (eds). Robbins and cotran pathologic basis of disease. 7th ed. Philadelphia, PA: Elsevier Saunders, 2005; 511–554.
21. La Perna L, Olin JW, Goines D, et al. Ultrasound-guided thrombin injection for the treatment of postcatheterization pseudoaneurysms. *Circulation* 2000; 102(19): 2391–2395.
22. Middleton WD, Dasyam A, Teefey SA. Diagnosis and treatment of iatrogenic femoral artery pseudoaneurysms. *Ultrasound Q* 2005; 21(1): 3–17.
23. Wadhwani R, Chaubal N, Sukthankar R, et al. Color Doppler and duplex sonography in 5 patients with thoracic outlet syndrome. *J Ultrasound Med* 2001; 20: 795–801.
24. Lee AD, Agarwal S, Sadhu D. Doppler Adson's test: predictor of outcome of surgery in non-specific thoracic outlet syndrome. *World J Surg* 2006; 30: 291–292.
25. Divittorio R, Bluth EI, Sullivan MA. Deep vein thrombosis: diagnosis of a common clinical problem. *Ochsner J* 2002. https://www.ncbi.nlm.nih.gov/pmc/articles/PMC3399231.
26. EBSCO Information Services. DynaMed [Internet]. Ipswich, MA: EBSCO Information Services, 1995. Record No. T920576, Evaluation of Deep Vein Thrombosis (DVT). https://www.dynamed.com/topics/dmp~AN~T920576.
27. Cronan JJ. Venous thromboembolic disease: the role of US. *Radiology* 1993; 186: 619–630.
28. Needleman L. Update on the lower extremity venous ultrasonography examination. *Radiol Clin North Am* 2014; 52: 1359–1374.
29. Kearon C, Ginsberg JS, Hirsh J. The role of venous ultrasonography in the diagnosis of deep vein thrombosis and pulmonary embolism. *Ann Intern Med* 1998; 129: 1044–1049.
30. Khilnani NM, Min RJ. Imaging of venous insufficiency. *Semin Intervent Radiol* 2005; 22(3): 178–184.

CHAPTER 9

Musculoskeletal Ultrasound

Kalvin Zee[1], Rebecca Lee[1], Lindsay Ellison[1], Jia-an Zhu[2], and Nena L. Mason[3]

[1] Rocky Vista University, College of Osteopathic Medicine, Ivins, Utah, USA

[2] Department of Ultrasound, Peking University People's Hospital, Beijing, China

[3] Geisel School of Medicine at Dartmouth, Hanover, New Hampshire, USA

Introduction

Ultrasound is a unique diagnostic tool with advantages of being affordable, portable, radiation-free, and low-cost. In practice, ultrasound offers dynamic imaging of normal anatomy and pathology of tendons, muscles, nerves, joints, and osseous structures [1, 2]. Because of these beneficial qualities, ultrasound is being used increasingly in the evaluation of musculoskeletal diseases [3–8]. Additionally, ultrasound can be used to guide tissue biopsy for the diagnosis of lesions and drainage of abscesses in the treatment of musculoskeletal pathologies. Ultrasound-guided procedures are introduced in Chapter 13 of this book.

General Indications for Musculoskeletal Ultrasound

Rheumatologists are increasingly using ultrasound to assess the extent of inflammation in joints [9, 10]. Depiction of the architecture of joints and related structures is particularly useful in sports medicine and rehabilitation [11–14]. In cases of trauma, point-of-care ultrasound (POCUS) is increasing diagnostic accuracy by providing real-time imaging of muscles and bones [12]. Ultrasound is also commonly used to distinguish solid structures from cystic (fluid-filled) ones due to its high imaging resolution and diagnostic accuracy [15].Ultrasound TechniquesUltrasound of the musculoskeletal system is best performed using a high frequency (10–14 MHz) linear array transducer. Generous portions of transducer gel, a solid gel standoff pad, or a water bath may be used to ensure that the target structure is approximately 2 cm from the surface of the transducer. This will help maximize image clarity and contrast based on the scanning frequency. Begin with a large depth of field, obtain the target image, and center it on the imaging screen. Decrease the depth of field as much as possible without losing image contrast, resolution, or excluding surrounding structures that are relevant to the target structure. When obtaining a target image with ultrasound, it is important to separate various probe maneuvers in order to obtain high-quality images quickly and accurately [16]. This is especially critical in musculoskeletal ultrasound due to the large variety of anatomical structures that will be encountered. While using a large depth of field, begin by sliding the probe across the patient until the largest target structures (bones or large muscle groups) are centered on the imaging screen. Next, if necessary, slowly rotate the probe to bring target structures into the desired orientation relative to one another. Finally, fan and/or rock the transducer to fine-tune the image. Optimize returning sound echoes by ensuring the angle of insonation is as close to 90° perpendicular to the target structure as possible to avoid anisotropy artifact [16].

Shoulder Joint

Indications The most common shoulder injury that is routinely evaluated clinically is rotator cuff tear, with the supraspinatus being the most commonly ruptured structure [17–20]. The anterior border of the supraspinatus provides the most support to the rotator cuff and, therefore, commonly receives the most damage in cases of shoulder injury [21–23]. Traditionally, magnetic resonance imaging (MRI) has been used to evaluate tears in the rotator cuff tendons. However, recent studies have provided evidence that ultrasound imaging can be equally accurate in the diagnosis of rotator cuff tears compared to MRI [24, 25].

Patient and Probe Position – Supraspinatus Tendon To acquire an image of the supraspinatus, the patient must first be seated with the hand of the affected shoulder positioned on their "back pocket." This gesture allows for simultaneous abduction, internal rotation, and extension of the shoulder joint (Fig. 9.1). Place the probe anteriorly and transversely over the anatomical neck of the humerus with the indicator oriented to the patient's right side (Fig. 9.1b).

Begin moving the transducer superiorly until three distinct structures (the supraspinatus tendon, the deltoid muscle, and the humeral head) are noted (Fig. 9.2). The supraspinatus tendon should appear dome-shaped, hyperechoic, and striated. The supraspinatus can be found superficial to the humeral head and deep to the deltoid. The deltoid will appear hypoechoic, with hyperechoic connective tissue in between the muscle fascicles. The thin hypoechoic bursa and surrounding peribursal fat should lie between the supraspinatus tendon and deltoid muscle. Fine-tune the image by slightly rotating the probe to ensure that the probe is positioned parallel to the length of the supraspinatus. Take care to maintain the direction of the sound beam at 90° to the tendon. This will help avoid the tendon appearing more hypoechoic than it really is due to anisotropy [1]. Ensure that there is abundant gel between the shoulder and the lateral end of the probe's footprint. One must take special care with patients who have more rounded shoulder joints, as the transducer's footprint will have a greater risk of losing contact with the skin [26]. A supraspinatus tear usually starts at the anterior supraspinatus, adjacent to the surface of the humeral head (Fig. 9.2), where it is the most vulnerable [23]. Both partial and full-thickness supraspinatus tears will appear hypoechoic to anechoic if fluid accumulation is present (Fig. 9.3). The size of the tear should be recorded.

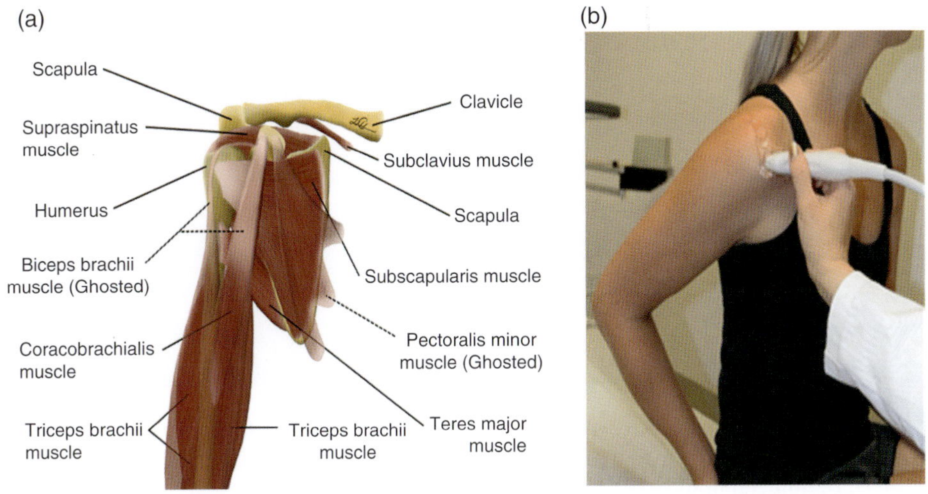

FIGURE 9.1 (a, b) Anatomy illustration of the shoulder (a) and how to perform an ultrasound scan of the supraspinatus (b).

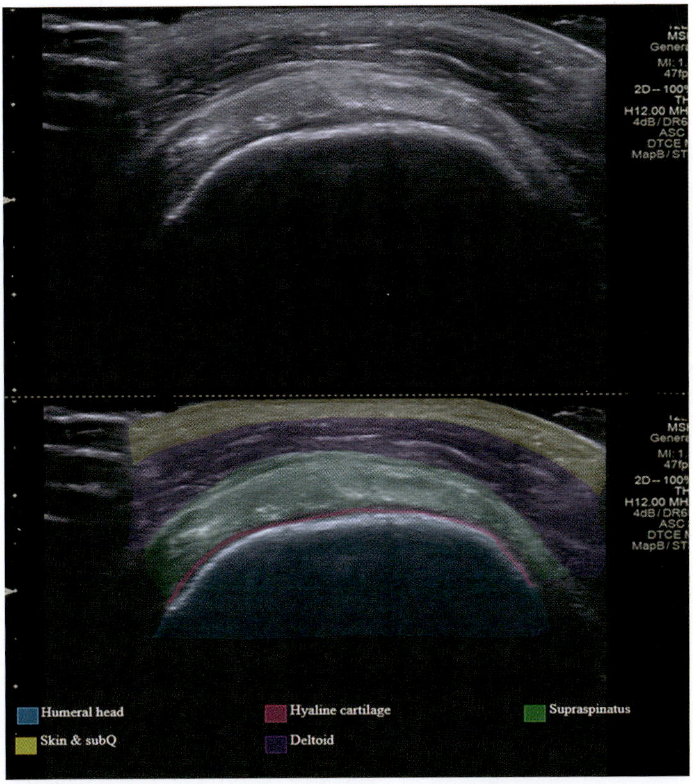

FIGURE 9.2 Labeled and unlabeled B-mode ultrasound images of the supraspinatus and surrounding structures.

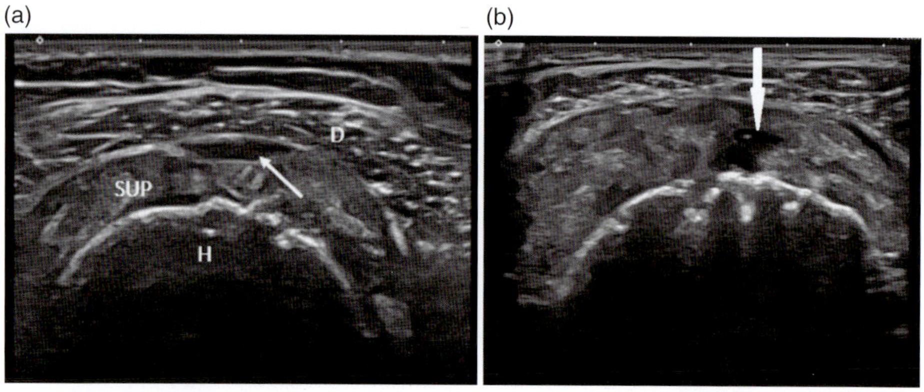

FIGURE 9.3 (a, b) Hypoechoic to anechoic fluid accumulation (white arrow) is present in partial (a) and full-thickness supraspinatus tears (b) in B-mode ultrasound images. D, deltoid muscle; H, humeral head; SUP, supraspinatus tendon.

Patient and Probe Position – Biceps Tendon To obtain a clear view of the tendon of the long head of the biceps, the patient must start in a seated position. The operator should then ask the patient to hold their upper arm to their side and bring their forearm parallel to their thigh, forming a right angle (Fig. 9.4a). The probe should be placed on the anterior surface of the humeral head with the indicator oriented toward the patient's right side. Slide the probe superiorly and inferiorly until a divot in the hyperechoic periosteal line is seen. This divot represents the intertubercular groove. Slight fanning may be necessary to note the anisotropy of the tendon of the long head of the biceps, which is an oval-shaped structure lying within the

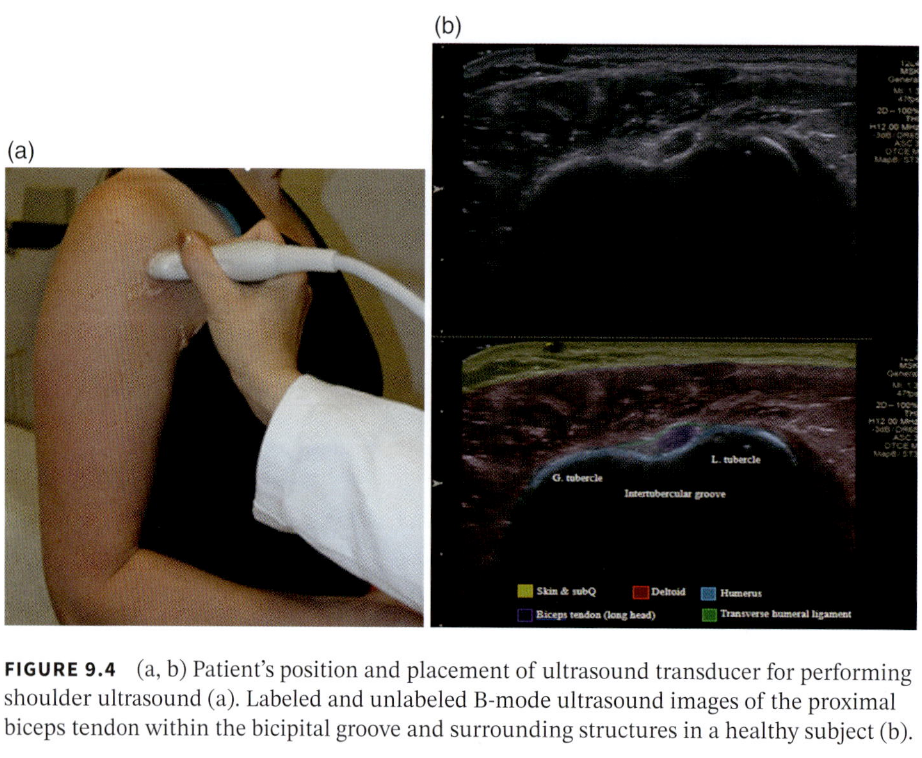

FIGURE 9.4 (a, b) Patient's position and placement of ultrasound transducer for performing shoulder ultrasound (a). Labeled and unlabeled B-mode ultrasound images of the proximal biceps tendon within the bicipital groove and surrounding structures in a healthy subject (b).

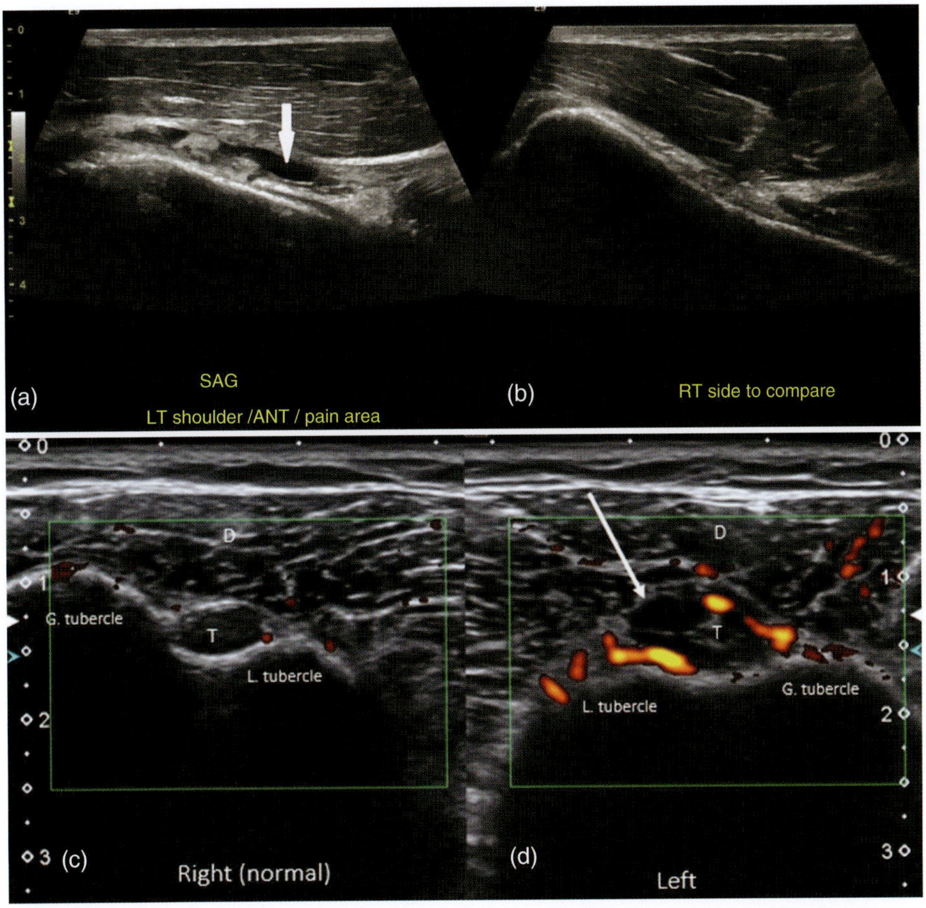

FIGURE 9.5 (a–d) Double image (side-by-side) is commonly used to detect pathology of biceps tendon by comparing the side with injury (a) and contralateral healthy side (b). In another case, a transverse plane image of the right biceps tendon appears normal (c). There is a small amount of fluid (d, white arrow) surrounding the proximal left biceps tendon, as well as a hypoechoic defect and hypervascularity in the tendon, suggesting a partial tear in the left proximal biceps tendon. D, deltoid; T, tendon.

intertubercular groove (Fig. 9.4b). Once the tendon is identified, slide the probe superiorly and inferiorly to examine the length of the tendon until it is no longer visible. A partially ruptured biceps tendon will appear as an oval, hyperechoic structure that is partially filled or surrounded by anechoic fluid. In contrast, a completely ruptured biceps tendon will retract from the intertubercular groove, presenting as an empty groove (Fig. 9.5).

Elbow Joint

Indications Patients with elbow injuries typically present with localized pain [27]. Tendon overuse syndromes and traumatic injuries are two of the most common causes of elbow pathologies [28]. Lateral epicondylitis is the most common cause of pain on the radial side of the elbow, as well as the most common tendon overuse syndrome [28, 29]. In fact, lateral epicondylitis affects 1–3% of the population in the age group of 40–60, often causing pain and difficulty performing daily activities among those affected [29]. Sonographic imaging of the origin of the common extensor tendon has been established as an accurate method to confirm lateral epicondylitis, rule out other lateral elbow injuries, and determine whether intervention is necessary [30, 31]. Traumatic injury can also affect the distal biceps tendon and typically presents as anterior elbow pain [27, 28]. Distal biceps tendon ruptures commonly occur among middle-aged men who weight train, particularly when a heavy load is placed on a flexed elbow [28, 32–34]. Ultrasound has been shown to be as accurate in the diagnosis of distal biceps tendon tears as MRI [32].

Patient and Probe Position – Common Extensor Tendon To view the common extensor tendon with ultrasound, the patient may place their palms together with their forearms resting on the table (Fig. 9.6). This "prayer position" allows for slight flexion and internal rotation of the patient's elbows. Palpate the patient's lateral epicondyle and follow the lateral humerus distally until a divot is felt. Place the probe parallel to the forearm on the previously found divot, at the radio-capitellar joint (Fig. 9.6). The transducer indicator should point toward the patient's shoulder. The common extensor tendon consists of the joined tendons of the extensor carpi radialis brevis, extensor carpi ulnaris, extensor digitorum, and extensor digiti minimi [26]. It should appear as a long, fibrillar, hyperechoic structure, with the radial collateral ligament located just deep to it. The radial and humeral heads should be found in the far-field of the image. The radial collateral ligament can be distinguished from the common extensor tendon by its bony attachment to the radial head. The deep surface of the radial collateral ligament also attaches to the flange of the elbow. The lateral flange is triangular in shape and sits between the radius and humerus (Fig. 9.6). Slight rotation of the probe clockwise or counterclockwise may maximize the echo signal and confirm that the probe is aligned with the common extensor tendon, instead of the deeper radial collateral ligament. In cases of lateral epicondylitis, the common extensor tendon will be damaged from a combination of myxoid and

(a) (b)

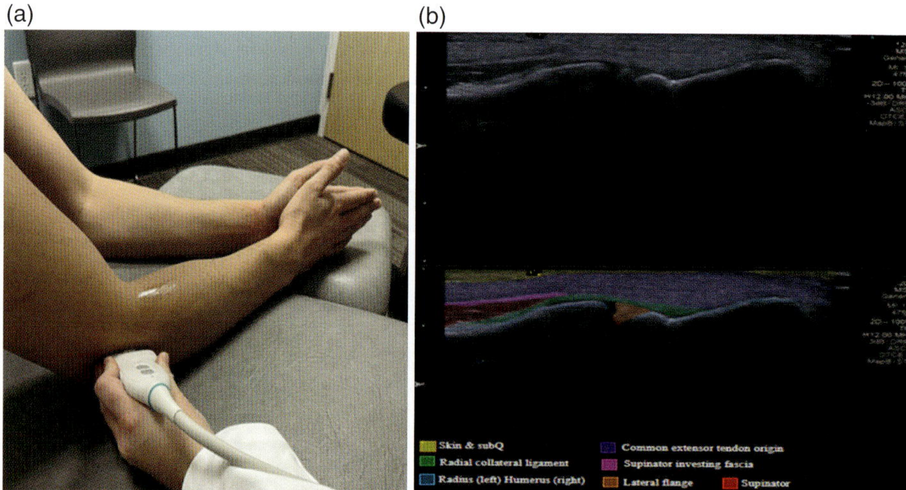

FIGURE 9.6 (a, b) How to perform an ultrasound scan of the common extensor tendon of the elbow joint (a). Labeled and unlabeled B-mode ultrasound images of the common extensor tendon of the elbow and surrounding structures (b).

hyaline degeneration, fibrosis, and calcification. Over time, as the elasticity in the common extensor tendon is lost, the risk of rupture increases [35]. A partial rupture of the common extensor tendon is most commonly seen in conjunction with lateral epicondylitis. In an acute injury, the partial rupture site will appear hypoechoic with a forming anechoic hematoma interlaced between the fibers. An acute, complete rupture will show a hematoma with an absent tendon, whereas a chronic rupture will show no hematoma [35].

Patient and Probe Position – Distal Biceps Tendon To view the distal biceps tendon with ultrasound, the patient's elbow must be supinated and flexed to approximately 25° (Fig. 9.7). Place the probe on the ulnar side of the forearm in the transverse plane, with the indicator oriented to the patient's right side. Rotate the probe clockwise so that it is at an angle of approximately 45° to the forearm, with the indicator pointing toward the lateral epicondyle. Locate the ulna, which will have a hyperechoic border and be slightly pointed. Sweep the probe anterolaterally until the radius is located and centered on the image. The radius should appear more rounded than the ulna. While maintaining visual on the radius, slowly slide the probe proximally until an echogenic, fibrillar structure that attaches to the radius is found. This is the distal biceps tendon. The transducer should be positioned parallel to the distal biceps tendon in order to visualize its long axis, which will appear as a series of straight, fibrillary, echogenic lines (Fig. 9.7). Superficial to the tendon is the pronator teres, which is a hypoechoic structure with echogenic connective tissue separating each muscle fascicle. Rotation of the probe slightly counterclockwise or clockwise may be performed until the tendon achieves maximal length. Confirm the tendon is

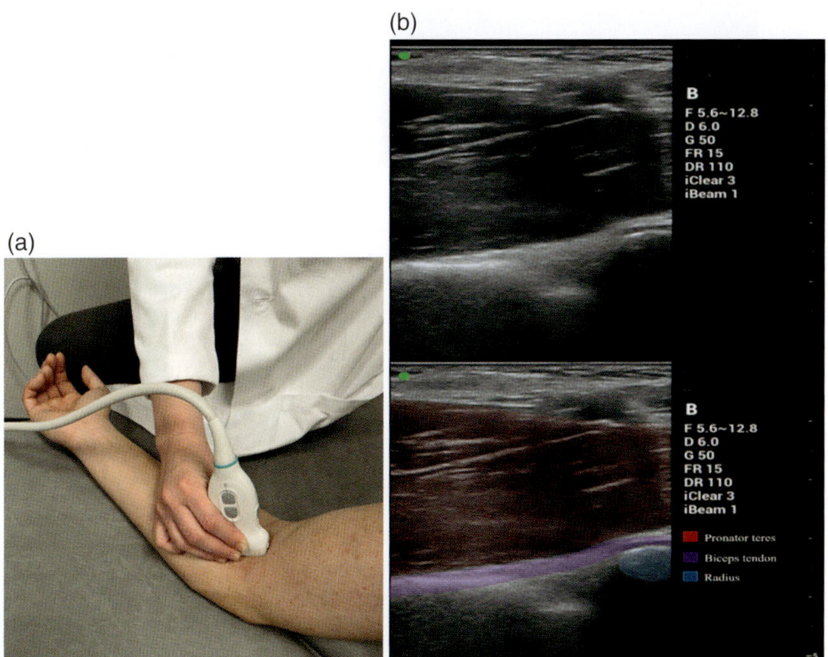

FIGURE 9.7 (a, b) How to perform an ultrasound scan of the distal biceps tendon (a); B-mode ultrasound of distal biceps tendon and surrounding structures (b).

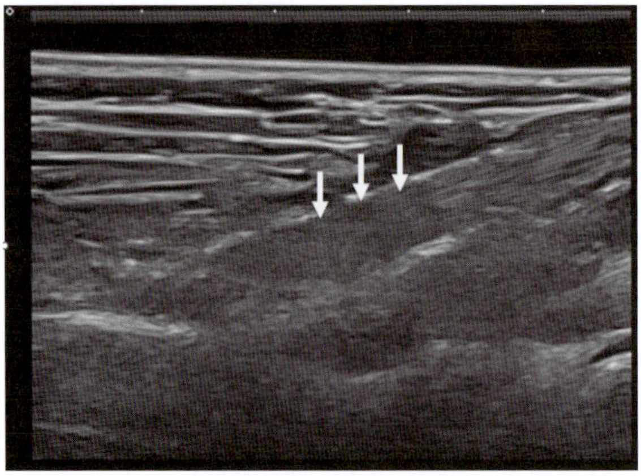

FIGURE 9.8 B-mode ultrasound image of longitudinal distal biceps tendon (white arrows) appears thickened, hypoechoic, and loss of parallel echogenic lines.

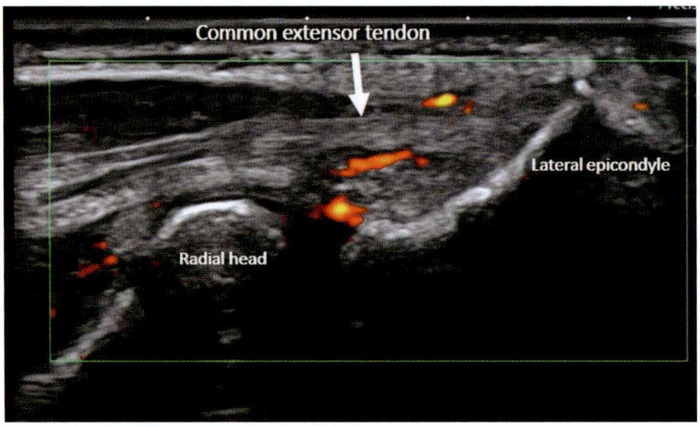

FIGURE 9.9 Hypervascularity in the longitudinal common extensor tendon on power Doppler image may indicate tendinosis.

the distal biceps tendon by directing the patient to supinate and pronate their wrist, which should cause the tendon to move at the radial head attachment site. A partially ruptured distal biceps tendon will appear hypoechoic against the hyperechoic tendon. A completely ruptured distal biceps tendon may appear hypoechoic, thickened, and lose parallel echogenic lines (Fig. 9.8). Hypervascularity in the common extensor tendon may indicate tendinosis (Fig. 9.9).

Wrist Joint

Indications Carpal tunnel syndrome is the most common peripheral nerve entrapment syndrome. Most cases of carpal tunnel syndrome are idiopathic [36, 37]. Patients with this disorder typically present with pain, numbness, and paresthesias in the hand, thumb, index, middle, and fourth fingers, due to compression of the median nerve in the carpal tunnel [38]. These symptoms are typically most severe at night and when gripping objects for extended periods [39]. Measuring the cross-sectional area of the median nerve can aid in assessing the severity of carpal tunnel syndrome [40]. Sonography can be used to measure the cross-sectional area of the median nerve as it travels through the carpal tunnel [41, 42].

Patient and Probe Position – Median Nerve Optimizing a nerve requires high-resolution ultrasound imaging. In order to image the ventral wrist and median nerve within the carpal tunnel, the patient rests their arm with their palm facing upward (Fig. 9.10). Place the probe transversely across the distal wrist crease. The indicator should be oriented toward the patient's right side. At this location, the median nerve will lie superficially in the carpal tunnel, just deep to the flexor retinaculum and superficial to the index finger portion of the flexor digitorum profundus (Fig. 9.10). The nerve itself will be oblong in shape with a hyperechoic exterior border. The interior of the nerve will consist of a mixture of hyperechoic and hypoechoic portions, giving it a "strawberry" like appearance. The pisiform can be found at the medial aspect of the carpal tunnel, while the trapezium will be located at the lateral-most aspect of the carpal tunnel. Once identified, the nerve can be traced along its length by moving the probe distally and proximally. If there is compression of the median nerve within the carpal tunnel, the nerve will appear abnormally flattened against the flexor retinaculum. The degree of nerve impingement can be quantified using sonographic measurements (Fig. 9.11) [41, 42].

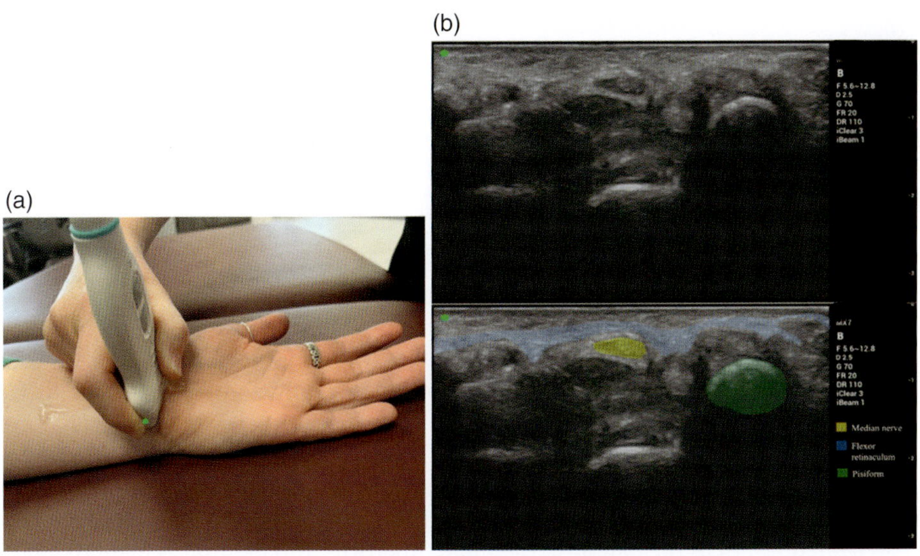

FIGURE 9.10 (a, b) How to perform an ultrasound scan of the median nerve within the carpal tunnel (a) and labeled and unlabeled B-mode ultrasound images of the median nerve within the carpal tunnel and surrounding structures (b).

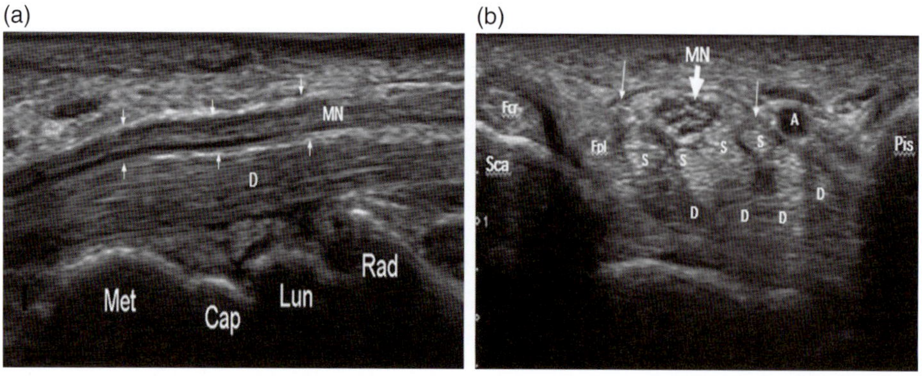

FIGURE 9.11 Normal medial nerve (MN) on longitudinal (a) and transverse (b) planes and median nerve in carpal tunnel syndrome. A, artery; D, flexor digitorum profundus tendon; Fcr, flexor carpi radialis; Fpl, flexor pollicis longus; Sca, scaphoid; Pis, pisiform; Cap, capitate; Met, metacarpal bone; Lun, lunate; Rad, radius. S, flexor digitorum superficialis tendon.

Knee Joint

Indications One of the most common knee injuries involves damage to both the medial collateral ligament (MCL) and the medial meniscus, resulting from a valgus force [43]. The incidence of such injuries is increased in patients who participate in sports or occupations that require squatting and kneeling [44]. Another common knee-related complaint is anterior knee pain due to patellar tendinosis, which is caused by overuse of the knee through movements like running and jumping [45, 46]. Both of these soft tissue and knee pathologies can be visualized with ultrasound. MCL and medial meniscus pathologies can be visualized by first sliding the transducer over the MCL to identify any changes in echogenicity, then placing the transducer along the medial joint line to view any changes to the medial meniscus [47]. Additionally, the operator can isolate the patellar tendon by sliding the probe superiorly and inferiorly, while monitoring for changes in echogenicity that may indicate tendon tear or tendinosis [48].

Patient and Probe Position – Patellar Tendon To image the patellar tendon with ultrasound, the patient is placed in a supine position with their hip extended and knee flexed to 30°. The transducer should be placed in the sagittal plane, just inferior to the apex of the patella, with the indicator pointing toward the patient's head (Fig. 9.12). Fanning the probe medially and laterally will allow the operator to visualize the entire structure. Alternatively, the transducer may be placed in the transverse plane with the indicator pointing to the patient's right side. From this position, the operator fans the transducer in a superior-to-inferior fashion in order to visualize the entire patellar tendon. The patellar tendon should span from the apex of the patella to the tibial tuberosity, broadening as it approaches these bony attachments (Fig. 9.12). While scanning the longitudinal plane of the patellar tendon, the operator should observe any abnormal changes in echogenicity and vascularity of the tendon (Fig. 9.13).

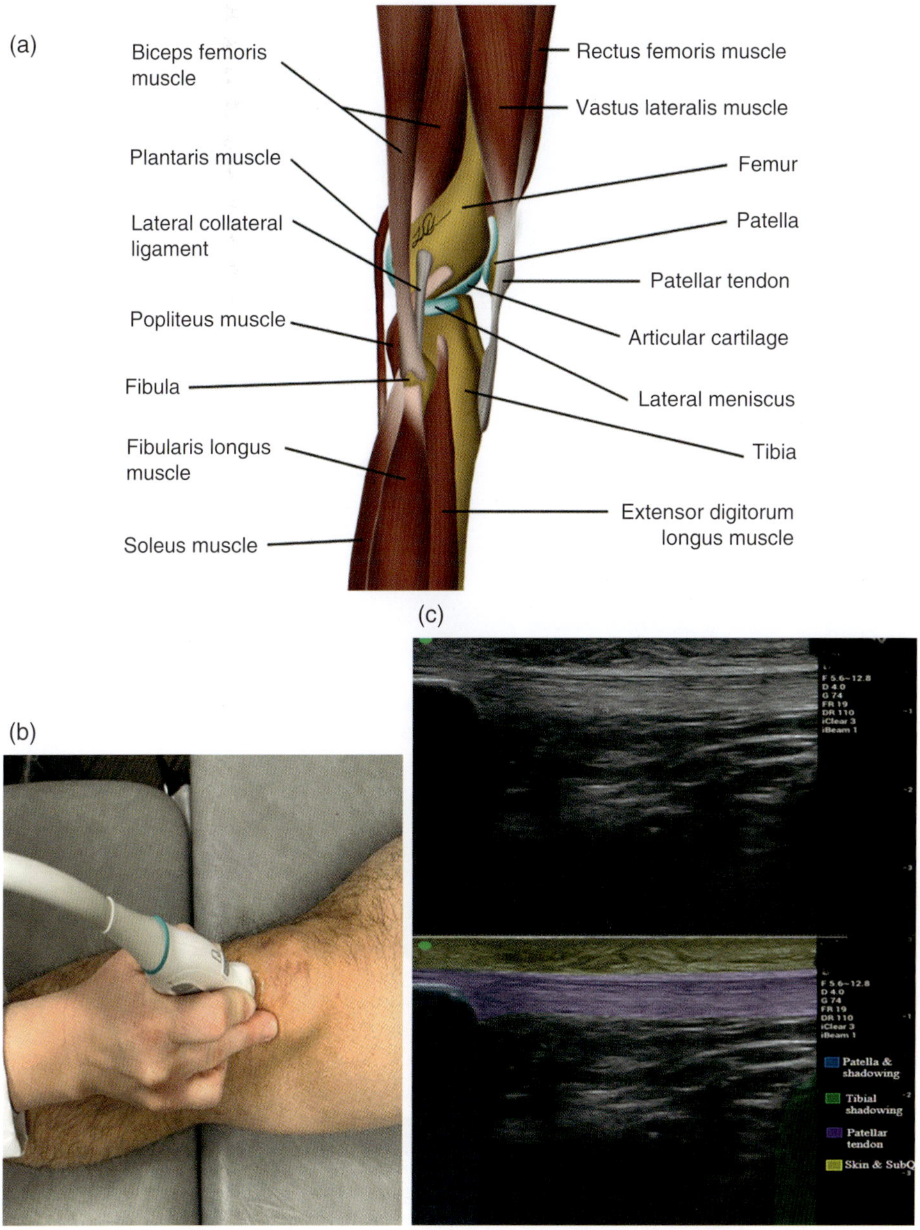

FIGURE 9.12 (a–c) Anatomy illustration of the knee (a); How to perform an ultrasound scan of the patellar tendon (b); unlabeled and labeled B-mode ultrasound images of the patellar tendon and surrounding structures in longitudinal plane (c).

Patient and Probe Position – MCL and Medial Meniscus To view the MCL using ultrasound, the patient is placed in a supine position with 10–15° of knee flexion and slight external rotation of the leg. The transducer is then placed on the medial aspect of the knee between the joint space of the femoral and tibial condyles with the indicator pointing superiorly (Fig. 9.14). The MCL should appear as a dense bundle of long, hyperechoic collagen fibers extending from the medial

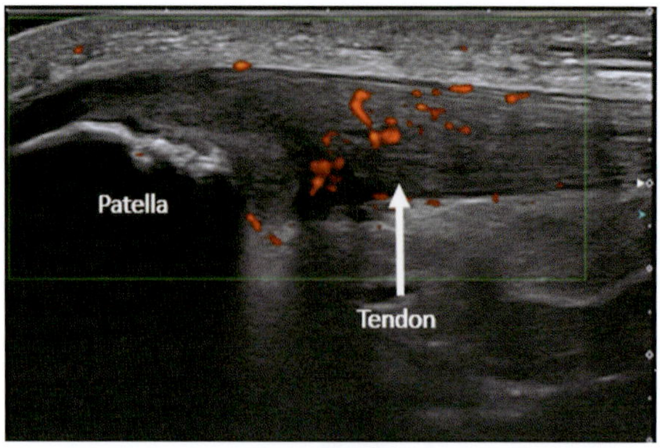

FIGURE 9.13 Patella tendon (white arrow) appearing thickened and hypervascular suggests tendinitis.

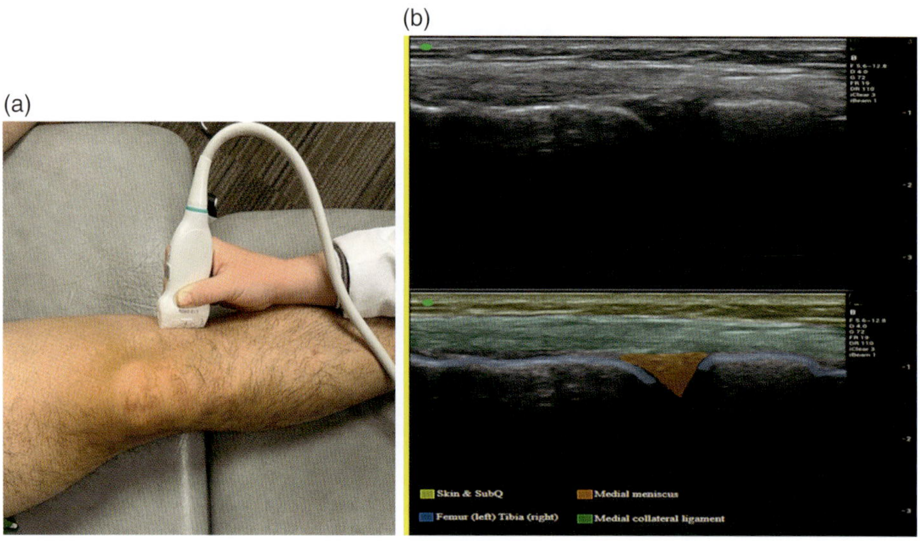

FIGURE 9.14 (a, b) How to perform an ultrasound scan of the MCL and medial meniscus (a); Labeled and unlabeled B-mode ultrasound images of the MCL, medial meniscus, and surrounding structures (b).

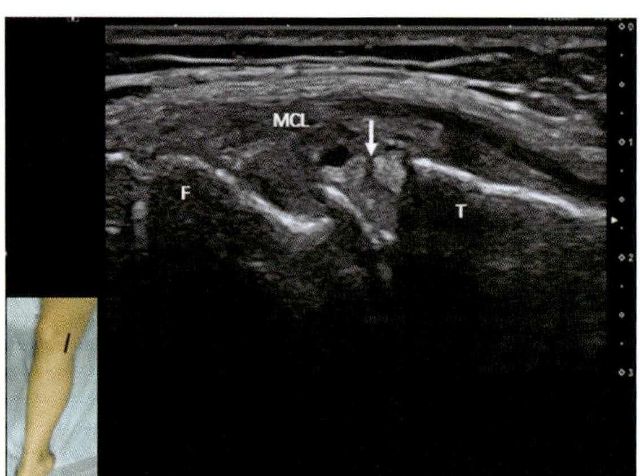

FIGURE 9.15 Transverse plane ultrasound image shows swelling of the medial meniscus (arrow) and medial collateral ligament (MCL). F, fibula; T, tibia.

femoral condyle to the proximal tibia (Fig. 9.14). To view the medial meniscus, slowly sweep the probe in an anterior to posterior fashion. The medial meniscus should appear as a small, triangular-shaped piece of echogenic tissue, located just lateral to the articular surface of the femur and tibia and pointing toward the joint space (Fig. 9.14). The "base" of the medial meniscus triangle will bulge outwards when the knee joint is fully extended and shift deeper into the joint space as the knee joint flexes. The meniscus will not bulge outwards, however, if there is a meniscal tear. Moreover, hypoechoic fluid will collect between the medial meniscus and MCL, implying a lack of attachment between the two structures (Fig. 9.15). Unfortunately, only the external portion of the meniscus may be visualized with ultrasound, as the internal portion will be obscured by the knee joint.

Summary

As demonstrated in this chapter, POCUS can be a highly valuable tool in the assessment of a wide variety of musculoskeletal diseases, including soft tissue, tendon, and ligamentous pathologies. Sonographic imaging was also highlighted for its efficacy in diagnosing overuse disorders and nerve entrapment syndromes, such as lateral epicondylitis and carpal tunnel syndrome, respectively. Lastly, this chapter detailed how damage to structures of the knee joint can be easily visualized with sonography, including the patellar tendon, medial meniscus, and MCL. While there is great utility in sonography, it should be noted that MRI and/or X-ray may be required after ultrasound examination for confirmation and further evaluation in some patients with acute and chronic MSK conditions.

Review Questions

1. Which transducer would be the most appropriate when performing an ultrasound of the musculoskeletal system?
   - **a.** 14 MHz, curved array
   - **b.** 12 MHz, curved array
   - **c.** 12 MHz, linear array
   - **d.** 8 MHz, linear array
   - **e.** 5 MHz, linear array
2. In order to achieve the highest quality image possible, the angle of insonation should be at an approximate _____ angle to the tendons and muscles.
   - **a.** 45°
   - **b.** 90°
   - **c.** 120°
   - **d.** 150°
   - **e.** 180°
3. In the carpal tunnel, the median nerve lies _______ to the flexor retinaculum and ________ to the flexor digitorum profundus.
   - **a.** Superficial, deep
   - **b.** Medial, lateral
   - **c.** Deep, medially
   - **d.** Deep, superficial
   - **e.** Lateral, superficial

4. Which of the following most accurately describes the appearance of nerves on ultrasound?
   a. A hyperechoic exterior and an interior that has hypoechoic and hyperechoic patches
   b. Anechoic throughout the structure
   c. Hyperechoic throughout the structure
   d. A hypoechoic exterior and an interior that has hypoechoic and hyperechoic patches
   e. Nerves cannot be visualized with ultrasound
5. Where are you most likely to find a tear in the rotator cuff?
   a. Posterior supraspinatus tendon, mid-substance tear
   b. Anterior supraspinatus tendon, adjacent to the greater tuberosity of the humerus
   c. Infraspinatus
   d. Subscapularis
   e. There is no pattern
6. How do you avoid hypoechogenicity of a tendon due to anisotropy?
   a. Remove the probe completely and add more gel
   b. Apply more pressure directly to the probe
   c. Rotate the probe in a counterclockwise or clockwise fashion
   d. Fan the probe back and forth in the short axis
   e. Use a phased array probe instead of a linear probe
7. A 38 year/old male presents with anterior elbow pain after his first CrossFit competition. What diagnosis do you suspect, and what view of ultrasound could you obtain to confirm?
   a. Lateral epicondylitis; long-axis view of the common extensor tendon with a lateral approach
   b. Radial nerve injury; short-axis view at the radial neck to examine the radial nerve
   c. Medial epicondylitis; short-axis view of the common flexor tendon with a medial approach
   d. Radial head fracture; short-axis view of the radial head with a lateral approach
   e. Distal biceps tendon rupture; a long-axis view of the distal biceps tendon with a medial approach
8. In lateral epicondylitis, also known as "tennis elbow," a rupture of the common extensor tendon is often seen due to structural damage from continuous stress. On B-mode imaging, why does there appear to be an anechoic chamber among the hypoechoic rupture site?
   a. The friction caused air trapping resulting in the anechoic chamber
   b. The anechoic chamber represents shadowing
   c. The anechoic chamber represents a hematoma from an acute injury
   d. The anechoic chamber is due to anisotropy
   e. The anechoic chamber represents a hematoma from a chronic injury
9. A 48-year-old female presents with knee pain. On exam, the patient exhibits reproducible anterior knee pain with jumping. What would be the most accurate description of ultrasound imaging?
   a. Hyperechoic structure spanning the patella to the tibial tuberosity
   b. Outward bulge of a structure upon knee extension
   c. It is unable to be visualized on ultrasound
   d. Anechoic material around the patellar tendon
   e. Hypoechoic exterior and an interior with hypoechoic and hyperechoic patches

10. What is a common injury sustained after a valgus force to the knee?

a. ACL tear

b. MCL + medial meniscus tear

c. Lateral meniscus tear

d. Patellar tendon rupture

e. Hamstring tear

Correct answers: 1, c; 2. b; 3. d; 4. a; 5. b; 6. d; 7. e; 8. c; 9. d; 10. b.

References

1. Lento PH, Primack S. Advances and utility of diagnostic ultrasound in musculoskeletal medicine. *Curr Rev Musculoskelet Med* 2008; 1: 24–31.
2. Hashefi M. Ultrasound in the diagnosis of noninflammatory musculoskeletal conditions. *Semin Ultrasound CT MRI* 2011; 32: 74–90.
3. Patil P, Dasgupta B. Role of diagnostic ultrasound in the assessment of musculoskeletal diseases. *Ther Adv Musculoskelet Dis* 2012; 4: 341–355.
4. Gupta Y, Rastogi R, Pratap V, et al. Role of high resolution ultrasonography (HRUS) in musculoskeletal diseases with its clinico-radiological correlation. *IJMRP* 2017. https://doi.org/10.21276/ijmrp.2017.3.3.067.
5. Bierig SM, Jones A. Accuracy and cost comparison of ultrasound versus alternative imaging modalities, including CT, MR, PET, and angiography. *JDMS* 2009; 25: 138–144.
6. Roll SC, Asai C, Tsai J. Clinical utilization of musculoskeletal sonography involving non-physician rehabilitation providers: a scoping review. *Eur J Phys Rehabil Med* 2016; 52: 253–262.
7. Özçakar L, Tok F, De Muynck M, Vanderstraeten G. Musculoskeletal ultrasonography in physical and rehabilitation medicine. *J Rehabil Med* 2012; 44: 310–318.
8. Ziegler DW. Orthopedic perspectives of musculoskeletal ultrasound. *Phys Med Rehabil Clin N Am* 2010; 21: 631–644.
9. Grassi W, Salaffi F, Filippucci E. Ultrasound in rheumatology. *Best Pract Res Clin Rheumatol* 2005; 19: 467–485.
10. Backhaus M, Burmester G, Gerber T, et al. Guidelines for musculoskeletal ultrasound in rheumatology. *Ann Rheum Dis* 2001; 60: 641–649.
11. Faltus J, Boggess B, Bruzga R. The use of diagnostic musculoskeletal ultrasound to document soft tissue treatment mobilization of a quadriceps femoris muscle tear: a case report. *Int J Sports Phys Ther* 2012; 7: 342–349.
12. Finnoff JT. The evolution of diagnostic and interventional ultrasound in sports medicine. *PM&R* 2016; 8: S133–S138.
13. Nwawka OK. Update in musculoskeletal ultrasound research. *Sports Health* 2016; 8: 429–437.
14. Perrier P, Leyral J, Thabouillot O, et al. Usefulness of point-of-care ultrasound in military medical emergencies performed by young military medicine residents. *BMJ Mil Health* 2019. https://doi.org/10.1136/jramc-2018-001132.
15. Tarrazo JS, Morales JC, Pujol JS, et al. Usefulness and reliability of point of care ultrasound in family medicine: focused ultrasound in neck and emergency. *Aten Primaria* 2019; 51: 367–379.
16. Bahner DP, Blickendorf JM, Bockbrader M, et al. Language of transducer manipulation: codifying terms for effective teaching. *J Ultrasound Med* 2016; 35: 183–188.

17. Kang Y, Lee JW, Ahn JM, et al. Instability of the long head of the biceps tendon in patients with rotator cuff tear: evaluation on magnetic resonance arthrography of the shoulder with arthroscopic correlation. *Skeletal Radiol* 2017; 46: 1335–1342.
18. Redondo-Alonso L, Chamorro-Moriana G, Jiménez-Rejano JJ, et al. Relationship between chronic pathologies of the supraspinatus tendon and the long head of the biceps tendon: systematic review. *BMC Musculoskelet Disord* 2014; 15: 377. https://doi.org/10.1186/1471-2474-15-377.
19. Vestermark GL, Van Doren BA, Connor PM, et al. The prevalence of rotator cuff pathology in the setting of acute proximal biceps tendon rupture. *J Shoulder Elb Surg* 2018; 27: 1258–1262.
20. Murthi AM, Vosburgh CL, Neviaser TJ. The incidence of pathologic changes of the long head of the biceps tendon. *J Shoulder Elb Surg* 2000; 9: 382–385.
21. Cudlip AC, Dickerson CR. Regional activation of anterior and posterior supraspinatus differs by plane of elevation, hand load and elevation angle. *J Electromyogr Kinesiol* 2018; 43: 14–20.
22. Rousseau T, Roussignol X, Bertiaux S, et al. Arthroscopic repair of large and massive rotator cuff tears using the side-to-side suture technique. Mid-term clinical and anatomic evaluation. *Orthop Traumatol Surg Res* 2012; 98: S1–S8.
23. Miller RM, Fujimaki Y, Araki D, et al. Strain distribution due to propagation of tears in the anterior supraspinatus tendon. *J Orthop Res* 2014; 32: 1283–1289.
24. de Jesus JO, Parker L, Frangos AJ, Nazarian LN. Accuracy of MRI, MR arthrography, and ultrasound in the diagnosis of rotator cuff tears: a meta-analysis. *AJR* 2009; 192: 1701–1707.
25. Gilat R, Atoun E, Cohen O, et al. Recurrent rotator cuff tear: is ultrasound imaging reliable? *J Shoulder Elb Surg* 2018; 27: 1263–1267.
26. Beggs I. *Musculoskeletal ultrasound*. Lippincott Williams & Wilkins, 2013.
27. Copas D, Talbot JC. Clinical assessment of the elbow. *Orthop Trauma* 2016; 30: 291–300.
28. Draghi F, Danesino G, De Gautard R, Bianchi S. Ultrasound of the elbow: examination techniques and US appearance of the normal and pathologic joint. *J Ultrasound* 2007; 10: 76–84.
29. Amroodi MN, Mahmuudi A, Salariyeh M, Amiri A. Surgical treatment of tennis elbow; minimal incision technique. *Arch Bone Jt Surg* 2016; 4: 366–370.
30. Connell D, Burke F, Coombes P, et al. Sonographic examination of lateral epicondylitis. *AJR* 2001; 176: 777–782.
31. Levin D, Nazarian LN, Miller TT, et al. Lateral epicondylitis of the elbow: US findings. *Radiology* 2005; 237: 230–234.
32. de la Fuente J, Blasi M, Martínez S, et al. Ultrasound classification of traumatic distal biceps brachii tendon injuries. *Skeletal Radiol* 2018; 47: 519–532.
33. Lacheta L, Siebenlist S. Anatomy, biomechanics, and pathology of the distal biceps tendon. *Operative Techniques in Sports Medicine* 2018; 26: 110–113.
34. Virk MS, DiVenere J, Mazzocca AD. Distal biceps tendon injuries: treatment of partial and complete tears. *Oper Tech Sports Med* 2014; 22: 156–163.
35. Kachrimanis G, Papadopoulou O. Acute partial rupture of the common extensor tendon. *J Ultrasound* 2010; 13: 74–75.
36. Padua L, Coraci D, Erra C, et al. Carpal tunnel syndrome: clinical features, diagnosis, and management. *Lancet Neurol* 2016; 15: 1273–1284.
37. Lewallen L, Rizzo M. Unusual causes of carpal tunnel syndrome. In: Duncan SFM, Kakinoki R (eds). *Carpal tunnel syndrome and related median neuropathies*. Springer, 2017; 97–108.
38. Wipperman J, Goerl K. Carpal tunnel syndrome: diagnosis and management. *Am Fam Physician* 2016; 94: 993–999.
39. Schick CW, Kaplan FTD. Differential diagnosis of carpal tunnel syndrome. In: Duncan SFM, Kakinoki R (eds). *Carpal tunnel syndrome and related median neuropathies*. Springer, 2017; 39–49.

40. Klauser AS, Ellah MMA, Halpern EJ, et al. Sonographic cross-sectional area measurement in carpal tunnel syndrome patients: can delta and ratio calculations predict severity compared to nerve conduction studies? *Eur Radiol* 2015; 25: 2419–2427.
41. Azami A, Maleki N, Anari H, et al. The diagnostic value of ultrasound compared with nerve conduction velocity in carpal tunnel syndrome. *Int J Reum Dis* 2014; 17: 612–620.
42. Nakamichi KI, Tachibana S. Ultrasonographic measurement of median nerve cross-sectional area in idiopathic carpal tunnel syndrome: diagnostic accuracy. *Muscle Nerve* 2002; 26: 798–803. https://doi.org/10.1002/mus.10276.
43. Phisitkul P, James SL, Wolf BR, Amendola A. MCL injuries of the knee: current concepts review. *Iowa Orthop J* 2006; 26: 77–90.
44. Raj MA, Bubnis MA. Knee meniscal tears. In: *StatPearls [Internet]*. StatPearls Publishing, 2019.
45. Wilson JJ, Best TM. Common overuse tendon problems: a review and recommendations for treatment. *Am Fam Physician* 2005; 72: 811–818.
46. Razek A, Fouda N, Elmetwaley N, Elbogdady E. Sonography of the knee joint. *J Ultrasound* 2009; 12: 53–60.
47. Ghosh N, Kruse D, Subeh M, et al. Comparing point-of-care-ultrasound (POCUS) to MRI for the diagnosis of medial compartment knee injuries. *J Med Ultrasound* 2017; 25: 167–172.
48. Baloch N, Hasan OH, Jessar MM, et al. "Sports Ultrasound," advantages, indications and limitations in upper and lower limbs musculoskeletal disorders. Review article. *Int J Surg* 2018; 54: 333–340.

CHAPTER 10

Extracranial Arteries

Valentina Bonnefil, Zoya Sandhu, and Jing Gao
Rocky Vista University, College of Osteopathic Medicine, Ivins, Utah, USA

Introduction

Extracranial artery ultrasound consists of imaging the carotid, subclavian, and vertebral arteries in the cervical region [1]. Changes in vessel wall properties and distensibility of the carotid artery have been considered as the window to arteriosclerotic and atherosclerotic disease in the heart and other parts of the arterial system. Ultrasound can be used to screen accumulation of cholesterol within the carotid arteries to help with early intervention in preventing cerebrovascular diseases [2]. In disease diagnosis, quantitative ultrasound measurements can be taken of the intima-media thickness, the size of atherosclerotic plaque, as well as lumen reduction of the arteries [3]. This is a simple and cost-effective imaging technique for both assessing risk of future ischemic stroke and the likely source of a stroke after such an event [4]. Additionally, the use of ultrasound can help identify other vascular pathologies in the neck region, such as subclavian steal syndrome (SSS), by visualizing blood flow directionality and velocity [5, 6]. Furthermore, the speed and accessibility of ultrasound are vital for the diagnosis of traumatic neck injury and time-sensitive pathologies, such as carotid artery dissection [7]. Following the development of portable and handheld ultrasound devices, Doppler and grayscale ultrasound are established approaches for identifying arterial pathologies in the cervical region, which can be performed in rural areas and clinical settings [8].

This chapter aims to introduce basic anatomy, ultrasound exam protocol, and ultrasound images of normal and common pathologies of extracranial arteries in the cervical region.

General Anatomy

Extracranial Carotid Artery

The right common carotid artery (CCA) is a branch of the subclavian artery, and the left is a direct branch of the arch of the aorta. They ascend bilaterally until a bifurcation at approximately the third cervical vertebra (CV3), which produces internal and external branches of the carotid artery (Fig. 10.1). The carotid body resides near the bifurcation of the common carotid. The carotid body functions as a chemoreceptor that senses blood oxygenation.The external carotid has eight main branches

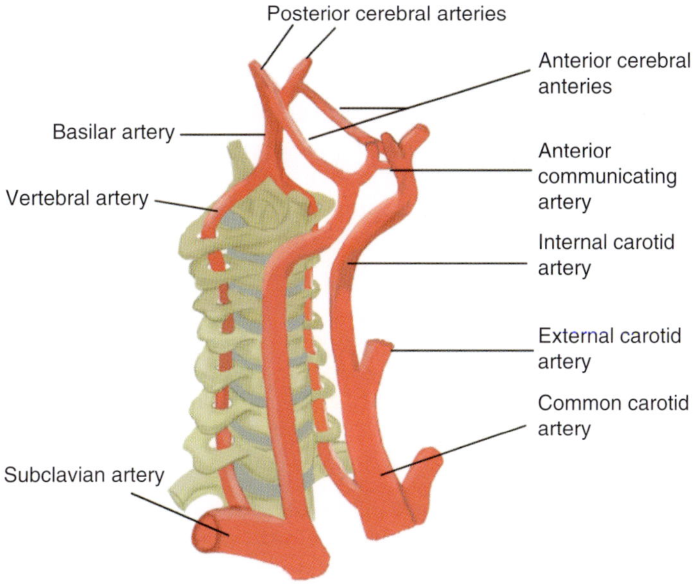

FIGURE 10.1 Anatomy of the carotid artery, subclavian artery, and vertebral artery.

supplying blood primarily to the face and neck. In ascending branching order, they are: superior thyroid artery, ascending pharyngeal artery, lingual artery, facial artery, occipital artery, posterior auricular artery, maxillary artery, and the superficial temporal artery [9].

The internal carotid enters the skull through the carotid canal, and it is a primary contributor to a large anastomosis, known as the circle of Willis, located at the base of the brain. The internal carotid artery (ICA) proceeds through the skull and then gives off several branches, including the ophthalmic and posterior communicating arteries, before bifurcating into the anterior cerebral artery and middle cerebral artery. The two anterior cerebral arteries are connected by the anterior communicating artery, and they also provide blood to the medial parts of the brain. The ophthalmic arteries provide blood to the eyes. The middle cerebral arteries provide blood to the lateral portions of the hemispheres [10].

Subclavian Artery and Vertebral Artery

The left subclavian artery is a branch of the aortic arch, and the right subclavian artery is a branch of the brachiocephalic trunk (Fig. 10.1). The subclavian artery enters the neck between the anterior and posterior scalene muscles. The artery is divided into three parts and described in relation to the anterior scalene muscle. The first part is medial to the anterior scalene muscle and gives off three branches (vertebral, internal thoracic, and thyrocervical trunk arteries). The second part is posterior to the anterior scalene muscle and has one branch (costocervical trunk). The third part is lateral to the anterior scalene and has one branch (dorsal scapular artery) [9].

The vertebral arteries are the first branches of the subclavian artery (Fig. 10.1). They provide blood supply to the neck and the cervical spinal cord. They ascend from approximately cervical vertebra 6 (CV6) to CV1 by traveling through transverse foramina until they reach the skull, where they enter through the foramen magnum and contribute to the circle of Willis. Then, they each provide bilateral branches known as the posterior inferior cerebellar arteries, which provide blood to the cerebellum. After the posterior inferior cerebellar arteries, the vertebral arteries join to form the basilar artery. The basilar artery gives off bilateral branches known as the anterior inferior cerebellar arteries. The basilar artery provides many smaller pontine arteries before providing two branches known as the superior cerebellar arteries and the posterior cerebral arteries, which provide blood to the occipital regions of the brain. The bilateral posterior communicating arteries connect the middle and posterior cerebral arteries [10].

Ultrasound Indications

Clinical Symptoms

- **TIA:** Transient Ischemic Attack (TIA) is an occurrence in which oxygenated blood flow is unable to reach the brain. However, the transient nature indicates that oxygenated blood flow returns to the area within a few minutes, and there is no permanent damage to the brain. Patients experiencing a TIA can present with changes in consciousness, attention, motor abilities, sensory abilities, and language difficulties. These symptoms will be resolved within 24 hours. A patient who presents with a TIA commonly requires a carotid ultrasound for a more accurate stroke risk assessment [4].
- **Stroke:** Stroke arises from a complete lack or reduction of oxygenated blood to the brain. In contrast with TIA, strokes are not transient. Occlusion of an artery is due to factors such as thrombosis or plaque formation. Patients experiencing a stroke will present with the same symptoms of a TIA, but the symptoms will not resolve within 24 hours. Ultrasound is a fast and robust tool to assess the cause of stroke, which could be an occlusion or severe stenosis in the carotid arteries [4].
- **Amaurosis fugax:** An occlusion in the ophthalmic artery that leads to temporary loss of vision in one or both eyes. This is often a warning sign of an impending stroke. There are several causes such as emboli. Emboli most often occlude the carotid artery on the same side as the symptoms [1].
- Unexplained neurological symptoms (e.g. numbness, tingling, and motor changes that may result from poor blood supply to the central nervous system) [11, 12].
- **Neck trauma:** Evaluate potential fracture of the cervical spine that may damage the extracranial arteries. Ultrasound can help determine the need for emergency surgical intervention [1].
- **Syncope (fainting), seizures, dizziness:** Ultrasound can be used to rule out carotid artery occlusion when determining the etiology of syncope [1].

Physical Examination

- Cervical bruit as high-pitched sound resulting from arteriovenous fistula (AVF) or arterial stenosis [4, 12, 13].
- Pulsatile neck masses are suspicious of complications such as AVF in patients underwent invasive procedures [11].

- **Evaluation of suspected subclavian steal syndrome**: Upon stenosis or occlusion of the subclavian artery proximal to the branching of the vertebral artery. This leads to a reversal of blood flow in the vertebral artery. This generally leads to insufficient oxygenated blood delivery to the brain [5, 6, 14, 15].
- **Suspected carotid artery dissection**: The innermost layer of the carotid artery tears, which leads to stroke and hemorrhage [7, 16].
- Hollenhorst plaque is visualized on retina fundoscopic examination and is an indication of ICA stenosis [17].

Medical and Family History

- Follow-up with patients with proven carotid disease for monitoring disease progression [3, 18].
- History of head and neck radiation: Radiation predisposes patients to neoplasms and damages coronary arteries. Ultrasound can be used to screen for masses and plaques in this region [1].
- Fibromuscular dysplasia: Fibromuscular dysplasia leads to arterial stenosis and aneurysm [1].
- Screening high-risk patients for developing atherosclerosis (hypertension, diabetes, hyperlipidemia) [3, 13, 19].
- Preoperative evaluation for cardiovascular surgical procedures (CABG, valve replacement) [1].

Ultrasound Techniques

Preparation: Resting for 5–10 minutes prior to the examination is requested.

Position: Patient is in a supine position with or without head turning away approximately 20° from the side being scanned. The patient should be stable in either position. Scanning is performed without head rotation with patients on a ventilator. Placing a pillow to support the neck may help improve the stability of the neck during the scanning [20].

Scanning protocol: Ultrasound gel is placed between the transducer and skin for ultrasound beam transmission. A linear array transducer (6–10 MHz) is suitable for carotid ultrasound.

Grayscale image: Common settings for carotid ultrasound include image depth of 3–5 cm, high frame rate, and resolution of grayscale image. Palpate for the carotid pulse lateral to the trachea. Longitudinal and transverse sections of the artery should include the artery from the proximal CCA at the aortic arch (left), and the innominate artery (right) to the distal ICA. Transverse (Fig. 10.2) and longitudinal (Fig. 10.3) scans of the artery are performed when the patient is comfortable and relaxed.

Longitudinal section: Place transducer vertically and slide the transducer until a lumen is identified. In comparison with the internal jugular vein, the CCA is located relatively anterior, toward the middle, and is incompressible. Continue to slide the transducer in a vertical plane to identify where the

(a) (b)

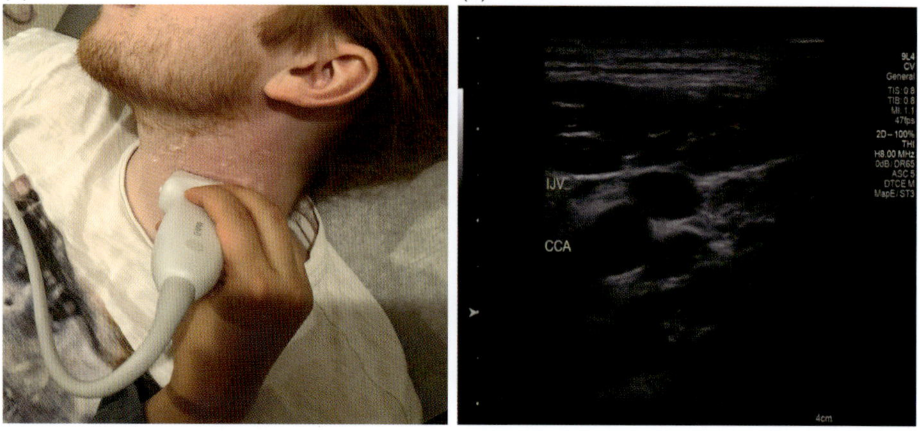

FIGURE 10.2 Transducer (a) and patient positioning for transverse image (b) of the common carotid artery. CCA, common carotid artery; IJV, internal jugular vein. The indicator on the transducer should be oriented toward the patient's right axilla for transverse images of the carotid artery. B-mode image (b) of the transverse plane of CCA and IJV.

(a) (b)

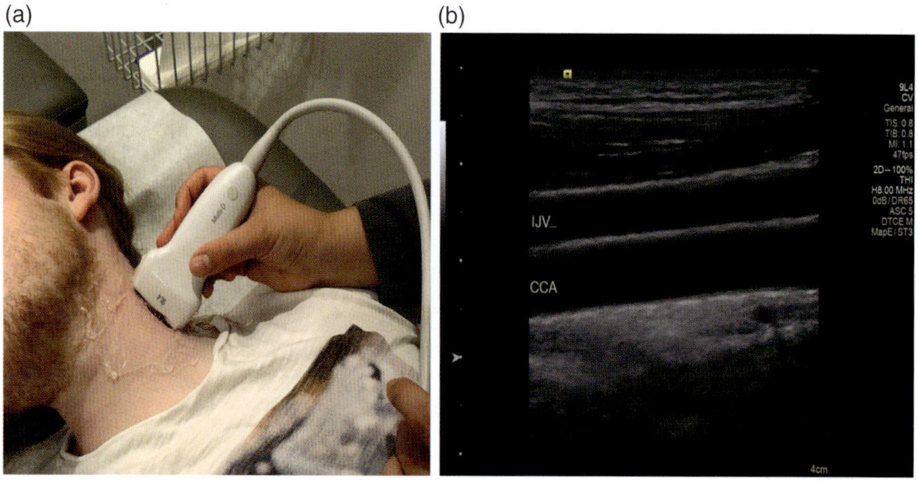

FIGURE 10.3 (a) Transducer and patient positioning for imaging the longitudinal plane of the carotid artery. The indicator on the probe should be oriented toward the patient's head for scanning the longitudinal carotid artery and vertebral artery. (b) B-mode image of the longitudinal plane of the common carotid artery (CCA) and internal jugular vein (IJV).

carotid bifurcates into the internal and external carotid arteries. Transverse section: once the carotid artery is identified, carefully rotate the transducer 90° with the arrow pointing to the right side of the patient. Ensure that the carotid remains in the plane.

Color flow imaging: Color flow imaging setting for arterial flow with moderate to high wall filter, high frame rate to minimize aliasing (Fig. 10.4). Color flow imaging displays the direction and the mean velocity of blood flow. It can be used to locate the region of lumen narrowing, high velocity, as the guidance to spectral Doppler to measure the maximum velocity at the stenotic artery.

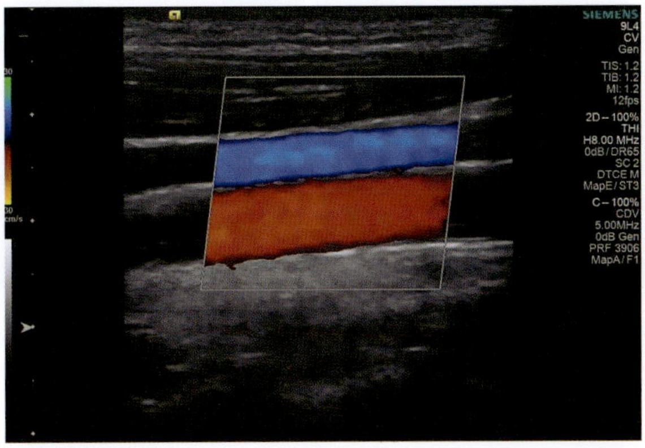

FIGURE 10.4 Color flow imaging of the longitudinal plane of the common carotid artery (red color representing cephalic blood flow toward the transducer) and internal jugular vein (blue color representing blood flow away from the transducer in this image).

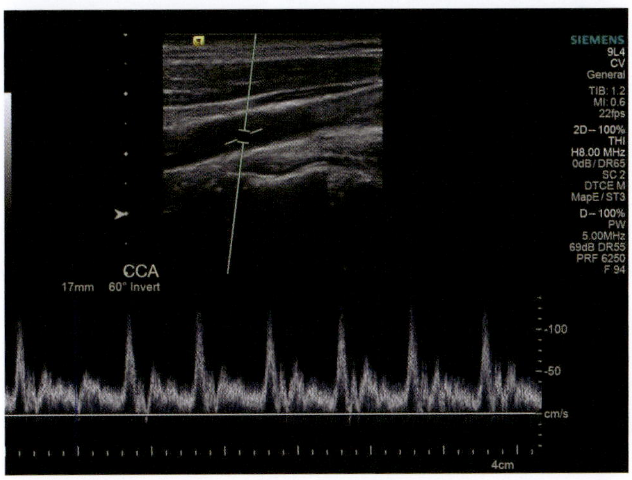

FIGURE 10.5 Spectral Doppler image of the longitudinal plane of the common carotid artery (CCA). The peak systolic velocity (PSV) value is lower than 230 cm/sec in a normal carotid artery. The patient may have a high risk for CVA if PSV >230 cm/sec. Special attention should be paid to correct Doppler angle to be less than 60°.

Spectral Doppler: Spectral Doppler sets the baseline, scale, and gain depending on the flow velocity in a sampled artery. Adjust the waveform amplitude to be able to display the maximum Doppler velocity and waveform clearly (Fig. 10.5). Doppler angle correction of less than 60° and Doppler gate placed in the center of the artery are recommended [19, 20].

Ultrasound of Normal Carotid and Vertebral Arteries

Color flow imaging is important for demonstrating the patency and flow direction of the CCA, CCA bulb/bifurcation (Fig. 10.6), ICA (Fig. 10.7), and vertebral artery (Fig. 10.8).

(a) (b)

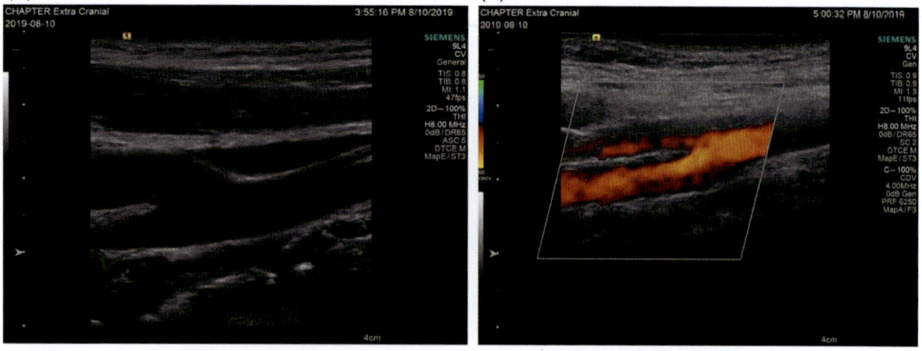

FIGURE 10.6 B-mode image (a) of longitudinal distal common carotid artery (CCA), CCA bulb, and CCA bifurcation. There is no atherosclerotic plaque present in the distal CCA or bulb region. Color flow imaging (b) of the common carotid artery bifurcation.

(a) (b)

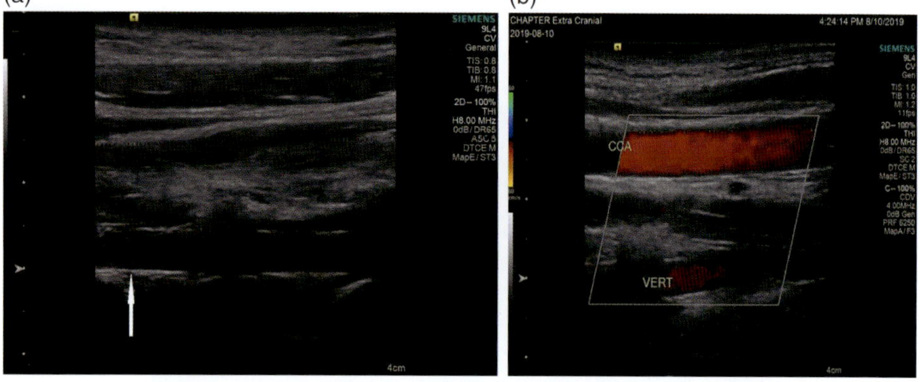

FIGURE 10.7 B-mode image (a) of the vertebral artery (white arrow). Color flow imaging (b) of the common carotid artery (CCA) and vertebral arteries (VERT) in the longitudinal plane. The direction of blood flow in the vertebral artery is the same as that in the common carotid artery (red color), which represents the cephalic direction of the blood flow in both CCA and VERT.

(a) (b)

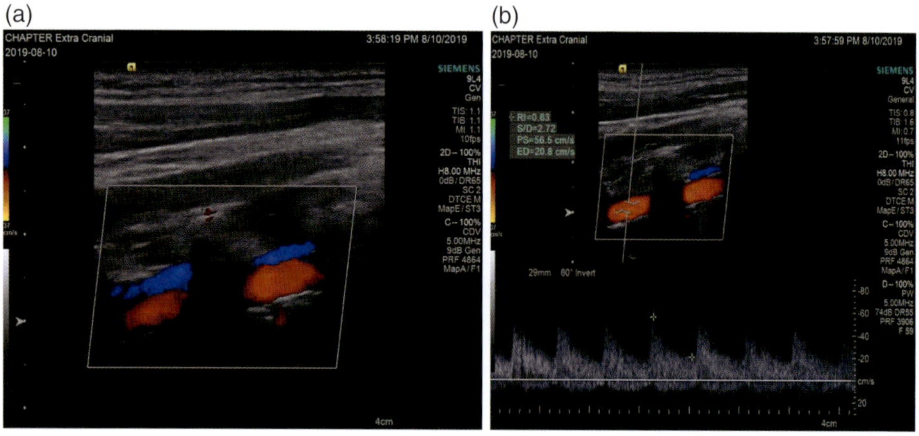

FIGURE 10.8 Color flow imaging (a) and spectral Doppler (b) of the vertebral artery and vein. Color flow imaging (inverted color code) of the longitudinal vertebral artery (red color) and vein (blue color). Color flow imaging demonstrates not only the patency of the vessels but also shows the cephalic direction of blood flow in the vertebral artery. The vessel with a blue color is the vertebral vein flowing away from the brain. Place the Doppler gate in the center of the artery with angle correction (<60°) to measure the maximum flow velocities (b). Normally, vertebral artery flow appears with low resistance, monophasic, and in a cephalic direction.

Ultrasound in Common Pathologies

Carotid Artery Intima Media Thickness (IMT) and Atherosclerosis

The measurement of IMT is considered a screening tool for predicting and detecting cardiovascular disease during cardiovascular risk assessments in patients who are asymptomatic but have known risk factors for developing cardiovascular disease in the future. An IMT of >0.9 mm is considered thickened and is a marker of asymptomatic organ damage [21]. An atherosclerotic plaque is considered to be present when the IMT is greater than 1.1 mm. IMT can be measured periodically in patients with known cardiovascular disease. IMT measurement can also be used to assess the efficacy of drug therapy such as the effectiveness of lipid-lowering medication [22, 23]. The lumen diameter of the carotid artery is the distance across a section of the artery. An IMT is measured in the posterior wall of the distal CCA (Fig. 10.9). A high-resolution grayscale image is requested to optimize the intima media clearly. Recently, measurement software (such as arterial health assessment designed by Siemens Healthineers) has been developed to quantify IMT automatically or semiautomatically (Fig. 10.9).

Carotid Artery Stenosis

When scanning for plaque within the carotid arteries, it is useful to classify the plaque in a standardized manner. The classification that is most used is the modified Dr. Gray-Weale, which identifies four distinct plaque types based on ultrasound morphology [24]. Type 1 is predominantly echolucent plaques that are associated with a higher risk of ischemic events [25]. Type 2 is >75% echolucent but with echogenic areas. Type 2 also confers a higher risk of ischemic cerebrovascular events. Type 3 is

(a) (b)

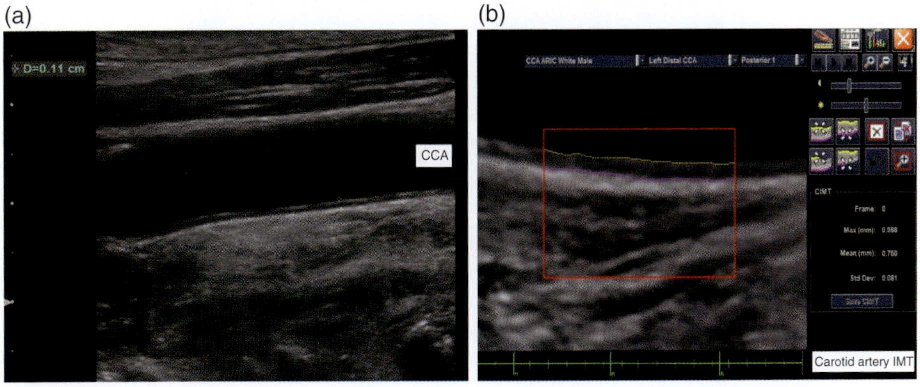

FIGURE 10.9 The intima-media thickness (IMT) is measured at the posterior wall of the distal carotid artery in B-mode image (a). Using artery health package (AHP, Siemens Medical Solutions) software, the IMT is estimated from the posterior wall of the common carotid artery (CCA). The mean IMT (0.76 mm) is the average of IMT measurements in 10 mm length of the posterior arterial wall (b).

predominantly echogenic with small areas (<25%) of echolucency and is less likely to result in embolic events and subsequent ischemic injury. Finally, Type 4 is all echogenic and confers the least risk for cerebrovascular accidents compared to the other plaque subtypes. Still, it should be noted that Type 4 does indicate increased aortic arterial stiffness [24]. Echolucent material is consistent with the lipid core and/or intraplaque hemorrhage, features which have been shown to be associated with a higher risk of future stroke [25]. In contrast, echogenic material is consistent with predominantly fibrous tissues. Types 1 and 2 are unstable plaques, often with a large lipid core and thin fibrous cap, making them more likely to rupture and dislodge, causing occlusion of smaller vessels in the brain. In contrast, types 3 and 4 have a larger fibrous capsule with a smaller lipid core, making them more stable.

In addition, it is important to classify the degree of stenosis. A reduction of arterial lumen can be visualized on color flow imaging (Figs. 10.10 and 10.11), and

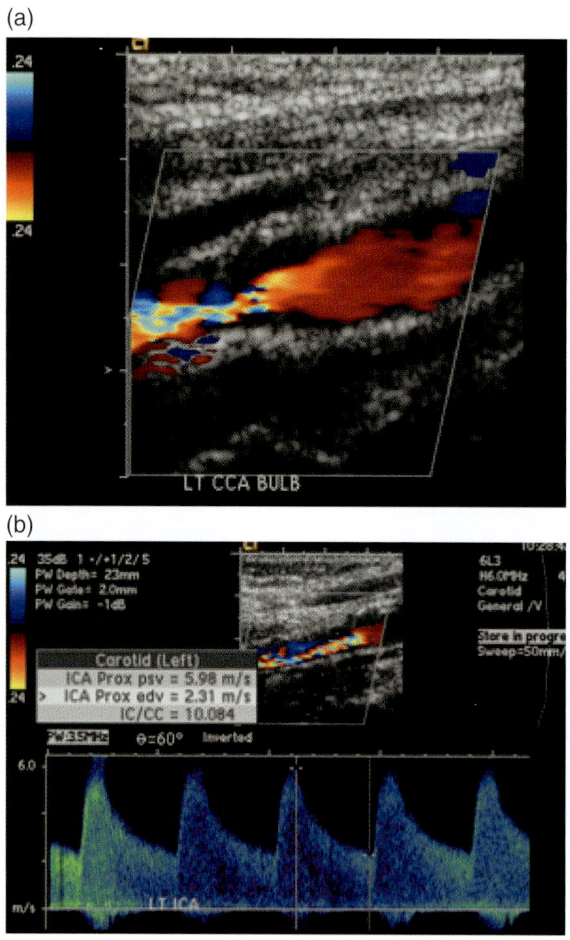

FIGURE 10.10 Color flow and spectral Doppler images present a severe carotid artery stenosis. Mixed red with green and blue colors in color flow imaging represent significantly turbulent and high velocity flow in the proximal internal carotid artery (ICA, a). Quantitative measure of high peak systolic velocity (PSV) 5.98 m/sec at the stenotic ICA (b) and substantially elevated ICA/CCA ratio of 10.084 (normal <3) demonstrates a severe stenosis in the left (LT) proximal ICA.

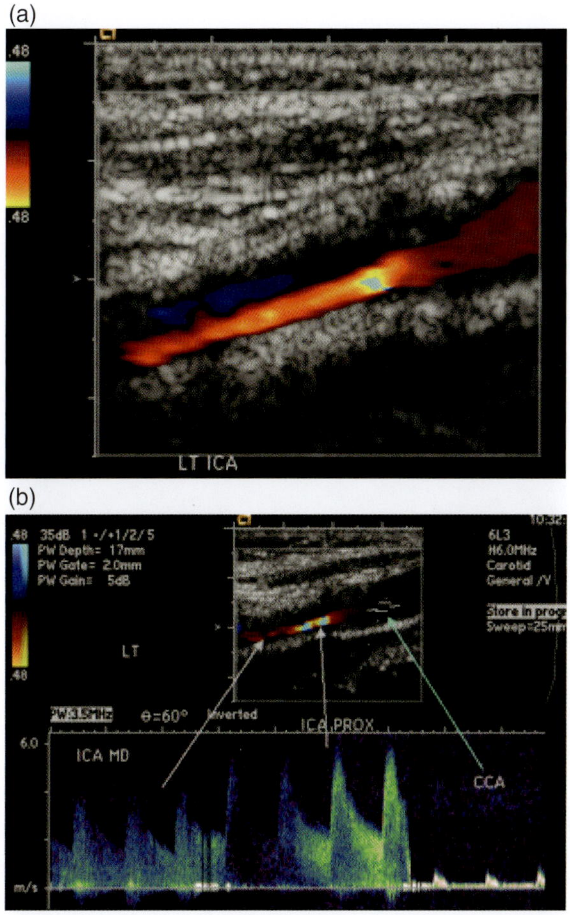

FIGURE 10.11 Using color flow imaging (a) as a guidance, the site of high flow velocity appears in the stenotic proximal internal carotid artery (ICA). Spectral Doppler (slow speed) can be used to trace the change in flow velocities from the normal common carotid (CCA) to the site of stenosis in the proximal ICA and distal to the stenosis (mid ICA). The Doppler spectrum displays the gradient of velocity difference between arterial segments with and without stenosis (b). LT, left; ICA MD, mid ICA.

the severity of arterial stenosis is determined by the peak systolic velocity (PSV) at the site of stenosis and the PSV ratio, which is PSV measured at the site of stenosis compared to PSV measured proximal to the stenosis (PSV ratio = PSV of ICA/PSV of CCA). In low degree stenosis (artery lumen reduction <40%), PSV ICA/CCA is <2, and PSV of ICA is <160 cm/sec. Moderate stenosis (artery lumen reduction 50–60%) shows increased flow on color flow imaging, PSV at the stenosis is around 210 cm/sec, and ICA/CCA ≥ 2. In hemodynamically relevant stenosis (artery lumen reduction >70%), there is a significant increase in PSV at the stenosis (>330 cm/sec) and ICA/CCA (>4) (Fig. 10.10) [26–28]. An interventional management such as endarterectomy and/or stent (Fig. 10.12) may be required in the patient with a hemodynamically significant stenosis [27, 28]. However, no surgical treatment has been proven to reduce the risk of future stroke in patients with complete arterial occlusion (Fig. 10.13).

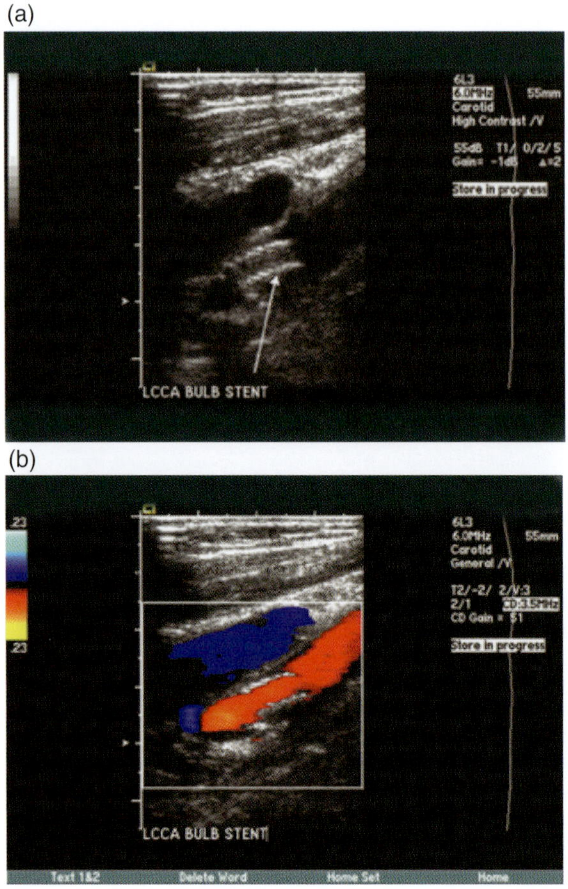

FIGURE 10.12 B-mode image (a) and color flow imaging (b) of the carotid artery with stent placement. Color flow imaging demonstrates that the stent (arrow) is patent. LCCA, left common carotid artery.

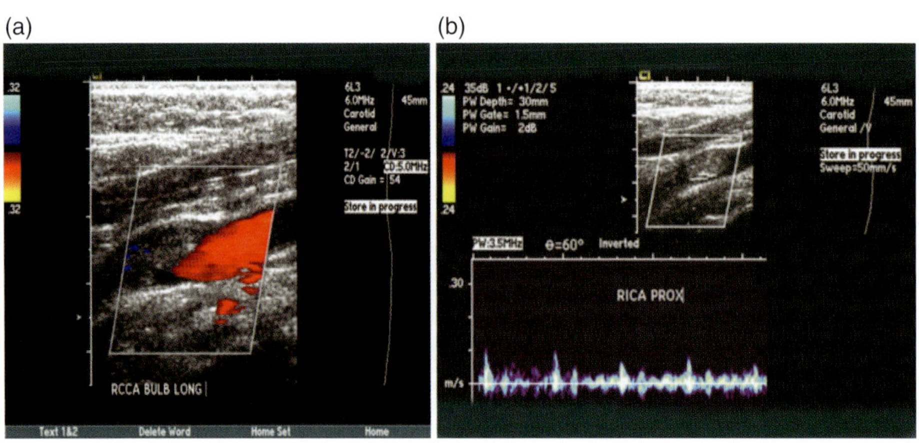

FIGURE 10.13 Color flow imaging (a) and spectral Doppler (b) demonstrate no flow in the right proximal internal carotid artery (RICA PROX). LONG, longitudinal; RCCA, right common carotid artery.

In occlusive carotid artery disease, no flow in the site of disease is demonstrated in color flow imaging and/or spectral Doppler images (Fig. 10.13). Collateral flow formation (arterialized external carotid artery and branch formation) may develop.

Carotid Artery Dissection

Carotid artery dissection occurs when the layers of the carotid artery wall separate, and hemorrhage extends into the vessel wall. This dissection can develop local thrombosis, which may impair blood flow to the brain and can potentially lead to stroke. Carotid artery dissection is one of the most common causes of stroke in young patients. Timely diagnosis of carotid artery dissection is crucial to decrease mortality rates and better patient outcomes. Ultrasound is noninvasive and fastest screening tool that can be used to identify carotid artery dissection [7]. Dissection flap can be visualized on B-mode and M-mode ultrasound images (Fig. 10.14). Magnetic resonance angiography (MRA) and computed tomographic angiography can further demonstrate the dissection site.

Vertebral Artery and Subclavian Steal Syndrome

SSS occurs when severe stenosis (or occlusion) in the subclavian artery results in decreased blood flow to the vertebral artery and axillary artery. As the degree of stenosis increases, the pressure decreases in the arm arteries distal to the stenosis. The pressure gradient that is developed because of the subclavian stenosis results in reversed blood flow in the vertebral artery distal to and ipsilateral to the subclavian artery stenosis [29].

A patient with unilateral upper limb claudication, with or without coldness of the hand or fingers, may be experiencing SSS. This phenomenon most commonly

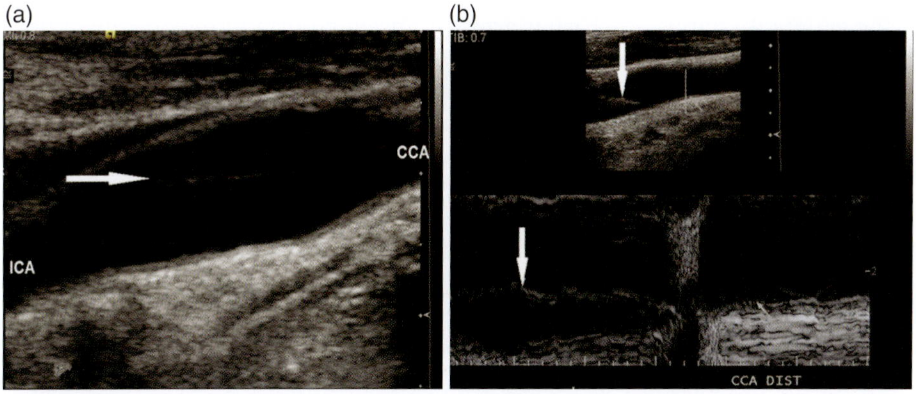

FIGURE 10.14 B-mode (a), M-mode (b) ultrasound images demonstrate a dissecting flap (large white arrows) in the common carotid artery (CCA) bulb in a 45-year-old woman with fibromuscular dysplasia. Carotid artery dissection was also demonstrated on magnetic resonance angiography. ICA, internal carotid artery.

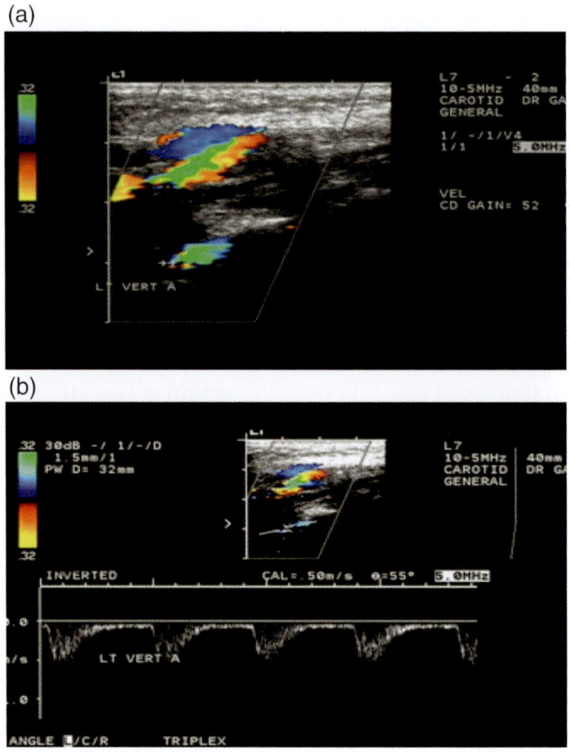

FIGURE 10.15 Retrograde flow appears in color flow (a) and spectral Doppler (b) images of the left vertebral (VERT) artery (longitudinal plane). An antegrade (cephalic) flow is in the carotid artery (red color), and retrograde flow is in the left vertebral artery. A, artery; LT, left.

occurs in the left upper extremity and is rarely seen in the right upper extremity. To supply oxygenated blood to the left upper limb, blood is stolen from the junction of the vertebral arteries, the basilar artery. Consequently, a retrograde blood flow in the ipsilateral vertebral artery (Fig. 10.15) develops for bypassing the segment of the occlusion at the proximal subclavian artery. Because SSS can cause decreased blood flow to the brainstem, cerebellum, and occipital lobes, patients can present with neurological complaints such as presyncope, dizziness, nausea, or lightheadedness [14].

Assessing the subclavian artery with ultrasound Doppler is a quick and noninvasive step in determining whether to recommend surgery or endovascular treatment for a patient with suspected SSS. When the subclavian stenosis is at least >50%, most patients will have intermittent or continuous reversal of flow in the vertebral artery. Doppler ultrasound is more sensitive than conventional angiography for detecting flow reversal [29, 30]. If a patient with significant symptoms, vertebral artery waveforms can be examined, and grayscale can be used to evaluate the severity of stenosis [31]. The transient early systolic deceleration followed by transient cessation of antegrade flow or a transient reversal of flow seen on color flow imaging is a characteristic of severe SSS [15]. Reversal flow in the distal vertebral artery can be observed using transcranial ultrasound via the occipital window approach (Fig. 10.16).

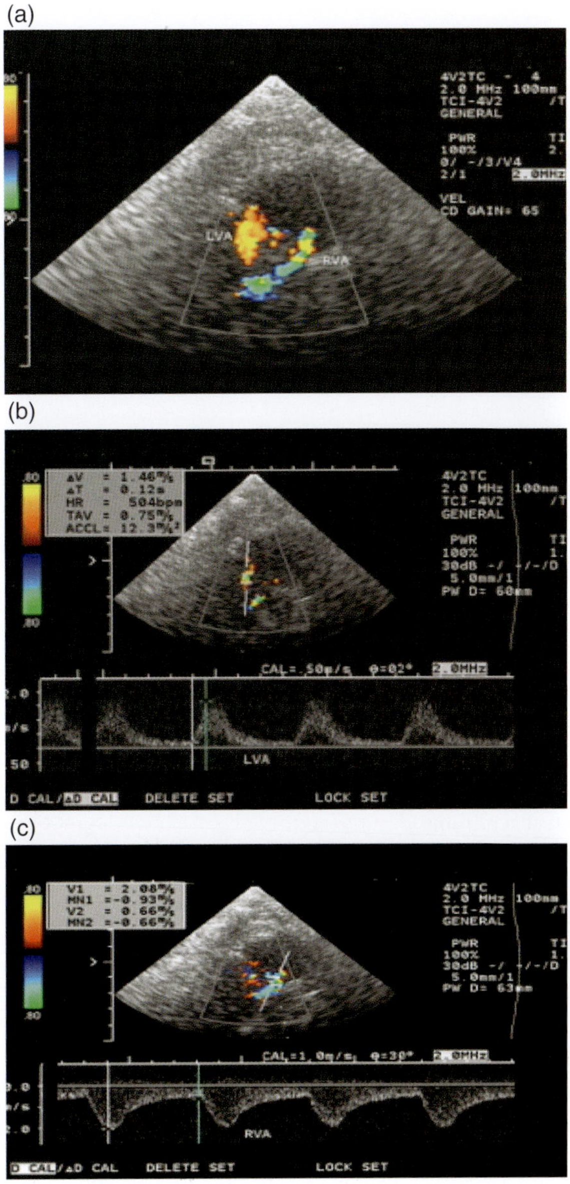

FIGURE 10.16 Transcranial ultrasound (via the occipital window approach) is performed on the same patient in Figure 10.15. Again, color flow (a) and spectral Doppler (b and c) show that the flow direction in the left vertebral artery (LVA, red) is retrograde, which differs from anterograde flow in the right vertebral artery (RVA, blue).

Summary

Extracranial ultrasound is an invaluable tool in the diagnosis of chronic atherosclerotic cardiovascular disease and for the evaluation of high-grade stenosis, occlusion, or dissection in the setting of TIA or ischemic stroke. The cervical vertebral arteries can also be evaluated for dissection and adequate perfusion via standard and widely available ultrasound techniques. Additionally, ultrasound can be an optimal technique to evaluate for SSS.

Review Questions

1. Identify a carotid artery that travels upward through carotid canal entering the skull and supplies the anterior and middle cerebral circulation.
   - a. Internal carotid artery
   - b. External carotid artery
   - c. Common carotid artery
   - d. Vertebral artery
2. What ultrasound technique is used for quantifying blood flow velocity in the CCA?
   - a. M-mode
   - b. Color Doppler
   - c. Grayscale
   - d. Spectral Doppler
3. What is the indication of intervention of carotid artery stenosis?
   - a. 30%
   - b. 50%
   - c. 70%
   - d. 90%
4. What pathology does a significant increase in intima media thickness of the common carotid artery present?
   - a. Aneurysm
   - b. Subclavian steal syndrome
   - c. Carotid artery dissection
   - d. Atherosclerosis
5. Where is the common site for developing atherosclerotic plaques?
   - a. Bifurcation of the common carotid
   - b. Bifurcation of the internal carotid
   - c. Circle of Willis
   - d. Vertebral artery
6. What is the best way to test if a vessel is internal jugular vein or carotid artery?
   - a. Power Doppler
   - b. Compression
   - c. Sway
   - d. Rotation
7. Who would be most at risk for a TIA?
   - a. 17-year-old high school athlete
   - b. 60-year-old smoker with high cholesterol
   - c. 40-year-old woman with a history of congenital heart disease
   - d. 2-year-old infant
8. What is the pathology when an intraluminal flaps are observed in the internal carotid artery on realtime B-mode ultrasound images?
   - a. Atherosclerosis of internal carotid
   - b. Carotid artery dissection

c. Subclavian steal syndrome

d. TIA

9. Which artery presents retrograde flow (color flow and spectral Doppler) in a patient with subclavian steel syndrome?.

   a. Internal carotid

   b. External carotid

   c. Common carotid

   d. Vertebral artery

10. What is the primary contributor of blood supply to the circle of Willis?

   a. Internal carotid

   b. External carotid

   c. Common carotid

   d. Vertebral artery

Correct answers: 1. a; 2. d; 3. d; 4. d; 5. a; 6. b; 7. b; 8. b; 9. d; 10. d.

References

1. AIUM practice parameter for the performance of an ultrasound examination of the extracranial cerebrovascular system. *J Ultrasound Med* 2016, 2016; 35(9): 1–11. doi.org/10.7863/ultra.35.9.1.
2. Shelat, AM. Carotid duplex: MedlinePlus medical encyclopedia. *MedlinePlus*, U.S. National Library of Medicine, 2018. http://www.medlineplus.gov/ency/article/003774.htm.
3. Grant EG, Benson CB, Moneta GL, et al. Carotid artery stenosis: grayscale and Doppler ultrasound diagnosis-society of radiologists in ultrasound consensus conference. *Radiology* 2003; 229: 340–346.
4. Transient Ischemic Attack (TIA). Mayo Clinic. Mayo Foundation for Medical Education and Research, 2019. http://www.mayoclinic.org/diseases-conditions/transient-ischemic-attack/symptoms-causes/syc-20355679.
5. Borstein NM, Norns JW. Subclavian steal: a harmless hemodynamic phenomenon? *Lancet* 1986; 2: 303–305.
6. Walker DW, Acker JD, Cole CA. Subclavian steal syndrome detected with duplex pulsed Doppler sonography. *Am J Neuroradiol* 1982; 3: 615–618.
7. Sturzenegger M, Mattle HP, Rivoir A, Baumgartner RW. Ultrasound findings in carotid artery dissection analysis of 43 patients. *Neurology* 1995; 45: 691–698.
8. Pseudoaneurysm: what causes it? *Mayo Clinic*, Mayo Foundation for Medical Education and Research, 2019. http://www.mayoclinic.org/tests-procedures/cardiac-catheterization/expert-answers/pseudoaneurysm/faq-20058420.
9. Hansen JT, Netter FH. Essential guide to netters anatomy. Singapore: Elsevier (Singapore) Pte Ltd, 2011.
10. Nguyen H, Duong H. Anatomy, head and neck, anterior, common carotid artery. StatPearls, 2019. https://www.ncbi.nlm.nih.gov/books/NBK546613.
11. Arteriovenous fistula. *Mayo Clinic*, Mayo Foundation for Medical Education and Research, 2018. http://www.mayoclinic.org/diseases-conditions/arteriovenous-fistula/symptoms.
12. Moneta GL, Edwards JM, Papanicolaou G, et al. Screening for asymptomatic internal carotid artery stenosis: duplex catena for discriminating 60% to 99% stenosis. *J Vasc Surg* 1995; 21: 989–994.
13. Waxman SG. Clin neuroanatomy. 28th ed. New York: McGraw-Hill, 2017.

14. Gomez CR. Subclavian steal syndrome. UpToDate, 2023. http://www.uptodate.com/contents/subclavian-steal-syndrome.
15. Kliewer MA, Hertzberg BS, Kim DH, et al. Vertebral artery Doppler waveform changes indicating subclavian steal physiology. *Am J Roentgenol* 2000; 174: 815–819.
16. Sidhu PS, Ray-Chaudhun K, Khaw KT. Case report: moyamoya disease mimicking a spontaneous internal carotid artery dissection on Doppler ultrasound. *Eur Radiol* 2000; 10: 149–153.
17. Bakri SJ, Luqman A, Pathic B, et al. Is carotid ultrasound necessary in the clinical evaluation of the asymptomatic Hollenhorst plaque? (an American ophthalmological society thesis). *Trans Am Ophthalmol Soc* 2013; 111: 17–23.
18. Salonen R, Salonen JT. Progression of carotid atherosclerosis and its determinants: a population-based ultrasonography study. *Atherosclerosis* 1990; 81: 33–40.
19. Tahmasebpour HR, Cooperberg PL, et al. Sonographic examination of the carotid arteries. *Radiographics* 2005; 25: 1561–1575.
20. Polak JF. Carotid ultrasound. *Radiol Clin North Am* 2001; 39: 569–589.
21. Simon A, Gariepy J, Chironi G, et al. Intima-media thickness: a new tool for diagnosis and treatment of cardiovascular risk. *J Hypertens* 2002; 20: 159–169. https://doi.org/10.1097/00004872-200202000-00001.
22. Goff DC Jr, Lloyd-Jones DM, Bennett G, et al. 2013 ACC/AHA guideline on the assessment of cardiovascular risk: a report of the American College of Cardiology/American Heart Association Task Force on Practice Guidelines. *J Am Coll Cardiol* 2014; 63: 2935–2959.
23. de Groot E, Jukema JW, Montauban van Swijndregt AD, et al. B-mode ultrasound assessment of pravastatin treatment effect on carotid and femoral artery walls and its correlations with coronary arteriographic findings: a report of the regression growth evaluation statin study (REGRESS). *J Am Coll Cardiol* 1998; 31: 1561–1567.
24. Zureik M, Jeanne-Marie TM, et al. Echogenic carotid plaques are associated with aortic arterial stiffness in subjects with subclinical carotid atherosclerosis. *Hypertension* 2003; 41: 519–527.
25. Gray-Weale AC, Grahan JC, Burnett JR, et al. Carotid artery atheroma: comparison of preoperative B-mode ultrasound appearance with carotid endarterectomy specimen pathology. *J Cardiovasc Surg* 1988; 29(6): 676–681.
26. Gupta A, Kesavabhotla K, Baradaran H, et al. Plaque echolucency and stroke risk in asymptomatic carotid stenosis: a systematic review and meta-analysis. *Stroke* 2015; 46: 91–97.
27. Saxena A, EYK N, Lim ST. Imaging modalities to diagnose carotid artery stenosis: progress and prospect. *Biomed Eng Online* 2019; 18(1): 66. https://doi.org/10.1186/s12938-019-0685-7.
28. von Reutern GM, Goertler MW, Bornstein NM, et al. Grading carotid stenosis using ultrasonic methods. *Stroke* 2012; 43: 916–921.
29. Komatsubara I, Kondo J, Akiyama M, et al. Subclavian steal syndrome: a case report and review of advances in diagnostic and treatment approaches. *Cardiovasc Revasc Med* 2016; 17: 54–58. https://doi.org/10.1016/j.carrev.2015.11.001.
30. Reivich M, Holling HE, Roberts B, Toole JF. Reversal of blood flow through the vertebral artery and its effect on cerebral circulation. *N Engl J Med* 1961; 265: 878–885.
31. Harper C, Cardullo PA, Weyman AK, Patterson RB. Transcranial Doppler ultrasonography of the basilar artery in patients with retrograde vertebral artery flow. *J Vasc Surg* 2008; 48: 859–864.

CHAPTER 11

The Endocrine System

Daniel Daskalakis[1], Andrew Fisher[1], Shane Kaysen[1], and Pintong Huang[2]

[1] Rocky Vista University, College of Osteopathic Medicine, Ivins, Utah, USA

[2] Department of Ultrasound in Medicine, the Second Affiliated Hospital, Zhejiang University School of Medicine, Hangzhou, China

Introduction

The endocrine system is a network of organs that communicate through molecules known as hormones. These hormones travel through the blood circulation to reach target organs that house specific receptors for these hormones. Once reaching the target organs, these hormones start a cascade of secondary messengers to maintain homeostasis and health of the organ. The principal organs involved in the endocrine system are the hypothalamus, pituitary gland, thyroid gland, parathyroid glands, pancreas, adrenal glands, ovaries, and testes, with the control center, or primary gland, being the pituitary gland. The pituitary sends the bulk of the messages (hormones) and participates in a multitude of feedback mechanisms to allow the organs to maintain their respective equilibrium [1].

In 2003, approximately 5% of the US population, roughly 16.5 million people, reported regularly taking medication for thyroid disease [2], but new data suggests these figures may be increasing. The incidence of thyroid cancer has increased from 5% in 1992 to 13% in 2016 [3]. High-resolution ultrasound is a very useful imaging technique to assess thyroid and parathyroid gland pathologies due to their superficial locations; however, ultrasound is not commonly used as the first imaging technique to assess the deeply located adult adrenal gland [4].

In this chapter, we will be focusing on the anatomy of the thyroid, parathyroid, and adrenal glands, as well as discussing techniques on how to perform an ultrasound scan of these endocrine glands. This chapter will also present ultrasound images with characteristics of normal glands and glands demonstrating pathological changes. Ultrasound of the ovaries and testes will be discussed in the gynecology (Chapter 6) and genitourinary (Chapter 7) chapters, respectively. Ultrasound-guided fine needle aspiration (FNA) of thyroid nodules will be introduced in Chapter 13 of this book.

General Anatomy

Thyroid

The thyroid gland lies within the infrahyoid compartment, anteromedially to the trachea and inferior to the cricoid cartilage, sitting just medial to the insertion of the sternocleidomastoid muscles [5]. It is medial to the carotid artery and internal jugular vein, both of which supply and drain the thyroid blood flow through their branches, respectively. The embryological development of the thyroid gland follows a descending pathway from the primitive tongue, down to the infrahyoid compartment. This migratory pathway can potentially give rise to anomalies such as pyramidal lobes and thyroglossal duct cysts. It is easiest to localize and palpate the thyroid by finding the space above the jugular notch of the manubrium and softly palpating the trachea on each of its sides. It is common practice to have the patient swallow to improve palpability for any abnormalities in the thyroid.

The thyroid gland is comprised of two main lobes located at each side of the trachea with an isthmus that connects the middle/lower lobes by draping across the midline of the trachea (Fig. 11.1). In approximately 10–40% of the population, there is a third lobe that extends from the isthmus. This is referred to as the pyramidal lobe and is normal in terms of functionality. The thyroid and its various lobes are all surrounded by the thyroid capsule [5]. This capsule is slightly hyperechoic on ultrasound imaging and serves as a landmark to easily differentiate the thyroid from the surroundings. The embryological development of the thyroid can also serve as a potential for an anomaly called ectopic thyroid tissue, which occurs when small fragments of thyroid tissue are lost during its migratory descent down the thyroglossal duct. These small fragments may stem from single cells or cell clusters that can

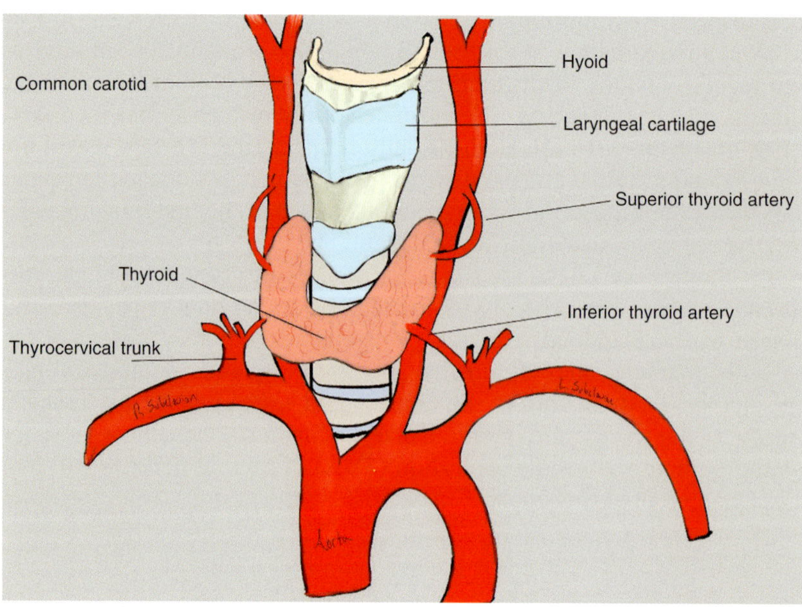

FIGURE 11.1 Anatomy illustration of the anterior neck. This gives a great depiction of the thyroid in its relationship with the surrounding structures.

grow into their own functional endocrine tissue. These ectopic fragments can be seen along the trachea and above the hyoid in some cases. Note that these may be physiologically active and may require investigation in patients with abnormal thyroid function [6].

Parathyroid Glands

The parathyroid glands are a collection of four small ovoid-shaped glands with yellow or brown color and are located on the posterior aspect of the thyroid gland. The parathyroid glands are typically found directly on the thyroid capsule but can be found within the capsule as well. They typically lie on the lateral aspects of each lobe as well as a pair of parathyroid glands inhabiting the upper and lower portions of their respective lobes (Fig. 11.2). The superior parathyroid glands are located above the level of the superior thyroid artery's intersection with the recurrent laryngeal nerve, and posterior to the recurrent laryngeal nerve. The inferior glands are typically found inferior to the inferior thyroid artery and anterior to the recurrent laryngeal nerve [5]. Knowledge of parathyroid anatomy is important because the normal parathyroid glands are not easily seen on B-mode ultrasound images due to their small size, and detection of pathologic findings is only possible when understanding the relation between the parathyroid and the thyroid glands. Be aware that the location and even the number of parathyroid glands can vary. Superior and inferior thyroid arteries provide blood supply to the thyroid and parathyroid glands. Venous blood drains to the plexus of anterior thyroid veins, and then returns through the superior, middle, or inferior thyroid veins to internal jugular and brachiocephalic veins [6, 7].

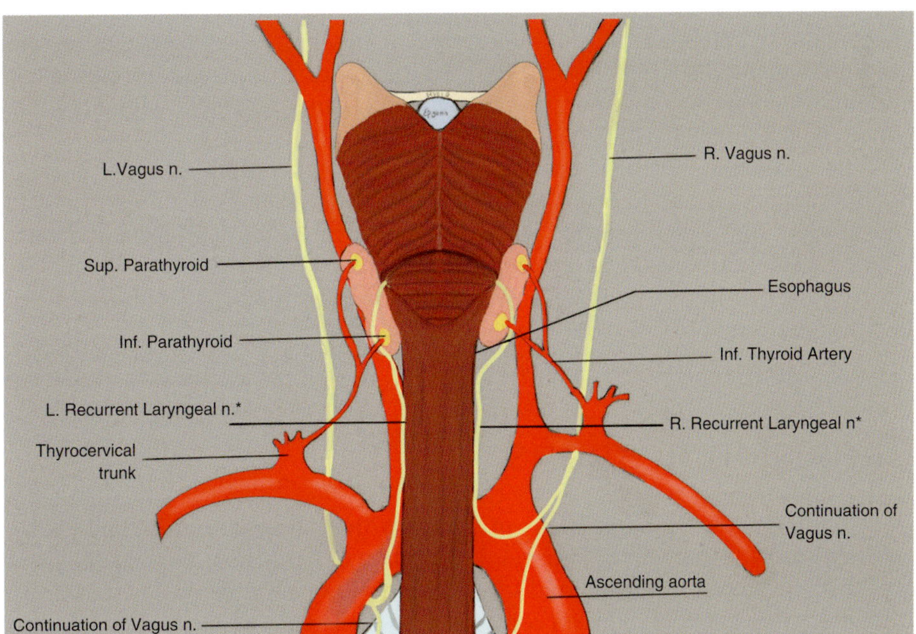

FIGURE 11.2 Anatomy of the parathyroid glands (posterior view).

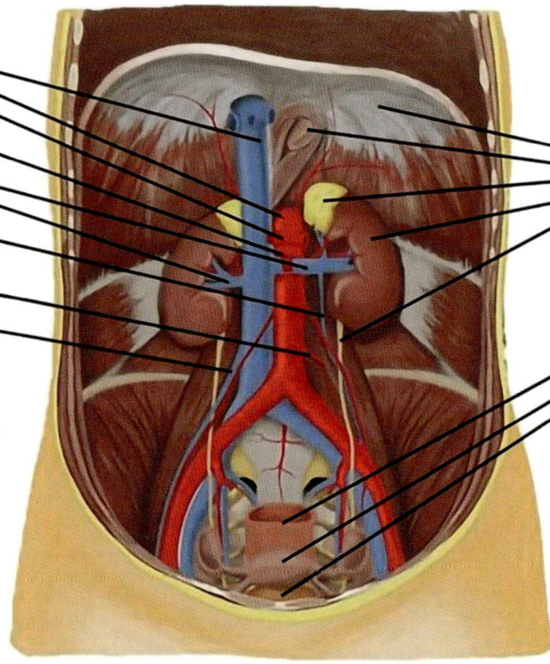

FIGURE 11.3 Anatomy of the adrenal glands.

Adrenal Glands

Adrenal glands are bilateral secretory organs located immediately superior to the upper pole of the kidneys (Fig. 11.3). To approximate the size of each adrenal gland, use the top half of the thumb. The adrenal glands themselves can be functionally divided into an outer part called the cortex and an inner medulla. The cortex secretes the hormones cortisol, aldosterone, and testosterone. The medulla produces the hormones epinephrine and norepinephrine, which are also called adrenaline and noradrenaline, respectively [8, 9].

The adrenal glands have one of the greatest blood supply rates per gram of tissue of any organ: up to 60 small arteries may enter each gland. Superior, mid, and inferior suprarenal arteries are branches of the abdominal aorta and renal artery, supplying blood flow to the adrenal glands. The right suprarenal vein drains into the inferior vena cava (IVC), and the left suprarenal vein drains into the left renal vein [10].

Clinical Indications

Ultrasound is the imaging modality of choice in the assessment of thyroid pathologies due to its advantages of high resolution, ease of performance, portability, and low cost. In addition, the thyroid's sensitivity to radiation makes performing a computed tomography (CT) scan contraindication. Therefore, ultrasound becomes the first-line imaging technique in diagnosis and follow-up of thyroid pathologies. Ultrasound of the endocrine system is primarily focused on the thyroid as it is the most accessible, easily distinguishable, and has a high relevance in the endocrine system. When thyroid disease is clinically suspected, ultrasound can be used to assess pathologies in the thyroid such as palpation of thyroid nodules, inspection of a goiter, blood tests (T3, T4, and TSH) indicating insufficient or overproduced thyroid hormones, family history of thyroid cancer, or history of radiation in the neck area [11].

Another clinical indication for ultrasound is for assessment of parathyroid glands, especially in suspicion of hyperparathyroidism. Patients with hyperparathyroidism may present with kidney calculi, gastrointestinal symptoms, loss of bone density, elevated parathyroid hormone (PTH), and elevated serum calcium levels. In secondary hyperparathyroidism, which develops in patients with hemodialysis or renal transplant, patients may have a nonspecific clinical appearance. Preoperative localization of abnormal parathyroid glands can be achieved using single or multiple imaging modalities (thin-section pre- and post-contrast-enhanced computed tomography, ultrasound, and dual-phase 99mTc-methoxyisobutylnitrile [MIBI] of the neck and chest) [12, 13].

Ultrasound is not commonly used to assess the adrenal glands in adults. Although computed tomography (CT) may be superior in imaging the adrenal glands in most instances, there are some pathologies of the adrenal gland that may be assessed with ultrasound. Some clinical indications for imaging the adrenal glands can include suspicions for adrenal lesions in the cortex and/or medulla. Adrenal hypofunction syndromes include adrenal insufficiency and adrenal atrophy caused by disorders of the pituitary, resulting in decreased adrenocorticotropic hormone (ACTH) production. Some hyperfunction pathologies include Cushing syndrome, which is an excess of cortisol secretion caused by pathologies such as adrenal hyperplasia, benign/malignant cortical neoplasms of the adrenal cortex. There are also medullary hyperfunctions that can be caused by medullary neoplasms [4, 14].

Ultrasound Techniques

Thyroid and Parathyroid

To image the thyroid and parathyroid glands, start by placing the patient in the supine position with a pillow under the shoulders to allow proper neck extension. With ultrasound gel, the operator places the transducer in the transverse and sagittal planes on the patient's neck, just above the sternal notch and between the distal attachments of the sternocleidomastoid muscles [11]. The thyroid appears as a relatively uniform structure in ultrasound images (Fig. 11.4).

A linear array transducer with 8–15 MHz (dependent on the depth of the thyroid glands) is suitable for scanning thyroid and parathyroid glands [12, 13]. Grayscale image and color flow imaging are basic imaging methods used to assess the morphology, homogeneity, and vascularity of the thyroid and parathyroid glands. Findings such as hyper or hypoechoic nodules could be suggestive of pathologic processes and would warrant further investigation, potentially even FNA. If nodules are found, the size and location of the nodules should be recorded. The thyroid should be maximally revealed to measure the thyroid and parathyroid glands in three dimensions (length, width, and anterior-posterior) accurately [11].

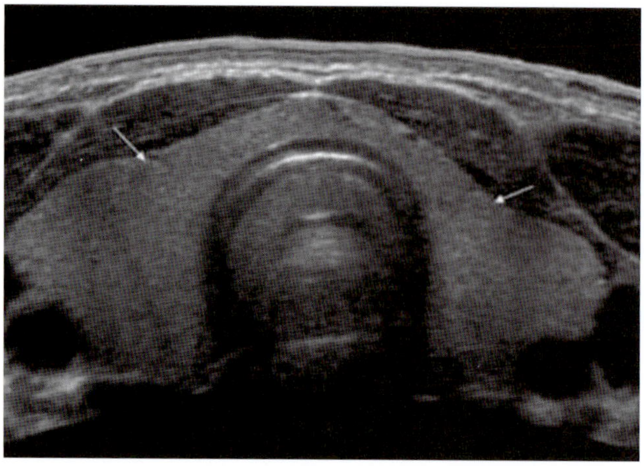

FIGURE 11.4 Transverse B-mode ultrasound image of normal thyroid gland (arrows).

Visualization of the parathyroid is a technical challenge due to its small size and deep location. Using the thyroid gland and peripheral vessels as landmarks, navigate around the thyroid into the lateral-medial, inferior-superior, and deeper aspects of each lobe [15]. In most cases, the parathyroid glands will be found near the thyroid capsule, and when parathyroid glands are enlarged, such as parathyroid adenomas [15].

Adrenal Glands

A curvilinear transducer with 3–5 MHz is used to image adrenal glands. Depth of the image is adjusted based on the patient's body habitus. Scanning is similar to imaging the kidneys; the supine and lateral decubitus positions are suitable, and the transducer is placed along the mid-axillary line to image the adrenal gland. The upper pole of the right kidney and the IVC are used as anatomic landmarks to search for the right adrenal gland. The upper pole of the left kidney and aorta are used to locate the left adrenal gland [4, 14]. In normal adults, it is challenging to optimize the triangle or wedge-shaped adrenal gland due to its small size and deep retroperitoneal location. An enlarged adrenal gland in adults and in neonates can be visualized in grayscale images. Generally, CT is superior to ultrasound in the assessment of adrenal gland pathologies [16, 17].

Common Pathologies

Thyroid Pathologies

Goiter Goiter is an abnormal enlargement of the thyroid gland found on physical examination and requires additional lab work to differentiate among the multiple possible etiologies. Goiters may be present in thyroid pathologies such as Grave's disease, Hashimoto's thyroiditis, and thyroid nodules. The ability to quickly screen

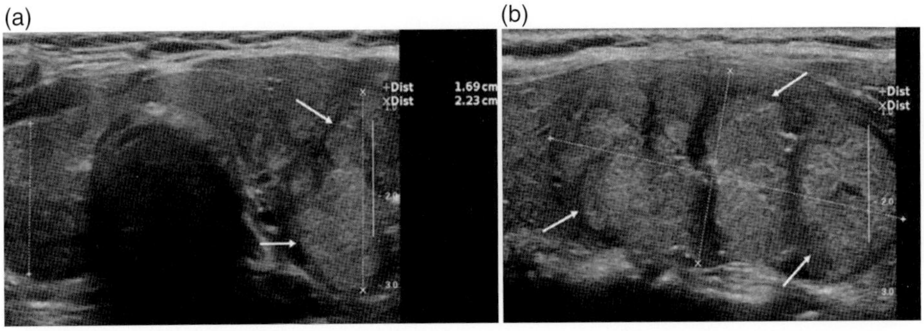

FIGURE 11.5 Multinodular goiter is present in the thyroid. Transverse (a) and longitudinal (b) B-mode ultrasound images show enlargement of the left lobe with multiple hyperechoic nodules (arrows).

the thyroid and recognize the changes specific to each pathology can be a tremendous advantage in differential diagnosis. It is important to note that not all thyroid enlargements are associated with an underlying pathology. One of the most common and historically relevant causes of thyroid enlargement, especially in the underdeveloped world, is iodine deficiency due to reduced dietary intake, and it should be considered when diagnosing thyroid disorders [18]. Multiple nodular goiters appearing with multiple hyperechoic nodules, with or without degeneration of the thyroid gland, are the most common cause of thyroid enlargement (Fig. 11.5).

Hashimoto's Thyroiditis Causes of thyroiditis include, but are not limited to, autoimmune disease, post-surgery, trauma, and other inflammatory causes. Hashimoto's thyroiditis is the most common type of thyroiditis [19]. If left untreated, it often results in hypothyroidism due to autoimmune destruction of the thyroid gland. Clinical manifestations of Hashimoto's thyroiditis include an enlarged thyroid gland (early stage), weight gain, cold sensitivity, dry skin, and fatigue [20]. Thyroid ultrasound can help provide additional morphologic imaging evidence to support a diagnosis of Hashimoto's in addition to laboratory tests [21].

Upon thyroid ultrasound, Hashimoto's will typically present with gland enlargement and diffuse small hypoechoic areas throughout the thyroid gland in the early stage of the disease. These findings can distinguish thyroiditis from possible malignant nodules or multinodular goiters. An increase in the vascularity on color flow imaging is a sign of an early stage of thyroiditis. In the late stage of thyroiditis, gland vascularity on color flow imaging can be normal (Fig. 11.6) or decreased vascularity [20]. Thyroid atrophy may appear as small-sized glands and hyperechoic echotextures in B-mode ultrasound in patients with long-term thyroiditis [22].

Grave's Disease and Hyperthyroidism Grave's disease is characterized as an autoimmune condition in which the body produces autoantibodies to the thyrotropin receptor on the thyroid gland, stimulating production and release of thyroid hormone. The consequent overstimulation of the thyroid leads to elevated thyroid hormone levels and hyperthyroidism [23].

Clinical manifestations of Grave's disease include thyroid enlargement, weight loss, heat intolerance, moist skin, anxiety, and peripheral tremors. If a visible or palpable goiter with suspicion of Grave's disease or hyperthyroidism, ultrasound can be used to add morphological information to the physical examination of the thyroid [20].

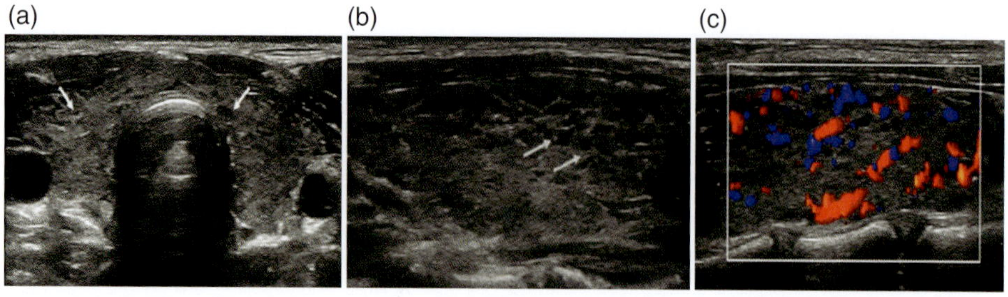

FIGURE 11.6 Thyroid ultrasound image recorded from a patient with Hashimoto's thyroiditis. Transverse plane of thyroid demonstrates diffuse, ill-defined, and hypoechoic areas in both left and right lobes (arrows) of the thyroid (a). Longitudinal images of the right lobe show multiple tiny hypoechoic nodules (white arrows) on B-mode ultrasound image (b) and mildly increased vascularity on color flow imaging (c).

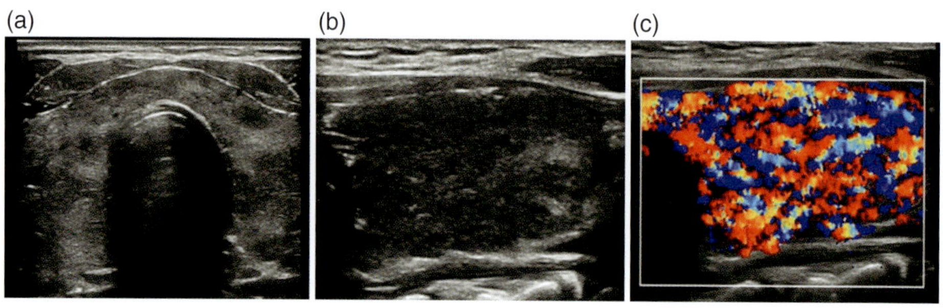

FIGURE 11.7 Thyroid with Grave's disease. (a) Transverse image of the thyroid gland shows mild enlargement of both thyroid lobes and the isthmus. The gland is diffusely hypoechoic and heterogeneous; (b) longitudinal image of the left lobe shows decreased echogenicity on B-mode image; (c) color flow imaging shows hypervascularity in the thyroid.

Grave's disease usually presents with the thyroid appearing diffusely enlarged and hypoechoic. Findings of increased vasculature and hyperemia throughout the thyroid may be suggestive of a Grave's disease (Fig. 11.7), and laboratory testing and clinical information are useful for a definitive diagnosis.

Toxic Adenoma and Multinodular Toxic Goiter The presence of a focal nodule with hypervascularity, as opposed to diffused nodules seen in Grave's disease, hints toward the possibility of a hormone-producing adenoma (single overproducing lesion) or multinodular toxic goiter (multiple overproducing lesions) [24]. Due to the underlying likelihood of a malignancy, thyroid scintigraphy is a useful tool to differentiate malignant (hot nodule) from benign (cold nodule) nodules and assess pathologies that may cause Grave's like symptoms. Fine needle aspiration cytology (FNAC) of the nodule may be required for further evaluation [25].

Benign Thyroid Nodules and Cyst Thyroid cysts and toxic adenomas are benign thyroid neoplasms [26]. Patients may present with a palpable thyroid mass, dysphagia, and/or signs of toxic adenomas (creating hormone independent of TSH stimulation) [27]. Ultrasound can provide details about its morphology and location and can assist in identifying cystic or solid thyroid lesions.

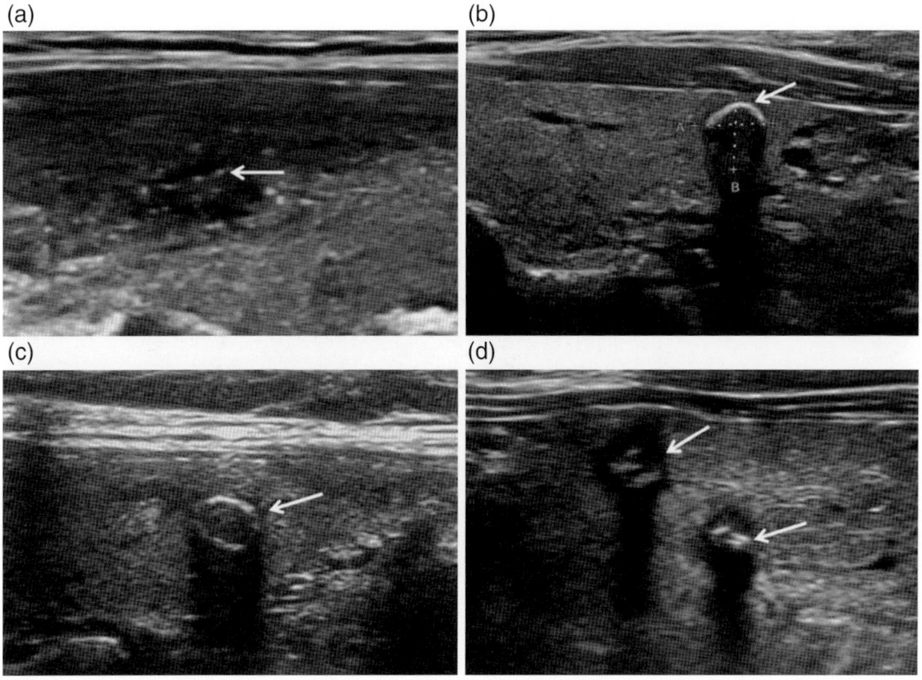

FIGURE 11.8 Thyroid nodules with variable types of calcifications (arrows). (a) Punctate microcalcifications; (b) peripheral calcification; (c) "eggshell" calcification; (d) macrocalcifications.

Using echogenicity alongside careful evaluation of additional characteristics such as calcification, echogenicity, shape, size, and vascularity, the operator can distinguish solid from cystic lesions and assess indications of thyroid malignancy [22].

Calcifications in a thyroid nodule appear hyperechoic. Hyperechoic structures are characterized by bright white crescents on the image surrounding the suspected nodule, also known as "halos" [21]. Acoustic shadowing may appear behind a large calcification (Fig. 11.8). Calcification patterns can help differentiate between benign or malignant nodules. Large calcifications (macrocalcification) with well-defined borders are usually suggestive of a benign lesion, whereas microcalcification (punctate microcalcifications) with irregular borders (Fig. 11.8) need further evaluation, such as FNA, with suspicion of malignancy [26].

These key features of both benign and malignant thyroid nodules can be instrumental in diagnosis, especially in terms of preventing unnecessary testing for a benign lesion. Cysts usually appear anechoic, colloid-filled, and possessing a "comet tail future" [28]. Honeycomb or sponge appearance nodules with microcystic spaces are indicators of benign nodules [29, 30].

Color flow imaging is also a key tool in the assessment of focal and diffuse thyroid pathologies. Varying intensity of color-coded Doppler signals can provide valuable information on the likelihood of malignancy versus a benign lesion. A focal nodule with high vascularity in color follow imaging may increase the chance of malignancy (Fig. 11.9).

Papillary Thyroid Carcinoma Papillary thyroid carcinoma (PTC) is the most common thyroid cancer [31]. This neoplasm should be considered if a hypoechoic mass is found with its border extending outside of the thyroid, and FNA

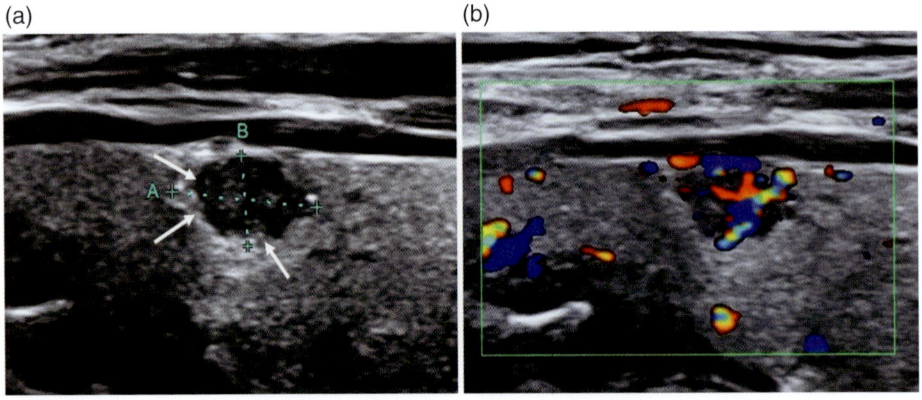

FIGURE 11.9 Multiple punctate calcifications (arrows) in a hypoechoic thyroid nodule in B-mode image (a). The nodule with hypervascularity displays in color flow imaging (b).

should be requested for a definitive diagnosis [32]. As discussed earlier, suspicion for malignancy should rise when a thyroid nodule appears as a solid aspect, marked hypoechogenic, taller-than-wide shape, irregular margin, extrathyroidal extension, microcalcification, and hypervascularity in ultrasound (Fig. 11.9).

Parathyroid Gland Pathologies

Primary Hyperparathyroidism Primary hyperparathyroidism is the hyperfunction of the parathyroid glands from oversecretion of PTH, which is commonly caused by adenoma, hyperplasia, and PTH carcinoma. 80% of patients are asymptomatic, and pathology is only detected by blood test [12]. Parathyroid adenomas and parathyroid hyperplasia inappropriately overproduce PTH, and a subsequent increase in blood calcium levels is seen. Hypercalcemia from bone breakdown ensues, causing pathological conditions (fractures). Common lab findings and clinical features of hyperparathyroidism include elevated serum levels of intact PTH, elevated serum calcium, abnormal bone density, and nephrolithiasis. Ultrasound of the parathyroid glands may be useful in detecting parathyroid adenomas, the most common (approximately 85%) cause of primary hyperparathyroidism [33].

Parathyroid adenomas in ultrasound images appear as round or multi-lobular hypoechoic nodules located in close proximity to the parathyroid glands (see anatomy section), with most cases having a single adenoma [33]. Adenomas are easily detectable once they reach 1 cm in diameter, but have the potential of growing much larger. Ultrasound can help determine if the adenoma is uninodular or multinodular. Color flow imaging may be used to show feeding vessels and vascularization of glands, which may help determine the likelihood of a hyperfunctional neoplasm (Fig. 11.10). FNA is not requested in most parathyroid adenomas unless an intrathyroid parathyroid adenoma is suspected.

Secondary Hyperparathyroidism Secondary hyperparathyroidism occurs secondary to the patient undergoing hemodialysis and/or post renal transplantation, due to the reaction of the parathyroid glands to a hypocalcemic state. The main pathologic changes seen in parathyroid glands are parathyroid hyperplasia, which commonly involves all four glands (Fig. 11.11). Secondary hyperparathyroidism may

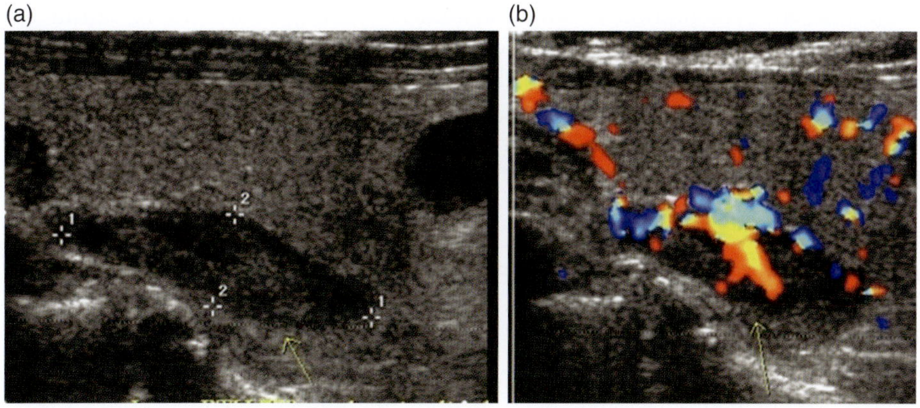

FIGURE 11.10 Longitudinal B-mode (a) and color flow imaging (b) of the thyroid and parathyroid glands (yellow arrow) taken from a 65-year-old woman with high serum calcium and high parathyroid hormone. The parathyroid gland is significantly enlarged and measures 1.1 cm (length) × 0.7 cm (anterior-posterior). Parathyroid gland is located deep to the thyroid, appearing hypoechoic in B-mode image. In addition, parathyroid adenoma and associated vessels are demonstrated in color flow imaging.

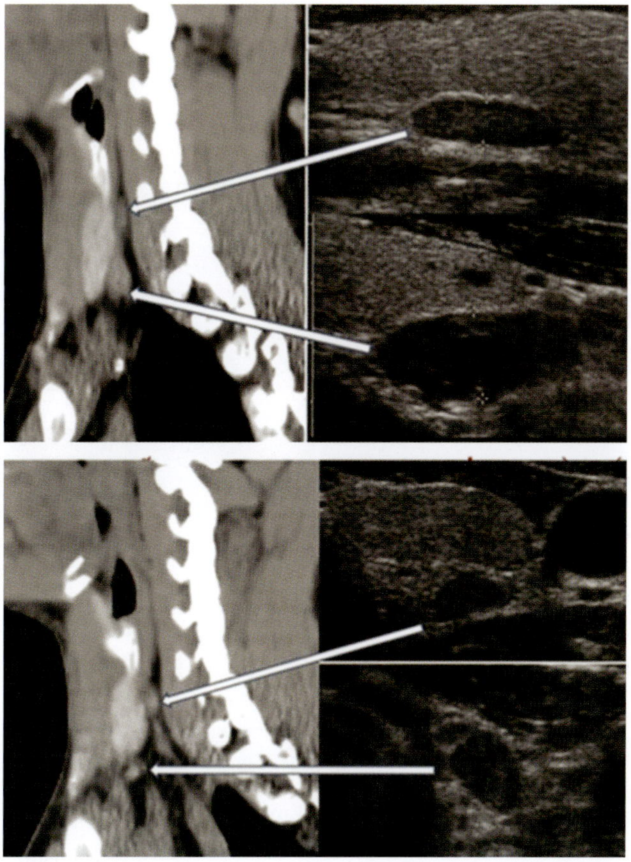

FIGURE 11.11 Thin-section CT (coronal view) and B-mode ultrasound of the thyroid and parathyroid glands are performed on a 56-year-old patient who has been on hemodialysis for eight years. Enlargement of all four parathyroid glands (arrows) is clearly visualized on both CT and ultrasound images.

have different presentations; serum calcium levels may be normal or minimally elevated. It may also be asymptomatic, with no renal calculus (different from primary hyperparathyroidism). CT and ultrasound can show enlargement of all glands in secondary hyperparathyroidism [15, 33]. The shape, echogenicity, and vascularity of parathyroid glands in secondary hyperparathyroidism appear similar to those in primary hyperparathyroidism.

Adrenal Glands Pathologies

Neuroblastoma Neuroblastoma is the second most common abdominal tumor in childhood, mainly occurring in children under five years of age [34]. Approximately 35% of neuroblastomas develop from the adrenal medulla, the rest from the sympathetic chain of the nervous system. Neuroblastomas may present as an asymptomatic abdominal mass or may show symptoms related to metastases or the secretion of catecholamines. Ultrasound is useful in assessing the extent of the local primary tumor and for the detection of liver metastases. Most neuroblastomas are very large and predominantly hyperechoic (Fig. 11.12). Neuroblastomas may appear as heterogeneous masses with calcification and hemorrhage [35].

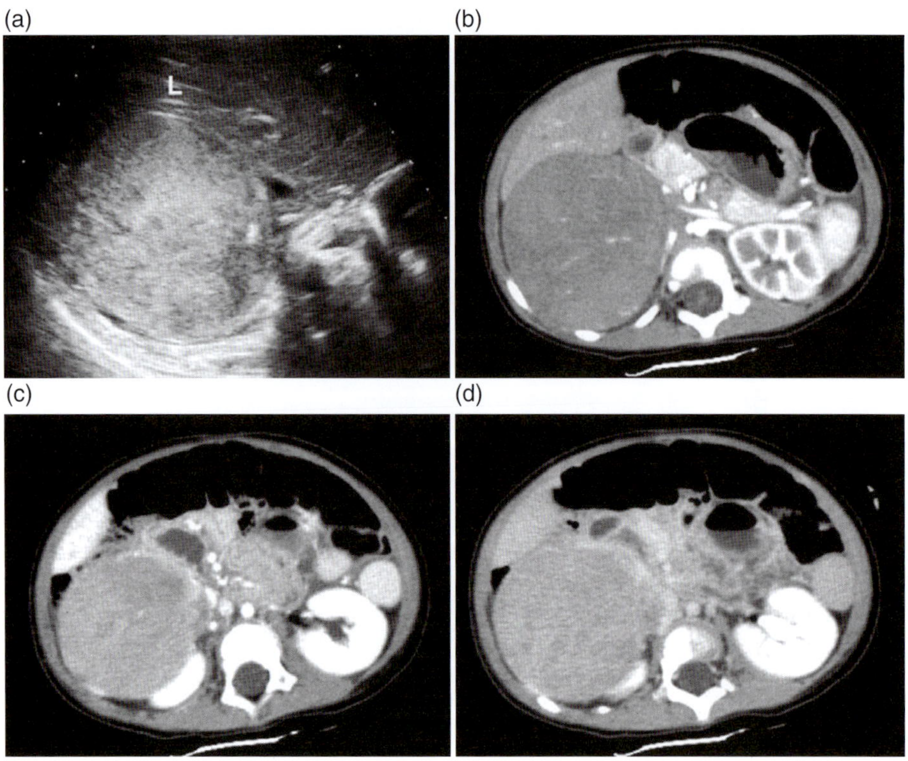

FIGURE 11.12 Neuroblastoma. (a) Transverse B-mode ultrasound image of the right upper abdomen demonstrates a large and hyperechoic solid mass in a 3-year-old girl; (b–d) contrast-enhanced CT demonstrates that the right adrenal mass is slightly enhanced in the artery phase (b), venous phase (c), and delay phase (d) with a round shape and well-defined margin. L, liver.

Adenoma of the Adrenal Cortex Adrenal adenomas represent the most common adrenal tumor; 10% of adrenal adenomas are bilateral, and their incidence increases with age. Adenomas are reported in patients with hypertension, diabetes, hyperthyroidism, and renal cell carcinoma [36]. Adenomas can be classified as either non-hyperfunctioning or hyperfunctioning. Most adenomas (90%) are non-hyperfunctioning and are often discovered incidentally in abdominal CT and MRI. Hyperfunctioning adenomas tend to present clinically with symptoms related to excessive production of hormones, including cortisol and aldosterone. Cushing's syndrome is caused by elevated ACTH production, which may come from a pituitary adenoma. It is characterized by truncal obesity, hirsutism, amenorrhea, hypertension, and weakness. Conn's syndrome results from the excessive secretion of aldosterone in about 70% of adrenal adenoma. Clinical features reveal hypertension, weakness, and tetany, and biochemical tests show hypokalemia, hypernatremia, and raised urine and serum aldosterone levels.

Adrenal adenomas may be discovered on ultrasound, which appear as small, round, well-defined solid masses (Fig. 11.13) [37]. However, differential diagnosis among various solid tumors and tumor-like lesions of adrenal glands is difficult with ultrasound alone. CT or MRI is necessary for further assessment [37].

Adrenal Hemorrhage in Neonates The neonatal adrenal gland undergoes a marked reduction in size following birth. The vessels in the primitive adrenal cortex become distended and are prone to hemorrhage. It is also reported that obstetric trauma, hypoxia, or coagulation disorders are related to adrenal hemorrhage in newborns. Infants usually show symptoms within 2–7 days of birth. Hemorrhage is more commonly seen on the right side, although up to 10% are bilateral [38]. Adrenal hematomas predominantly occur in the medulla. However, in some circumstances, the cortex may be stretched or disrupted, resulting in periadrenal hemorrhage. Clinical manifestations of neonatal adrenal hemorrhage are abdominal mass [38].

Ultrasound imaging is a routine method in the assessment of the adrenal glands in neonates. Acute adrenal hematomas are often anechoic but may be more reflective

(a) (b)

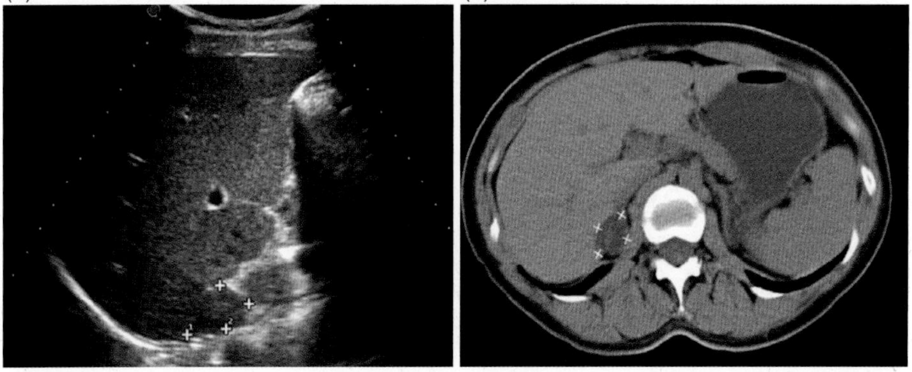

FIGURE 11.13 Adrenal adenoma. (a) B-mode ultrasound in transverse plane shows a small, solid right adrenal mass between the liver and upper pole of right kidney (between calipers); (b) CT scan demonstrates the classic low attenuation lesion in the right adrenal gland, indicating an adrenal adenoma (between calipers).

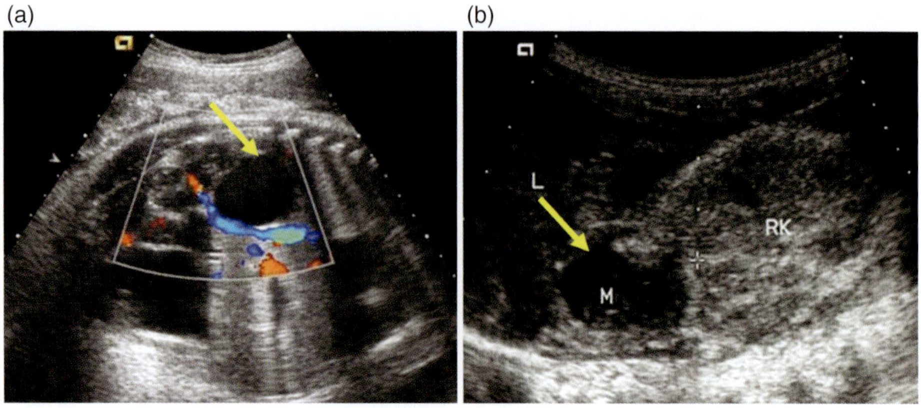

FIGURE 11.14 (a) Prenatal (third trimester) color flow imaging shows an anechoic, avascular area (yellow arrow) located in the fetal right adrenal gland region (between the liver and upper pole of the right kidney); (b) Follow-up B-mode ultrasound shows an increase in echogenicity and heterogeneity in the adrenal region (yellow arrow) after birth. L, liver; M, mass in the right adrenal region; RK, right kidney.

due to fibrin strand formation (Fig. 11.14). Hematomas may become smaller and lose reflectivity with clot liquefaction and will usually resolve with time, rarely requiring any intervention.

Summary

Ultrasound has proven to be a valuable imaging modality that is routinely used in assessing pathologies in endocrine organs. Ultrasound imaging is useful in assessing morphology and vascularity in the differentiation between malignant and benign thyroid nodules. Preoperative localization of abnormal parathyroid glands can be achieved using ultrasound and other imaging modalities such as thin-section neck CT with and without intravenous contrast or sestamibi (MIBI) scan. Although ultrasound is not the first-line imaging modality to visualize adrenal gland in adults, some large-sized neoplasms of the adrenal gland can be revealed in ultrasound and confirmed using a CT scan. Ultrasound is the first imaging modality of choice to assess adrenal hemorrhage in neonates.

Review Questions

1. An important feature for distinguishing thyroid carcinoma from Hashimoto's thyroiditis on ultrasound is
   - **a.** Degree of calcification
   - **b.** Increased vascularity
   - **c.** Hyperechoic focal nodule
   - **d.** Hypoechoic focal nodule with punctate calcifications

2. In ultrasound images, parathyroid gland(s) in a patient with hyperparathyroidism may appear
   - **a.** Multiple small, calcified nodules
   - **b.** A single large hypoechoic nodule where the parathyroid glands are suspected
   - **c.** Multi-lobular hypoechoic thyroid nodules
   - **d.** Highly vascular nodules appear throughout the thyroid
3. What ultrasound scanning frequency should be used to scan thyroid and parathyroid?
   - **a.** 1–5 MHz
   - **b.** 10–15 MHz
   - **c.** 30–40 MHz
   - **d.** 2–5 MHz
4. What does an increased vascularity in the thyroid gland indicate?
   - **a.** Thyroid abscess
   - **b.** Grave's disease
   - **c.** Thyroid cyst
   - **d.** Normal thyroid tissue
5. What would be suggested if calcifications extend beyond the border of the thyroid?
   - **a.** Papillary thyroid carcinoma
   - **b.** Benign nodule
   - **c.** Normal thyroid
   - **d.** Graves
   - **e.** Hashimoto's
6. How many parathyroid glands are there typically near the right lobe of the thyroid?
   - **a.** 1
   - **b.** 2
   - **c.** 3
   - **d.** 4
7. Where might you find ectopic thyroid?
   - **a.** Along the esophagus
   - **b.** Along the cervical vertebrae
   - **c.** Along the trachea
   - **d.** Along the common carotid arteries
8. What patient position is suitable for performing thyroid ultrasound?
   - **a.** Prone
   - **b.** Left lateral decubitus
   - **c.** Supine
   - **d.** Right lateral decubitus
9. Thyroid papillary carcinoma is highly suspected if
   - **a.** There is a decrease in vasculature of the surrounding tissue
   - **b.** A well-defined calcified mass is noted
   - **c.** A small, regularly shaped hypoechoic nodule is found
   - **d.** Borders of the nodule are found to extend beyond the thyroid tissue

10. Which is **NOT** an indication to suspect Hashimoto's?

- **a.** Goiter
- **b.** Cold sensitivity
- **c.** Dry skin
- **d.** Weight loss
- **e.** Gained weight

Correct answers: 1. d; 2. b; 3. b; 4. b; 5. a; 6. b; 7. c; 8. c; 9. d; 10. d.

References

1. National Evaluation Systems Inc. The endocrine system [and] instructor's guide: the endocrine system. In: Health occupations education module: instructional materials in anatomy and physiology for Pennsylvania health occupations programs. Amherst, MA: National Evaluation Systems Inc, 1980.
2. Helfand M. Screening for thyroid disease: systematic evidence review. Medicare coverage of routine screening for thyroid dysfunction, 2003. https://www.ncbi.nlm.nih.gov/books/NBK221542/.
3. Powers AE, Marcadis AR, Lee M, et al. Changes in trends in thyroid cancer incidence in the United States, 1992 to 2016. *JAMA* 2019; 322: 2440–2441.
4. Mayo-Smith WW, Boland GW, Noto RB, Lee MJ. State-of-the-art adrenal imaging. *Radiographics* 2001; 21: 995–1012.
5. Moore KL, Agur AMR, Dalley AF II, Moore KL. Chapter 9, Parathyroid. In: Moore's essential clinical anatomy. 6th ed. Wolters Kluwer, 2019; 1029–1031.
6. Miller FR. Surgical anatomy of the thyroid and parathyroid glands. *Otolaryngol Clin N Am* 2003; 36(1): 1–7.
7. Judith ER, Saba B. Anatomy of the pituitary, thyroid, parathyroid and adrenal glands. *Surgery (Oxford)* 2011; 9: 403. https://doi.org/10.1016/j.mpsur.2011.06.006.
8. Friedman TC. Adrenal gland. In: Benjamin IJ, Griggs RC, Wing EJ, Fitz JG (eds). Andreoli and Carpenter's Cecil essentials of medicine. 9th ed. Philadelphia, PA: Elsevier Saunders, 2016; chap 64.
9. Standring S. Suprarenal (adrenal) gland. In: Standring S (ed.). Gray's Anatomy. 41st ed. Philadelphia, PA: Elsevier, 2016; chap 71.
10. Mirilas P, Skandalakis JE, Colborn GL, et al. Surgical anatomy: the embryologic and anatomic basis of modern surgery. New York, New York, USA: McGraw-Hill Professional Publishing, 2004. ISBN 978-960-399-074-1.
11. Chaudhary V, Bano S. Thyroid ultrasound. *Indian J Endocrinol Metab* 2013; 17: 219–227. https://doi.org/10.4103/2230-8210.109667.
12. Haciyanli M, Lal G, Morita E, et al. Accuracy of preoperative localization studies and intraoperative parathyroid hormone assay in patients with primary hyperparathyroidism and double adenoma. *J Am Coll Surg* 2003; 197: 739–746.
13. Sukan A, Peyhan M, Aydin M, et al. Preoperative evaluation of hyperthyroidism: the role of dual-phase parathyroid scintigraphy and ultrasound imaging. *Ann Nucl Med* 2008; 22: 123–131.
14. Carir E, Aydin NE, Samdanci E, et al. Cystic adrenal lymphangioma–report of two cases and review of the literature. *J Pak Med Assoc* 2012; 62: 962–964.
15. Sung JY. Parathyroid ultrasonography: the evolving role of the radiologist. *Ultrasonography* 2015; 34(4): 268–274. https://doi.org/10.14366/usg.14071.
16. Chira RI, Chira A, Manzat-Saplacan R-M, et al. Adrenal glands transabdominal ultrasonography - pictorial essay. *Med Ultrason* 2017; 19: 318–323. https://doi.org/10.11152/mu-978.

17. Decmann Á, Perge P, Tóth M, Igaz P. Adrenal myelolipoma: a comprehensive review. *Endocrine* 2018; 59: 7–15. https://doi.org/10.1007/s12020-017-1473-4.
18. Eastman CJ, Zimmermann MB. The iodine deficiency disorders. In: Feingold KR, Anawalt B, Boyce A, et al. (eds). Endotext [Internet]. South Dartmouth, MA: http://MDText.com, Inc., 2000. https://www.ncbi.nlm.nih.gov/books/NBK285556.
19. Pishdad P, Pishdad GR, Tavanaa S, et al. Thyroid ultrasonography in differentiation between graves' disease and Hashimoto's thyroiditis. *J Biomed Phys Eng* 2017; 7: 21–26.
20. Fitzgerald PA. Thyroiditis. In: Papadakis MA, McPhee SJ, Rabow MW (eds). Current Medical Diagnosis and Treatment 2020. New York: McGraw-Hill Professional Publishing. ISBN 978-960-399-074-1.
21. Jameson JL. Principles of endocrinology. In: Jameson JL (ed.). Endocrinology: adult and pediatric. Elsevier, 2016. https://doi.org/10.1016/b978-0-323-18907-1.00001-9.
22. Blum M. Ultrasonography of the thyroid. Endotext [Internet], 2015. https://www.ncbi.nlm.nih.gov/books/NBK285555.
23. Latif R, Morshed SA, Zaidi M, Davies TF. The thyroid-stimulating hormone receptor: impact of thyroid-stimulating hormone and thyroid-stimulating hormone receptor antibodies on multimerization, cleavage, and signaling. *Endocrinol Metab Clin N Am* 2009; 38(2): 319–341. https://doi.org/10.1016/j.ecl.2009.01.006.
24. Medeiros-Neto G. Multinodular Goiter. In: Feingold KR, Anawalt B, Boyce A, et al. (eds). Endotext [Internet]. South Dartmouth, MA: http://MDText.com, Inc., 2000. https://www.ncbi.nlm.nih.gov/books/NBK285569.
25. Bahn RS, Castro R. Approach to the patient with nontoxic multinodular goiter. *J Clin Endocrinol Metab* 2011; 96: 1202–1212.
26. Liu YI, Kamaya A, Desser TS, Rubin DL. A Bayesian classifier for differentiating benign versus malignant thyroid nodules using sonographic features. *AMIA Annu Symp Proc* 2008; 2008: 419–423.
27. Cotran RS, Abbas AK, Kumar V, et al. Robbins and Cotran pathologic basis of disease. Philadelphia, USA: WB Saunders Company, 2015.
28. Perros P, Boelaert K, Colley S, et al. Guidelines for the management of thyroid cancer. *Clin Endocrinol* 2014; 81: 1–122. https://doi.org/10.1111/cen.12515.
29. Moon WJ, Jung SL, Lee JH, et al. Benign and malignant thyroid nodules: US differentiation–multicenter retrospective study. *Radiology* 2008; 247: 762–770.
30. Kim BM, Kim MJ, Kim EK, et al. Sonographic differentiation of thyroid nodules with eggshell calcifications. *J Ultrasound Med* 2008; 27: 1425–1430.
31. Siegel RL, Miller KD, Jemal A. Cancer statistics. *CA Cancer J Clin* 2019; 69: 7–34. https://doi.org/10.3322/caac.21551.
32. Hahn SY, Han BK, Ko EY, et al. Ultrasound findings of papillary thyroid carcinoma originating in the isthmus: comparison with lobe-originating papillary thyroid carcinoma. *AJR* 2014; 203: 637–642.
33. Johnson NA, Tublin ME, Ogilvie JB. Parathyroid imaging: technique and role in the preoperative evaluation of primary hyperparathyroidism. *AJR* 2007; 188: 1706–1715.
34. Lonergan GJ, Schwab CM, Suarez ES, Carlson CL. Neuroblastoma, ganglioneuroblastoma, and ganglioneuroma: radiologic-pathologic correlation. *Radiographics* 2002; 22(4): 911–934.
35. Hwang SM, Yoo SY, Kim JH, Jeon TY. Congenital adrenal neuroblastoma with and without cystic change: differentiating features with an emphasis on the value of ultrasound. *AJR* 2016; 207(5): 1105–1111.
36. Ambos MA, Bosniak MA, Lefleur RS, Mitty HA. Adrenal adenoma associated with renal cell carcinoma. *AJR* 1981; 136: 81–84.
37. Kim KW, Kim JK, Choi HJ, et al. Sonography of the adrenal glands in the adult. *J Clin Ultrasound* 2012; 40: 357–363.
38. Paterson A. Adrenal pathology in childhood: a spectrum of disease. *Eur Radiol* 2002; 12: 2491–2508.

CHAPTER 12

FAST/EFAST and Emergency Medicine

Jason Lee[1], Raymond Kwong[1], Andy Nigh[1], Ning Guo[2], and Yuan-Yi Zheng[2]

[1] Rocky Vista University, College of Osteopathic Medicine, Ivins, Utah, USA

[2] Department of Ultrasound, Shanghai Sixth People's Hospital, Shanghai Jiaotong University School of Medicine, Shanghai, China

Introduction

Ultrasonography was first introduced during World War II and, since then, has become an important diagnostic tool in patient care [1]. Originally used as an imaging modality exclusively in radiology, ultrasound is now being broadly utilized in many medical specialties [2]. One medical specialty that has vastly increased the use of ultrasound and contributed to its improvement is emergency medicine [2]. Ultrasound's appeal in emergency medicine, especially bedside ultrasound, is due to its availability, accuracy, portability, affordability, and quick results as a method to obtain a wide variety of diagnostic exams [3, 4]. In this chapter, we will highlight several applications of ultrasound in emergency medicine, including its indications, important anatomy, ultrasound techniques, and examination protocols.

FAST/EFAST

Focused assessment with sonography for trauma (FAST) is an ultrasound examination commonly used in emergency and post-trauma situations. The term FAST, coined in 1996, describes a standardized set of ultrasound examinations used when evaluating trauma patients [1]. The FAST exam is a rapid exam that lasts no more than four minutes [5]. It focuses on screening and evaluating bleeds within the torso [2]. Specifically, it evaluates the pericardial and peritoneal spaces for fluid following traumatic injury, such as blunt trauma and penetrating injuries [3].

Another common form of ultrasound used in emergency settings is the extended focused assessment with sonography in trauma (EFAST). EFAST expands upon FAST by providing additional evaluation of the hemithorax by helping to identify pneumothorax and hemothorax [5]. Due to its broader scope and ability to be used in place of a portable chest X-ray, the EFAST exam is quickly becoming incorporated into trauma protocol [3].

FAST/EFAST exam has become a standard of care in trauma management, especially in trauma patients with unstable conditions in rural regions [6]. Although the FAST/EFAST exam cannot replace other radiological imaging modalities, such as X-ray and CT, it still plays an important role in the triaging of patients when deciding whether they require immediate surgical intervention, further investigation, or observation [7]. Although the FAST exam is limited in the assessment of intestines compared with CT, its sensitivity ranges 28.1–100% and the specificity ranges 94.1–100% in detecting peritoneal bleeding [8].

Indications

The general indication for use of the FAST/EFAST exam is evaluating for the presence of traumatic free fluid, such as blood, in the pericardial, peritoneal, or pleural cavities [9]. Any mechanism of injury or symptoms that might suggest the presence of bleeding is an indication for the FAST/EFAST exam [10]. For example common situations include blunt or penetrating trauma to the abdomen or thorax and undifferentiated shock or hypotension. Some symptoms that may indicate further investigation include hypotension, tachycardia, and jugular vein distention [11]. There are no absolute contraindications for the use of the FAST/EFAST exam. However, the exam should be avoided if it would delay or interfere with a patient with clear indications for emergent surgical intervention [3, 9].

Ultrasound Techniques

A 3.5–5 MHz phased-array transducer is ideal for performing the FAST/EFAST exam [6]. Although it cannot provide a high-resolution image or as wide a view as using curvilinear or linear array transducers, it is able to fit into an intercostal space; therefore, minimizing rib shadow when scanning [11]. However, a high-frequency transducer may be preferred when performing the examination of the chest or a pediatric patient [5]. A curvilinear array transducer can also be used as it allows for a higher resolution image and a wider scanning area, but it is more likely to produce rib shadow when scanning the chest and heart [11].

Exam Protocol

The entire exam will be done with the patient supine [3]. The FAST exam will involve scanning the four following areas: right upper quadrant (RUQ), subxiphoid (pericardium), left upper quadrant (LUQ), and suprapubic (pelvis) [5]. The EFAST exam includes these four areas as well as an anterior thoracic view [9]. Each area allows the visualization of several parts of the torso where fluid collection is common (Fig. 12.1).

Right Upper Quadrant (RUQ) Scanning the RUQ allows visualization of the hepatorenal recess (Morison's pouch), the right paracolic gutter, the hepatodiaphragmatic area, and the caudal edge of the left liver lobe [3]. The most important

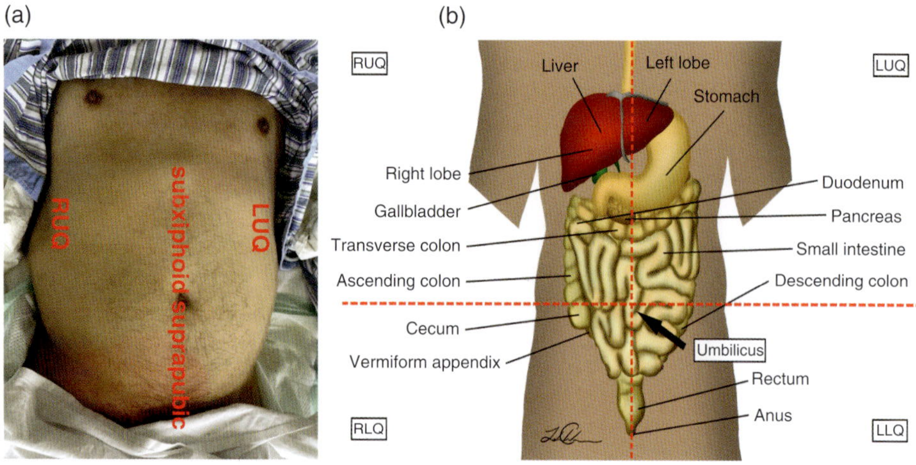

FIGURE 12.1 (a, b) FAST scanning protocol: LLQ, left lower quadrant; RLQ, right lower quadrant; LUQ, left upper quadrant of the abdomen; RUQ, right upper quadrant of the abdomen.

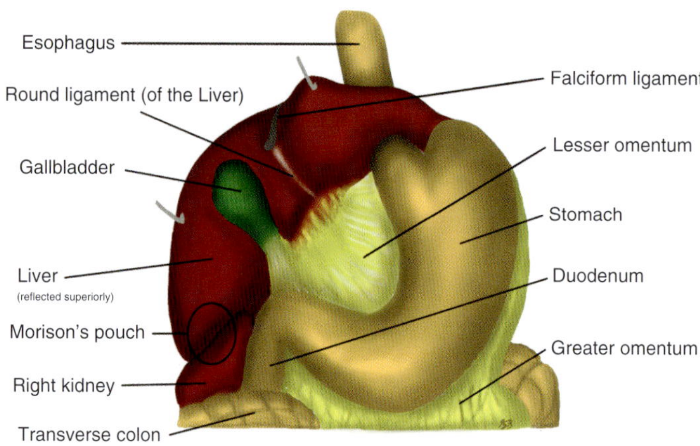

FIGURE 12.2 Illustration of the upper abdomen and Morison's pouch.

region within the RUQ (Fig. 12.2) is the hepatorenal recess (Morison's pouch), which is located between the interface between the liver and right kidney [11]. This is a potential space; therefore, there will be no fluid under normal conditions (Fig. 12.3b). Fluid accumulation in this space indicates a pathology and can be visualized as an anechoic stripe separating the liver and kidney and perihepatic with grayscale ultrasound (Fig. 12.3c) [11].

The following instructions describe the scanning protocol of RUQ [11, 12]:

1. Place the probe on the patient's right side on the midaxillary line between ribs 8 and 11 with the transducer indicator toward the patient's head (Fig. 12.3).
2. Rotate the probe to an oblique angle to fit it into the intercostal space (8–11).
3. If done correctly, this should provide an image containing the patient's liver and kidney interface (Morison's pouch). A positive test presents as a black (anechoic)

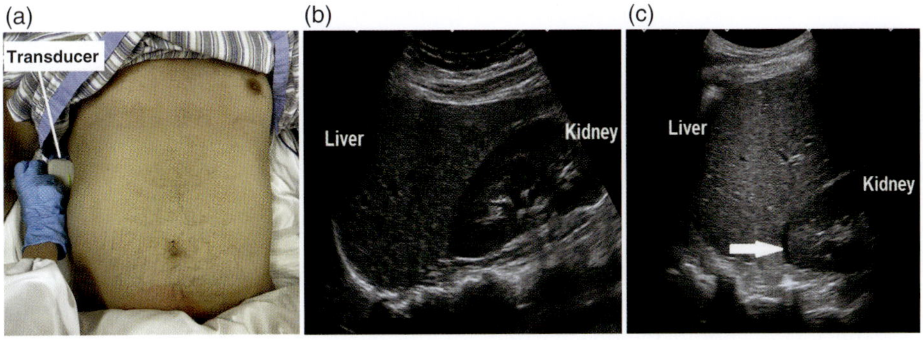

FIGURE 12.3 Placing the transducer on the right midaxillary line between ribs 8–11 (a). Normal hepatorenal recess (b) and abnormal hepatorenal recess (c. anechoic stripe – white arrow) on B-mode ultrasound images.

space between the liver and kidney. The size of the anechoic space depends on the amount of free fluid.

Besides Morison's pouch, it is also important to visualize the space between the liver and diaphragm as it is also susceptible to fluid accumulation. This space can be viewed at the same time and with the same scanning protocol used for Morison's pouch.

Subxiphoid (Subcostal) The subxiphoid view (Fig. 12.4) evaluates the pericardial space [3]. Specifically, it examines if there is any fluid accumulation surrounding the heart, as well as assessing cardiac contractility [5]. A normal pericardium will show a single hyperechoic line surrounding the heart (Fig. 12.4b). Fluid as an anechoic stripe appearing in the pericardium suggests a pericardial effusion (Fig. 12.4c) [6]. Although this scan can also be used to evaluate heart chamber size and global cardiac function, the main purpose of this scan is to assess pericardial effusion [11].

Identifying fluid accumulation in the pericardial space is crucial for the diagnosis of cardiac tamponade [12]. Cardiac tamponade occurs when pressure is applied to the heart because of pericardial fluid buildup. If the right atrial or right ventricular

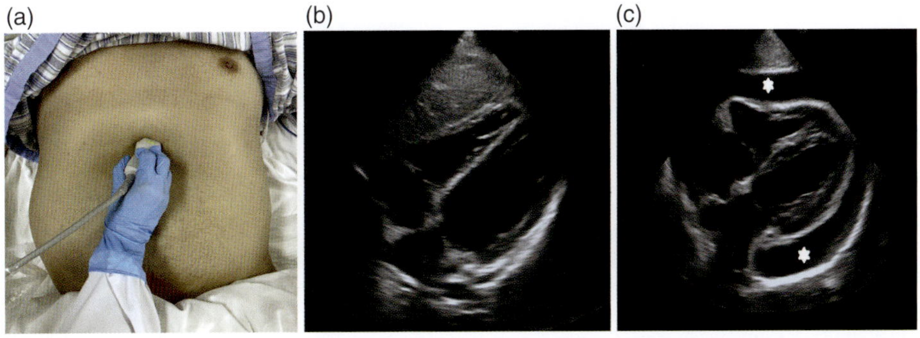

FIGURE 12.4 Placing the transducer below the xiphoid process (a). Normal pericardial space (b) and pericardial effusion (c, white stars) can be identified in B-mode images.

pressure becomes less than the pressure applied by the fluid, the chambers of the heart will not adequately fill. Consequently, cardiac output and ejection fraction will decrease [13].

The following instructions describe the scanning protocol of the subxiphoid view [11, 12]:

1. Locate the patient's xiphoid process by palpating the sternum and following inferiorly until you feel a soft drop-off. The bone before the drop-off is the xiphoid process.
2. Place the transducer just below the xiphoid process
3. The image should include portions of the left lobe of the liver as well as a coronal section of the heart, including its four chambers. The transducer can also be placed slightly to the right of the xiphoid process, directed toward the left shoulder, or flattened to the patient's abdomen with a pincer grip.

Left Upper Quadrant (LUQ) The LUQ scan (Fig. 12.5) is also known as the perisplenic view, as it allows visualization of the spleen and the perisplenic space, below the diaphragm, as well as the hepatorenal recess [9]. Similar to the other scans, a normal ultrasound image shows a thin or flushed space between the spleen-kidney or spleen-diaphragm interfaces (Fig. 12.5b) while a pathologic image will show a widened anechoic stripe indicating free fluid (Fig. 12.5c) [11]. This view has a technical challenge due to the smaller size of the spleen, its posterior positioning, and air from the stomach obscuring the LUQ.

The following instructions describe the scanning protocol for imaging LUQ [11, 12]:

1. Place the transducer on the patient's left posterior axillary line between ribs 6th and 9th (Fig. 12.5). This can easily be done by placing your knuckles on the exam table. This allows avoiding the stomach air and allows the spleen to act as an acoustic window for imaging the kidney.
2. Rotate the probe to an oblique angle to fit it into an intercostal space.

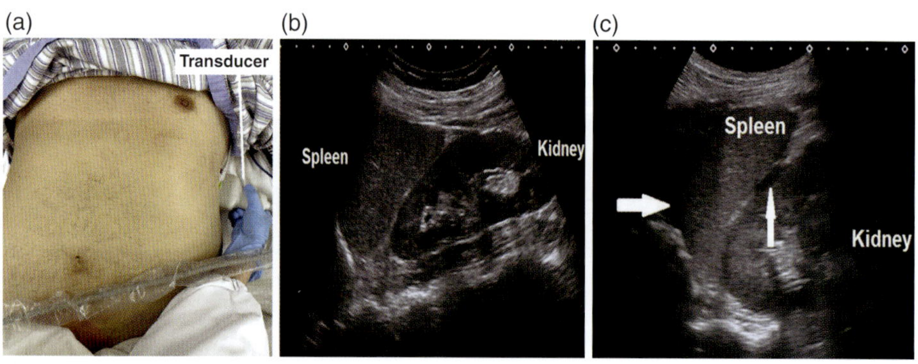

FIGURE 12.5 (a–c) Placing the transducer on the left posterior axillary line between ribs 6–9 (a). Normal perisplenic space (b) and minimal fluid in perisplenic space (c, anechoic stripe-white arrow) can be observed on B-mode ultrasound images.

3. The diaphragm, left kidney, and spleen should be imaged. If all three structures are not visible, try moving the probe superiorly one or two intercostal spaces while maintaining the same angle. Valsalva maneuver may help to improve the visualization of the spleen.

Suprapubic (Pelvis) The suprapubic view provides visualization of any free fluid within the pelvis. The pelvis should be imaged in both a longitudinal and transverse plane and is best done with a fluid-filled bladder [9]. In a male patient, fluid accumulation will typically present as an anechoic space posterior and superior to the bladder in the rectovesicular space (Fig. 12.6). In a female patient, the fluid will accumulate most often in the rectouterine pouch (Fig. 12.7), also known as the pouch of Douglas [11].

The following instructions describe the scanning protocol of suprapubic ultrasound [11, 12]:

1. **Longitudinal view:** Placing the transducer midline 2 cm above the patient's pubic symphysis, that is the cartilaginous joint between the right and left pubic bone midline.

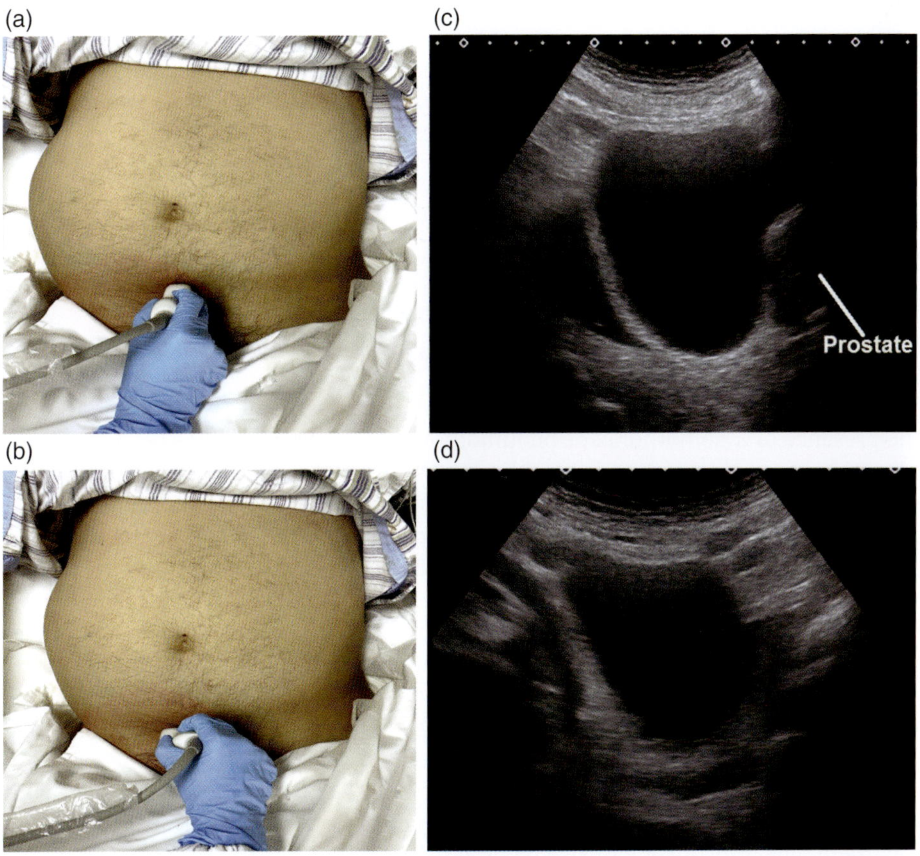

FIGURE 12.6 (a–d) Placing the transducer at suprapubic region longitudinally (a) and transversely (b) to perform pelvic ultrasound. Male pelvis, rectovesicular space can be imaged longitudinally (c) and transversely (d).

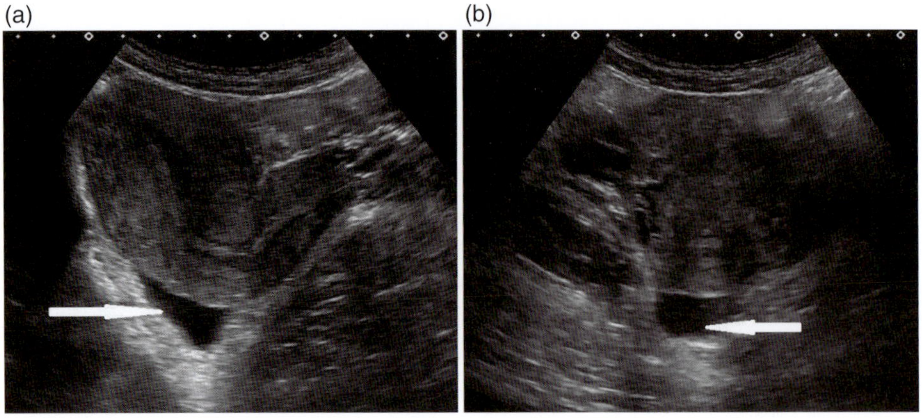

FIGURE 12.7 (a, b) A small amount of free fluid (white arrow) appears in longitudinal (a) and transverse (b) planes of a female pelvic ultrasound.

2. **Transverse view:** Placing the transducer midline 2 cm above the patient's pubic symphysis. In this plane, a common technical error in scanning male patients occurs when the probe is pointed too caudally, resulting in the prostate appearing alongside the bladder. The sound beam from the transducer should point deep into the pelvis to observe the retrovesicular space behind the bladder.

Other Pathologies in EFAST

Hemothorax and Pneumothorax

The anterior thoracic view is a part of the EFAST exam and allows for evaluation of the presence of a hemothorax or pneumothorax [3]. Ultrasound has been proven to be superior in comparison to a portable chest X-ray (PCXR) in evaluating a hemothorax, as it is able to detect a smaller volume of pleural fluid, 50–100 mL versus 175 mL. A hemothorax will appear as an anechoic space superior to the diaphragm [11].

A diagnosis of pneumothorax can be achieved in two different ways. First, as the visceral and parietal pleura slide against one another on B-mode image, they create an artifact known as the "ants marching" sign [5]. A lack of this artifact suggests a pneumothorax [3]. Second, normal lung sliding on M-mode image creates another artifact known as the "seashore" sign (Fig. 12.8a). Presence of a pneumothorax causes a lack of this artifact, replacing it with a "barcode" or "stratosphere" sign (Fig. 12.8b) on M-mode ultrasound image [3].

Unlike the other four areas, the anterior thoracic scan is best performed with a high-frequency transducer, either a phased-array or curvilinear transducer, but a low-frequency transducer can also be used [9]. The depth of the scan should also be set to a maximum of 4 cm unless the patient is extremely obese [11]. The scan should also be performed using both M-mode and B-mode methods. M-mode allows for the evaluation of pleural motion, while B-mode provides ultrasound artifacts and real-time observation of the lung sliding [5].

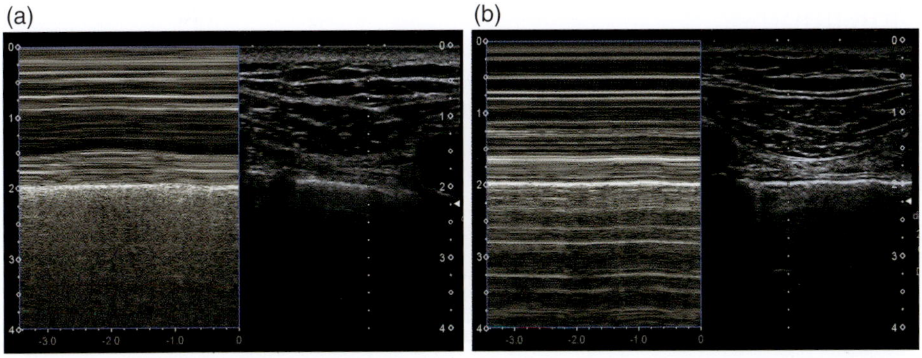

FIGURE 12.8 (a, b) With M-mode ultrasound, "seashore" sign (a) indicates normal, and "barcode" sign (b) suggests pneumothorax.

The following instructions describe the scanning protocol for lung ultrasound [11, 12]:

1. Place the transducer longitudinally, with the indicator pointing toward the patient's head, in the 3rd and 4th intercostal space at the right midclavicular line or the left anterior axillary line.
2. Move the transducer longitudinally until a rib can be seen on both sides of the image.
3. Observe the pleural movement on B-mode and record it with M-mode image.

Abdominal Aortic Aneurysm (AAA)

The aorta enters the abdominal region through the diaphragm around the vertebral level of T12. It then descends inferiorly and bifurcates into the common iliac arteries around the vertebral level of L5 (umbilicus) [14]. An abdominal aortic aneurysm (AAA) is considered when the aorta is dilated with its diameter >3 cm. AAAs often present with a classic triad of hypotension, abdominal or back pain, and a pulsatile abdominal mass [15]. Nonspecific symptoms can also occur such as syncope, weakness, and neurologic changes in the lower extremities [14]. However, because most patients with AAA are asymptomatic, they are often an incidental finding or go underdiagnosed and continue to expand until they rupture [16].

An AAA rupture is a life-threatening event with a mortality rate ranging from 80 to 90% [16]. Even with such a high risk of death, a ruptured AAA can present simply as hypotension. The early diagnosis and repair of an AAA directly improve the patient's outcomes [14]. It is, therefore, important to recognize risk factors for developing an AAA and take them into consideration when determining the diagnosis [15]. Ultrasound has been proven to be an effective method as it is a rapid, accessible, noninvasive, and reproducible method of assessment for the presence of an aneurysm, follow-up the progression, and determination of risk for rupture [17].

Indications

Indications for evaluation of an AAA are based on common symptoms such as abdominal, back, or chest pain, pulsatile abdominal mass, renal colic, syncope, or hypotension, and medical history of the patient [14]. Certain risk factors such as age older than 65 years, male sex, and smoking history may also indicate a need for screening [15]. It is recommended that a one-time screening for AAA be performed with men aged 65–75 years without smoking by the US Preventive Services Task Force [18]. The use of ultrasound does not have any absolute contraindications; however, it should be avoided if it would delay or interfere with a patient with clear indications for emergent surgical intervention [9]. Ultrasound may also be less effective in imaging the abdominal aorta in obese patients or those with increased bowel gas [19].

Ultrasound Techniques

A 2–5 MHz curvilinear probe or 1–5 MHz phased-array probe may be used [20].

Exam Procedure

The following instructions describe the protocol for scanning abdominal aorta [14, 20]:

1. Begin the examination with the patient supine.
2. Place the transducer just below the xiphoid process. The exam should be repeated with both transverse and longitudinal planes.
   a. Three portions of the aorta (proximal, middle, and distal) will be scanned from below the xiphoid process until the bifurcation and common iliac arteries.
   b. As the aorta is scanned, measurements of diameter should be taken. A normal diameter of the aorta measures <3 cm.
3. Once the transducer is placed transversely, identify the vertebral body, aorta, and IVC (Fig. 12.9a). The vertebral body appears horseshoe-shaped with a

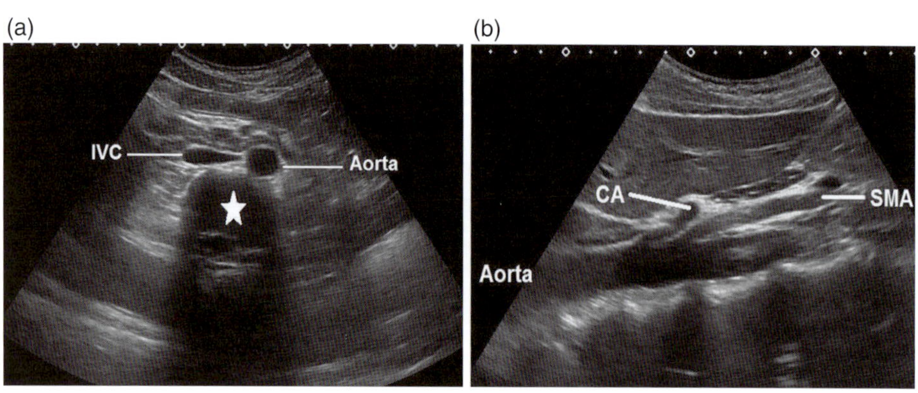

FIGURE 12.9 Transverse plane of the abdominal aorta (Aorta) and inferior vena cava (IVC) anterior to vertebral body (*) (a). Longitudinal plane of the abdominal aorta and its branches of celiac trunk (CA) and superior mesenteric artery (SMA) (b).

hyperechoic anterior surface and a posterior shadow. The aorta lies in the anterior and slightly left of the vertebral body. The inferior vena cava lies anterior and slightly right of the vertebral body.

4. Continue to scan longitudinally, the celiac trunk (the first branch) and superior mesenteric artery (the second branch) off the aorta can be revealed in the proximal portion (Fig. 12.9b), and then the aortic bifurcation at the vertebral level of L5.

Acute Appendicitis

Introduction

The appendix is a blind-ending pouch located on the inferior portion of the large intestine (cecum) near the junction of large and small intestine in the RLQ [21]. Acute inflammation of the appendix is referred to as acute appendicitis. Acute appendicitis classically presents with the triad of RLQ pain, fever, and vomiting [22]. Abdominal pain is the most common symptom, but patients also frequently present with nausea, anorexia, vomiting, and diarrhea or constipation [23]. Perforation or rupture of the appendix is possible and is the most common abdominal emergency [24]. Because of the unpredictability of rupture along with the nonspecific or overlapping symptoms with other diseases, acute appendicitis can be difficult to diagnose [24]. Ultrasound has a reported sensitivity of 67–100% and specificity of 95–98% for diagnosing appendicitis [25]. In addition, ultrasound can provide a quick, affordable, and noninvasive solution for diagnosing appendicitis without radiation exposure [22].

Indications

Indications for evaluation of appendicitis with ultrasound are based on presenting symptoms as described above, clinical presentation, detailed history, and physical examination [22]. The use of ultrasound does not have any absolute contraindications; however, it should be avoided if it would delay or interfere with a patient with clear indications for emergent surgical intervention [9].

Ultrasound Techniques

A high-frequency linear probe can be used or a curvilinear probe if more depth is required. Appendicitis can be diagnosed via sonographic criteria that include the following: a tubular structure that is >6 mm in diameter, noncompressible, and lacks peristalsis [21].

The following instructions describe the protocol of scanning the appendix [25]:

1. Begin with the patient supine and have them bend their knees in to help relax the abdominal wall muscles.
2. Place the transducer in the RUQ and pay special attention to image the area with maximal tenderness.

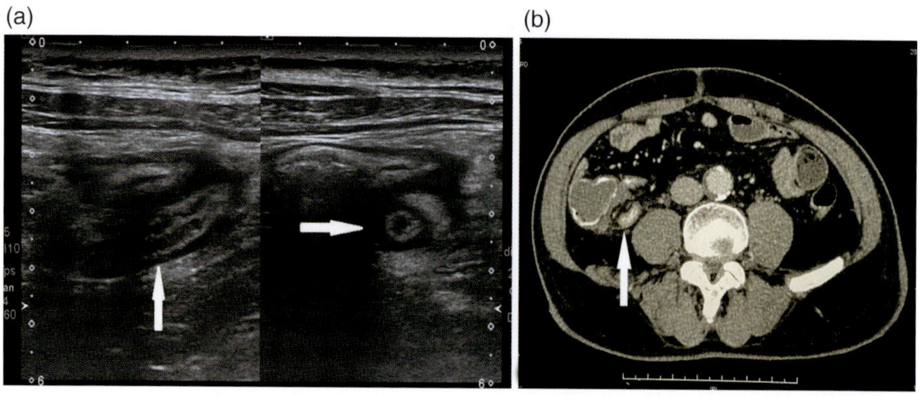

FIGURE 12.10 B-mode ultrasound (a) and CT (b) images of appendicitis (white arrows).

3. Move inferiorly to the RLQ until the cecum and terminal ileum are seen, and subsequently the appendix (Fig. 12.10a) and surroundings to assess the possibility of perforation.
4. Once the appendix has been identified, record it in two planes to ensure tubular shape and measure the thickness of the wall and diameter of the appendix.
5. Scan the entire appendix to its tip for signs of inflammation.

Acute Cholecystitis

Introduction

The gallbladder plays an important role in digestive system. It serves as a storage reservoir for bile, which is released by the liver and used for digesting fatty foods. It is located posterior to the liver and is attached to the vertical segment of the duodenum in the RUQ via various ducts. It may lie posterior to the costal margin and therefore require some maneuvering to get better access for imaging [26].

Acute cholecystitis is the result of inflammation of the gallbladder. Cholecystitis commonly presents with RUQ pain that radiates to the right shoulder, fever, nausea, and vomiting [27]. A serious but very rare complication of cholecystitis is perforation or rupture of the gallbladder, which can lead to infection of the peritoneum and is an emergency condition. The most common cause of cholecystitis is obstruction of the cystic duct due to gallstones [28]. Evaluation and diagnosis of cholecystitis should be focused on identifying the possible cause. Ultrasound is the preferred initial diagnostic tool for the diagnosis of cholecystitis due to its availability and higher sensitivity compared to other imaging modalities [27, 29].

Indications

Indications for evaluation of cholecystitis are based on symptoms as described above and clinical presentation [26]. If results are unclear or insufficient with ultrasound, a follow-up CT should be performed [30]. The use of ultrasound does not have any absolute contraindications; however, it should be avoided if it would delay or interfere with a patient with clear indications for emergent surgical intervention [9].

Ultrasound Techniques

A curved linear probe provides a wide/clear image and an increase in tissue penetration [29]. An alternative to a curved linear probe is a phased-array probe. Phased array probes are better able to fit in between ribs and provide a decrease in likelihood of rib shadowing. However, the image resolution of phased array is inferior to that of curvilinear array transducer [29].

A normal gallbladder is typically 6–7 cm in length and 2–3 cm in width and is fluid (bile) filled [31]. Diagnosing cholecystitis involves sonographic findings of gallstones, which will appear hyperechoic with posterior shadowing (Fig. 12.11). In addition to identifying gallstones, other diagnostic criteria include gallbladder wall thickness greater than 3 mm, presence of pericholecystic fluid, and a positive sonographic Murphy's sign [29].

The following instructions describe the protocol of gallbladder ultrasound [29, 32]:

1. Place the transducer in a transverse plane near the midline and inferior to the costal margin in the RUQ (Fig. 12.11). Due to the view of the gallbladder being obscured by the ribs, the patient may be required to take a deep inspiration and hold to have the diaphragm push the gallbladder into view. A normal gallbladder should appear as an anechoic pouch against the liver (Fig. 12.11).
2. The gallbladder should be viewed in both the transverse and longitudinal orientations, and the thickness of the gallbladder is measured on the transverse plane.

(a)

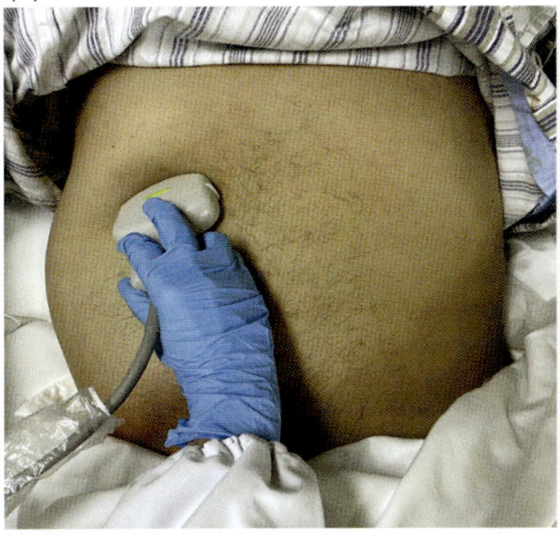

(b)

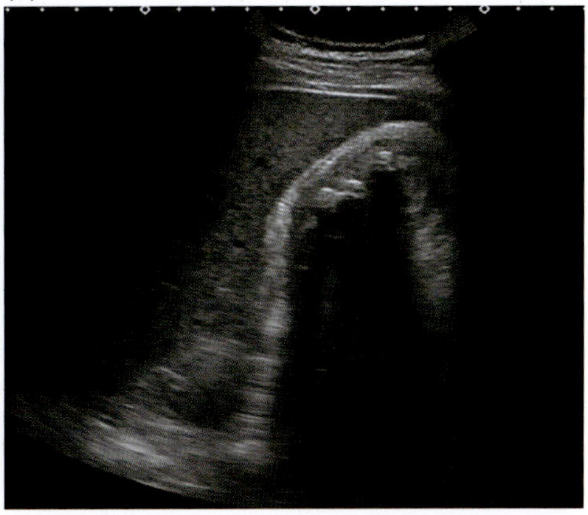

FIGURE 12.11 Imaging gallbladder can be done through an intercostal or subcostal approach (a). Gallbladder wall appears thickened and multiple stones with acoustic shadowing in the gallbladder on B-mode ultrasound image (b).

3. Look for evidence of gallstones and other signs of cholecystitis. If gallstones have been identified, the patient should rotate their torso. An absence of movement may indicate impacted stones as the source of inflammation [33].

Summary

The topics discussed in this chapter are some commonly used ultrasound exams in emergency medical care, and there are many applications of ultrasound in clinical patient care introduced in other chapters of this book. As technology continues to develop, the use of ultrasound will expand and play an even greater role in emergency settings.

Review Questions

1. Which of the following is not an area scanned in the FAST exam?
   - **a.** Splenorenal recess
   - **b.** Pericardium
   - **c.** Hepatorenal space
   - **d.** Cervical lymph nodes
2. The hepatorenal space (Morison's pouch) is viewed between what ribs?
   - **a.** Ribs 1–5
   - **b.** Ribs 2–7
   - **c.** Ribs 8–11
   - **d.** Ribs 11–12
3. The aorta passes through the diaphragm at what vertebral level?
   - **a.** T6
   - **b.** T8
   - **c.** T10
   - **d.** T12
4. What bony landmark is used to help locate the correct scanning position for viewing the pericardium?
   - **a.** Ribs 6–10
   - **b.** Xiphoid process
   - **c.** Sternum
   - **d.** Clavicle
5. Radiation of pain to which part of the body would support the suspicion of cholecystitis?
   - **a.** Left arm
   - **b.** Groin
   - **c.** Right shoulder
   - **d.** Lower back

Correct answers: 1. d; 2. c; 3. d; 4. b; 5. c.

References

1. Pariyahdath M, Snead G. Emergency ultrasound in adults with abdominal and thoracic trauma. *UpToDate*. www.uptodate.com. Published 2019.
2. Michalke JA. An overview of emergency ultrasound in the United States. *World J Emerg Med* 2009; 3: 85–90.
3. Bloom BA, Gibbons RC. Focused assessment with sonography for trauma (FAST). Treasure Island, FL: StatPearls, 2019.
4. Nelson BP, Chason K. Use of ultrasound by emergency medical services: a review. *Int J Emerg Med* 2008; 1: 253–259.
5. Giraldo-Restrepo JA, Serna-Jiménez TJ. The FAST and extended FAST examinations. *Colomb J Anesthesiol* 2015; 43: 299–306.
6. Richards JR, McGahan JP. Focused assessment with sonography in trauma (FAST) in 2017: what radiologists can learn? *Radiology* 2017; 283: 30–48.
7. Rowell SE, Barbosa RR, Holcomb JB, et al. The focused assessment with sonography in trauma (FAST) in hypotensive injured patients frequently fails to identify the need for laparotomy: a multi-institutional pragmatic study. *Trauma Surg Acute Care Open* 2019; 4(1): e000207. https://doi.org/10.1136/tsaco-2018-000207.
8. Savatmonkorngul S, Wongwaisayawan S, Kaewlai R. Focused assessment with sonography for trauma: current perspectives. *Open Access Emerg Med* 2017; 9: 57–62.
9. AIUM Practice Guideline. AIUM practice guideline for the performance of focused assessment with sonography for trauma (FAST) examination. *J Ultrasound Med* 2014; 33: 2047–2056.
10. Menaker J, Blumberg S, Wisner DH, et al. Use of the focused assessment with sonography for trauma (FAST) examination and its impact on abdominal computed tomography use in hemodynamically stable children with blunt torso trauma. *J Trauma Acute Care Surg* 2014; 77: 427–432.
11. Dawson M, Mallin M. FAST/EFAST. In: *Introduction to bedside ultrasound*. Vol 1. Lexington, Kentucky, USA: Emergency Ultrasound Solutions LLC, 2013; 2–21.
12. Jang T. Focused assessment with sonography in trauma. Medscape Web Site. https://emedicine.medscape.com/article/104363-overview#a2. Published 2017.
13. Jensen JK, Poulsen SH, Mølgaard H. Cardiac tamponade: a clinical challenge. *E-J Cardiol Pract* 2017; 15: 17–27.
14. Keisler B, Carter C. Abdominal aortic aneurysm. *Am Fam Physician* 2015; 91: 538–543.
15. Dawson M, Mallin M. AORTA. In: *Introduction to bedside ultrasound*. Vol 3. Lexington, Kentucky, USA: Emergency Ultrasound Solutions LLC, 2013; 49–63.
16. Medical Advisory Secretariat. Ultrasound screening for abdominal aortic aneurysm. *Ont Health Technol Assess Ser* 2006; 6: 1–67.
17. Creditt AB, Joyce M. Abdominal aortic aneurysm ultrasound. *Clin Ultrasound* 2018; 1: 135–147.
18. U.S. Preventative Services Task Force. Abdominal aortic aneurysm: screening. U.S. Preventative Services Task Force Web Site. https://www.uspreventiveservicestaskforce.org/uspstf/recommendation/abdominal-aortic-aneurysm-screening. Published 2019.
19. Sparks AR, Johnson PL, Meyer MC. Imaging of abdominal aortic aneurysms. *Am Fam Physician* 2002; 65: 1565–1570.
20. Jang T. Beside ultrasonography evaluation of abdominal aortic aneurysm. Medscape Web Site. https://emedicine.medscape.com/article/1977715-overview. Published 2017.
21. Fu J, Zhou X, Chen L, Lu S. Abdominal ultrasound and its diagnostic accuracy in diagnosing acute appendicitis: a meta-analysis. *Front Surg* 2021; 8: 707160. https://doi.org/10.3389/fsurg.2021.707160.
22. Daga S, Kachewar S, Lakhkar DL, et al. Sonographic evaluation of acute appendicitis and its complications. *West Afr J Radiol* 2017; 24: 152–156.

23. Craig S. Appendicitis. Medscape Web Site. https://emedicine.medscape.com/article/773895-overview. Published 2018.
24. Mostbeck G, Adam JE, Nielsen MB, et al. How to diagnose acute appendicitis: ultrasound first. *Insights Imaging* 2016; 7: 255–263.
25. Löfvenberg F, Salö M. Ultrasound for appendicitis: performance and integration with clinical parameters. *Biomed Res Int* 2016. https://doi.org/10.1155/2016/5697692.
26. Dawson M, Mallin M. RUQ. In: *Introduction to bedside ultrasound*. Vol 6. Lexington, Kentucky, USA: Emergency Ultrasound Solutions LLC, 2013; 110–118.
27. Acute Cholecystitis. radiopaedia.org. https://radiopaedia.org/articles/acute-cholecystitis?lang=us.
28. Pinto A, Reginelli A, Cagini L, et al. Accuracy of ultrasonography in the diagnosis of acute calculous cholecystitis: review of literature. *Crit Ultrasound J* 2013; 5: S11.
29. Bloom A. Cholecystitis workup. Medscape Web Site. https://emedicine.medscape.com/article/171886-overview. Published 2019.
30. Alshargi AO, Al-sallami SE, Hejazi HAM, Alahdal AIO. Accuracy of ultrasound in diagnosis of cholecystitis. *Egypt J Hosp Med* 2018; 73: 7146–7152.
31. Oluseyi KYH. Ultrasound determination of gall bladder size and wall thickness in normal adults in Abuja, North Central Nigeria. *Arch Int Surg* 2016; 6: 214–218.
32. Huang AA, Lin KW, Liu KL, et al. Diagnostic performance of ultrasound in acute cholecystitis: a systematic review and meta-analysis. *World J Emerg Surg* 2023; 18: 54. https://doi.org/10.1186/s13017-023-00524-5.
33. Navarro SM, Chen S, Situ X, et al. Sonographic assessment of acute versus chronic cholecystitis: an ultrasound probability stratification model. *J Ultrasound Med* 2023; 42: 1257–1265. https://doi.org/10.1002/jum.16138.

CHAPTER 13

Ultrasound-Guided Procedures

Mateen Razaan[1], Jonathan Hansen[1], Mikala Russell[1], Wei Zhang[2], and Wen He[2]

[1] Rocky Vista University, College of Osteopathic Medicine, Ivins, Utah, USA

[2] Department of Ultrasound, Beijing Tiantan Hospital, Capital Medical University, Beijing, China

Introduction

Ultrasound-guided invasive interventions play an important role in patient care for diagnostic and therapeutic purposes [1, 2]. In order to perform procedures successfully, clinicians should familiarize themselves with the basic technology and instrumentation for ultrasound imaging, as well as safety requirements. Furthermore, clinicians who use ultrasound imaging to guide procedures should understand and follow standard protocols, including but not limited to, obtaining informed consent, optimal room setup, preliminary scanning, needle visualization, documentation, and post-procedure care. Understanding the indications and contraindications for each ultrasound-guided procedure is necessary in the application of ultrasound imaging for specific procedures. In addition, the knowledge of the anatomy, physiology, and pathophysiology of the targeted organs and tissues is critical in the practice of each procedure [2]. Clinicians should also be able to recognize additional imaging modalities as they pertain to the procedural planning and diagnoses being investigated.

In this chapter, we discuss several common ultrasound-guided procedures that may be performed as point-of-care in clinical settings.

Indications and Contraindications

Indications

Common indications for ultrasound-guided procedures include diagnostic aspiration/biopsy to provide tissue samples for histopathologic determination of the disease, and therapeutic drainage of abscess, ascites, and effusions in the pericardial, peritoneal, and pleural spaces [1–3]. Ultrasound is used during these procedures as a guide to ensure precision, reduce risk for complications, and improve diagnostic and therapeutic efficacy. Other common procedures performed using ultrasound guidance include vascular access, peripheral nerve blocks in pain management, joint injection, and cyst aspirations.

Contraindications

General contraindications involving the performance of the procedure include known allergies to the injected material (if used) and lack of consent by the patient. Relative contraindications include risk of bleeding due to coagulopathy or concurrent anticoagulant therapy, infection at the entry site, or other pathologies that increase the likelihood of complications from the invasive procedure. The risk of complications due to bleeding is determined by coagulation status, proximity to vessels, depth of target, compressibility of bleeding site, and proximity to critical structures such as the spinal cord. The risk of bleeding complications can be reduced by best practices such as applying local pressure, use small gauge needle, needle visualization throughout the procedure, and post-procedure monitoring for bleeding. Additionally, underlying medical conditions that may be adversely affected by the intervention, or local dermatologic reactions, are also relative contraindications [4].

Periprocedural Management

Procedure Preparations and Post-procedure Observation

The same standards regarding all other interventional procedures apply to ultrasound-guided procedures, including review of prior imaging (if available), collection of medical history, and performing a thorough physical exam to screen for specific contraindications. Procedures should be performed in facilities with adequate equipment, trained personnel, and with appropriate procedural setup [3]. Informed consent must be obtained (in accordance with federal law and state regulation, as well as with local practice standards) and must encompass a discussion of the procedure, alternatives, and risks and benefits.

Appropriate procedural setup involves assistant personnel as needed, table height adjustment, machine placement, a transducer grasp allowing for positioning that is comfortable and minimizes movement for both patient and clinician, and adequate exposure of the target region. The clinician must ensure that he/she is on the same side as the target region and must allow for transducer manipulation with the nondominant hand and needle manipulation with the dominant hand, with supplies for the procedure within easy reach of the dominant hand.

As with all ultrasound-guided procedures, there is a risk of infection, and the procedure should be performed in accordance with the facility's infection control guidelines [5, 6]. The specific methods to reduce the risk of contamination and infection are generally dictated by practice-specific factors. The selected methods used during the procedure should be documented.

It is a common practice to keep a patient for observation anywhere from 3 to 6 hours after an ultrasound-guided procedure. Vital signs are to be measured with patients being closely monitored. Standard discharge documentation should be taken and properly explained to patients by the institution (clinic).

Ultrasound Techniques

Either a stationary (Fig. 13.1a) or portable (Fig. 13.1b) ultrasound scanner can be used.

Transducer

Proper transducer selection is determined based on the depth of the target organ (tissue). High-frequency (>10 MHz) linear array transducers provide better resolution for superficial structures and are useful for procedures in the neck, body wall, and extremities. Low-frequency transducers (1–5 MHz), such as curvilinear transducers, are appropriate for procedures involving deeper structures that necessitate a deeper penetration, such as for the viscera of the abdomen. Lastly, phased array probes (1–5 MHz) allow for being placed in a narrowed acoustic window (space), useful for procedures involving the chest and heart via intercostal or subxiphoid approach [4].

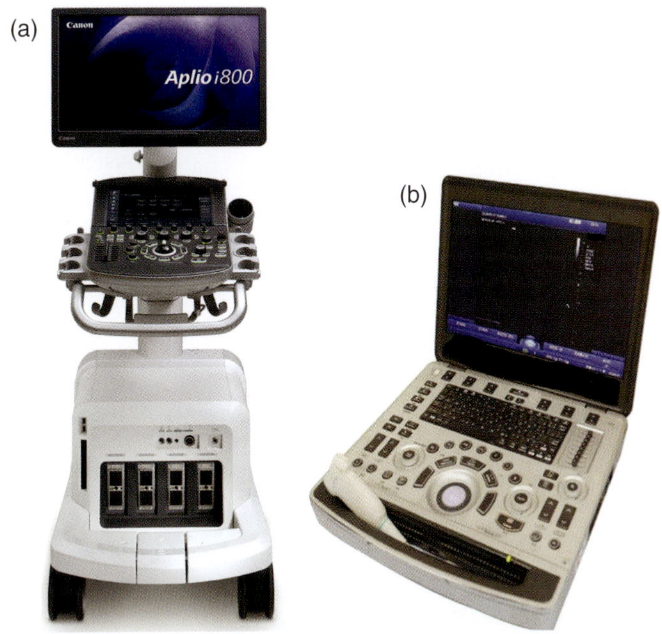

FIGURE 13.1 (a, b) Images of stationed ultrasound scanner (a) and portable ultrasound machine (b). Source: Courtesy of Canon Medical Systems USA, Inc.

Preliminary Scanning Techniques

Once a transducer is selected, preliminary diagnostic scanning allows for proper procedural planning. The scan is intended to identify the target tissue for the procedure and to survey the surrounding structures that may determine needle choice, entry point, needle trajectory, and site marking. The preliminary scan may show anatomic variations and/or associated and nonassociated pathologic findings, upon which the clinician must make a clinical assessment before proceeding with the procedure. If the findings require adjustment of the original plan, appropriate authorization must be obtained prior to continuing with the procedure.

Needle Tracking

Once the transducer is placed in the appropriate location and anesthesia has been administered according to practice-specific standards, the clinician should utilize the information acquired from the preliminary scan to advance the needle through the skin to the target.

A useful ultrasound artifact, as described in Chapter 1, is the "comet tail" artifact produced by the needle (Fig. 13.2). Accurate and safe use of ultrasound for procedures requires an appreciation of commonly seen ultrasound artifacts displaying the location of the needle [7].

In-Plane Approach

The in-plane approach involves parallel orientation of the long axis of the transducer and the needle shaft. In this way, the needle shaft and tip are visualized throughout the procedure, as shown in (Fig. 13.3a). The angle of the needle, relative to the transducer face, is modified depending on the thickness of soft tissues and depth of the target. A larger angle may make it more challenging to maintain adequate

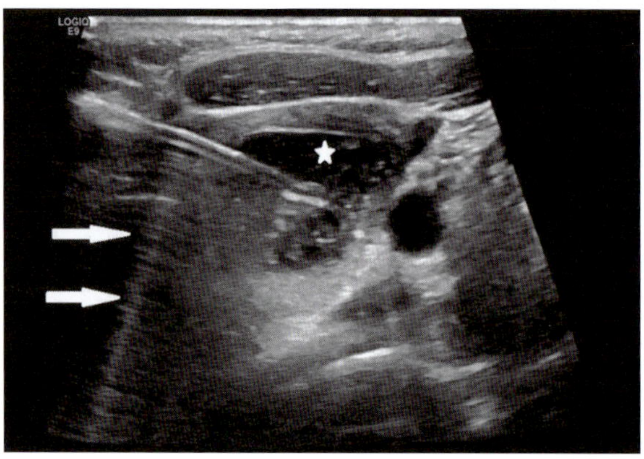

FIGURE 13.2 A B-mode ultrasound image shows the needle in an abscess (*) and "comet tail" artifact (arrows) deep to the needle.

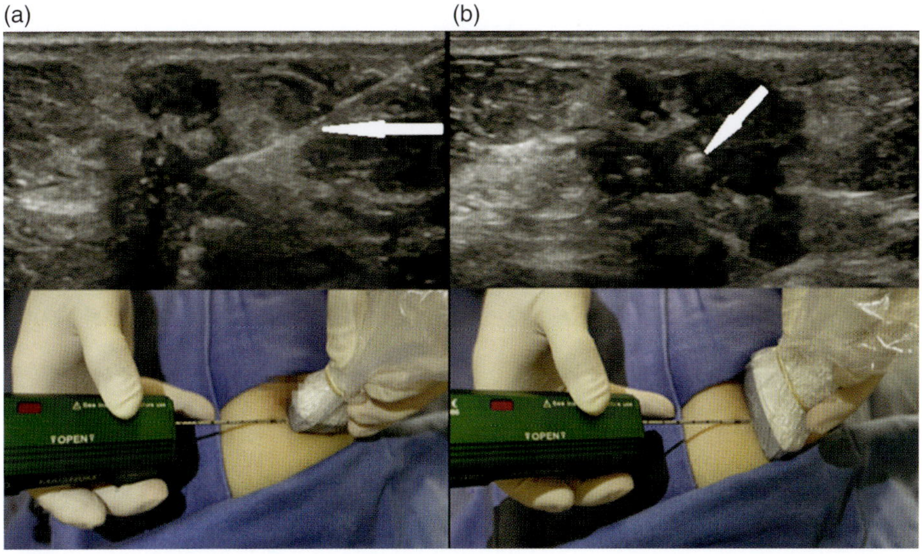

FIGURE 13.3 (a, b) (a) In-plane ultrasound view. (b) Out-of-plane view. Arrow - needle.

visualization of the needle shaft and tip. This technique is useful for superficial regions with minimal subcutaneous tissue [7, 8].

Out-of-Plane Approach

The out-of-plane approach involves perpendicular orientation of the long axis of the transducer and the needle shaft. The needle is visualized as a "dot" and represents a point along the shaft or the needle tip, depending on the relationship between the transducer and the needle. In this plane, the needle is advanced only to the point at which the "dot" first appears (Fig. 13.3b), which represents the needle tip. The "walk-down" maneuver, in which the first needle pass is typically shallow, is often used here. After the first pass, the needle is successively partially withdrawn, angled more steeply, and then advanced toward the target depth. This plane is useful for superficial regions with minimal surrounding soft tissue, and for intravascular needle or catheter placement [7]. This approach allows for simultaneous visualization of structures adjacent to the needle [8].

It is essential for clinicians performing ultrasound-guided procedures to be competent in both plane approaches, though they may favor one over the other. Some clinicians switch from one view to another during a procedure to provide orthogonal imaging of the needle; this helps them assess and confirm the needle location and its relationship with the target region as well as the surrounding structures [7].

Transducer Manipulation and Beam Steering

In order to maintain optimal visualization of the needle during ultrasound-guided procedures, the clinician must ensure his/her own position optimizes visualization while minimizing risk. The clinician may anchor the hand holding the transducer on the patient and use the table to support his/her elbows and arms. Thereafter, the clinician can utilize a variety of maneuvers involving the transducer and the needle to allow for further visualization.

1. Transducer translation, rotation, and fanning.
2. Needle jiggling (be careful with cutting needles), rotation, and larger needle gauge.
3. Visualization of the needle tip to inject anesthetic, saline, or contrast for the distribution of injectate and perform hydrodissection.
4. Beam steering to alter the angle of the ultrasound beam without moving the probe, which is accomplished by adding time delay to the transmission and reception of the ultrasound beam [9].

It is important to note that there are four major pitfalls and technical errors that may lead to increased complications during ultrasound-guided procedures. The four main errors to avoid are listed below. Many of these errors involve not keeping track of where the needle tip location is in the ultrasound image.

1. Inappropriately looking at the ultrasound image for gross adjustments, instead of looking directly at the transducer and needle.
2. Inappropriate use of in-plane versus out-of-plane needle approaches.
3. During in-plane approaches, not scanning across the needle shaft to ensure the tip of the needle is visualized (misalignment results in a false tip image as the needle shaft exits the sound beam).
4. Not appreciating the fact that tissue planes can cause refraction that distorts or alters the view of the distal end of the needle.

Common Ultrasound-Guided Procedures

Ultrasound-Guided Vascular Access

Transverse method (Fig. 13.4) – Place the ultrasound probe perpendicular to the artery (vein). Puncture the skin at a 90° angle, being sure to position the needle to the point on the probe that corresponds with the center of the screen. Upon proper orientation of the needle and transducer, the echoes representing the needle will enter the screen from the center. It is important to ensure that the probe is perpendicular to the artery (vein) so that the needle, transducer, and vessel are all properly aligned [10].

Longitudinal method (Fig. 13.5) – Place the ultrasound probe parallel to the artery (vein). Puncture the skin parallel to the ultrasound probe while aiming for the exact center of the probe. The needle will be visible either on the left or right side of the ultrasound screen, depending on the orientation of the probe [10]. Once the needle is inserted, the needle-guidewire-catheter unit is slowly advanced until blood return is visible. The guidewire is then advanced with the practitioner's dominant hand. Lastly, the catheter is advanced over the guidewire, and the guidewire and needle are removed. Secure the catheter with sutures or with a sterile dressing [11].

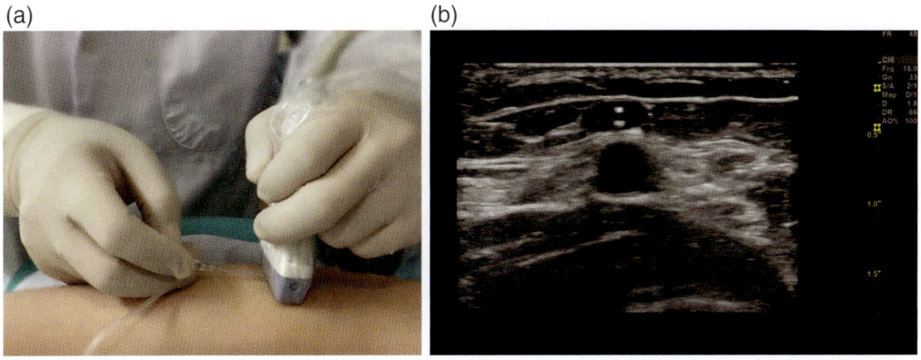

FIGURE 13.4 (a, b) Transverse method: transducer orientation (a) and ultrasound image (b).

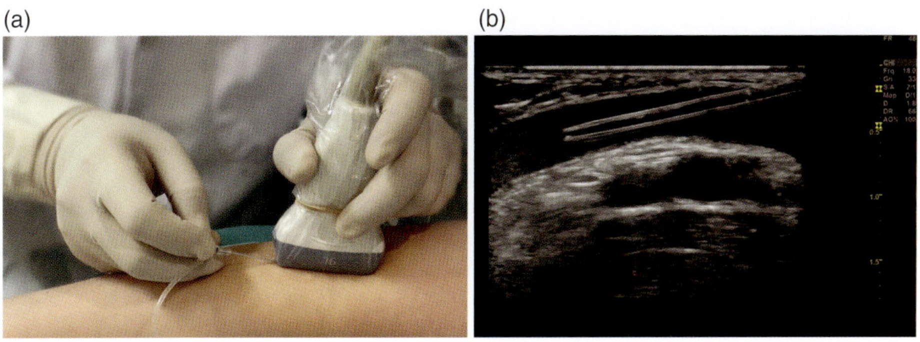

FIGURE 13.5 (a, b) Longitudinal method: transducer orientation (a) and ultrasound image (b).

Arterial Access

Using ultrasound to assist in placing a catheter into an artery allows practitioners to continuously monitor blood pressure, as well as take frequent blood samples for diagnostic purposes, for example, arterial blood gas analysis. Arterial catheters are conventionally placed using palpation of anatomic landmarks and pulses, but such palpation may be difficult in patients that are hypotensive, morbidly obese, or in patients who are atherosclerotic. Ultrasound use in arterial catheter placement provides the following advantages: visualization of real-time landmarks, monitoring location of the needle, improvement in first-attempt success rates, and reduction of procedure-related complications, including infections, hematomas, arteriovenous fistula, and significant pain for the patient [10, 11].

Equipment Recommended equipment for ultrasound-guided arterial catheter placement includes [10–12]:

- Ultrasound machine with linear (5–15 MHz) probe
- Arterial line kit
- Insertion needle with guidewire
- Sterile sleeve and ultrasound gel

- 2% chlorhexidine for skin preparation
- Sterile towels and drapes over the insertion site
- Sterile gloves, gown, and mask
- 1% Lidocaine with 5-cc syringe and 25-gauge needle
- Sutures, sterile gauze, sterile dressing

Patient Position Patient should be supine with the target artery visible to the provider. The practitioner should hold the ultrasound probe in his or her non-dominant hand to ensure comfort so that the remainder of the procedure can be completed with the practitioner's dominant hand [10].

Procedure Be sure to preserve sterile technique throughout the procedure to limit the risk of bloodstream infections. Prep the extremity being used for arterial vascular access with chlorhexidine and full sterile draping. Place the sterile sleeve over the ultrasound probe. The ultrasound probe is placed on the artery either where the pulse is palpated or by assessing anatomic landmarks if a pulse cannot be palpated. The artery will appear anechoic and can be distinguished from nearby veins due to pulsation, yet veins may display transmitted pulsations. Definitive pulsated pressures can be confirmed with color and spectral Doppler that can display arterial flow. Lidocaine is then injected to achieve local anesthesia. Either in-plane or out-of-plane methods can be used to guide arterial catheter placement [10].

Internal Jugular Vein Cannulation

Using ultrasound to guide needle insertion during internal jugular vein cannulation has proven to improve success and reduce complications in patients, where vein cannulation is most often found to be difficult. Some examples of these difficulties would be patients who are uncooperative, obese patients, or patients with shorter necks. Ultrasound guidance also helps avoid complications such as insertion failure, hematomas, pneumothorax, arterial puncture, and hemothorax [13].

Equipment (for control and peripheral venous access) [13]

- Ultrasound machine with a linear transducer (8–12 MHz), sterile sleeve, and gel
- Central line kit with intravenous catheter (size and length based upon diameter and depth of vein) (Peripheral venous catheters of appropriate size)
- Sterile drapes, gloves, gown, surgical mask, and cap
- Topical antiseptic
- Local anesthetic
- Isotonic saline and/or heparin for flushing the catheter
- Transparent adhesive dressing, tape
- Intravenous tubing and connectors
- Connective tubing and IV fluid
- Skin preparation materials

Patient Position If the patient is able to tolerate, place in Trendelenburg position (patient flat, supine with legs elevated higher than the head at about 15°) to maximize the internal jugular vein size and minimize possible complications. If the patient is unable to tolerate Trendelenburg position, maneuvers such as having "Valsalva" may help increase the vein diameter. The patient's head may be rotated slightly in order to reduce the overlap between the internal jugular vein and carotid artery in tolerant patients and those without cervical trauma. The operator should be positioned at the head of the bed throughout the procedure [13].

Procedure Before beginning the procedure and sterile preparations, pre-scan the patient. During the scanning, the extent of the internal jugular vein should be fully visualized in order to assess the anatomy and patency of the vein. After inspecting the internal jugular vein, choose a point of access to set up a sterile field around this access point. After sterile preparation of the site, the transducer starts the procedural scan in a transverse view. The chosen site should be where the internal jugular vein is lateral to the carotid artery and as close as possible to the surface of the skin. The anterior approach is most commonly used by inserting the needle at the apex of the triangle formed by the sternal and clavicular heads of the sternocleidomastoid muscle. Note the distance from the surface of the skin to the center of the vessel, which can be used to determine the distance from the transducer to penetrate the lumen of the vessel. Once blood return is observed, the ultrasound transducer may be placed aside to continue with the procedure [13].

Peripheral Venous Access

Ultrasound guidance for peripheral venous access can be utilized in patients whose venous access is difficult to achieve by landmark palpatory techniques [13].

Patient Position When gaining venous access, using vessels in the upper extremity is preferred. If possible, place the patient in a supine position. Place the extremity with the venipuncture site on a stable surface below heart level to allow venous dilation [13].

Procedure Commonly used veins may be found in the upper arm, antecubital fossa, or forearm. When available, superficial veins are preferred, as they are not typically close to other neurovascular structures. Potential vessels should be evaluated not only for depth and patency, but also for proximity to surrounding structures and the course that the vessel travels. A vein depth of about 5 mm is usually ideal for venous access. A rubber tourniquet may be utilized to distend the vessel and improve the ability of the catheter to puncture the vein without exiting the posterior wall. The site should be chosen and prepared by cleaning with an antiseptic agent while using clean gloves. An appropriate-gauge catheter of suitable length should be employed; length greater than 1.75 in. is usually recommended.

The site may be anesthetized by using a topical or injectable local anesthetic. Ultrasound guidance in peripheral veins utilizes an out-of-plane, in the short axis of the vessel. After ensuring the transducer is centered over the vein, insert the needle and advance slowly. If the needle tip is not easily identified, do not move the needle; move the probe to find the needle tip and redirect as needed. Successful ultrasound guidance is achieved when the operator pays special attention to the needle tip rather than the shaft to avoid penetrating the vein.

Blood return may be noted at the hub when the needle has successfully punctured the venous endothelium. Advance the needle tip to the center of the lumen of the vein. Once the catheter tip is appropriately placed, the catheter should be advanced, and the needle should slide out easily. Once the catheter is placed, the catheter should be flushed and secured [13].

Paracentesis

A paracentesis is performed for both diagnostic and therapeutic purposes. Abdominal fluid may be obtained to evaluate for infection or malignancy. Large volume ascites can be drained to relieve associated discomfort or dyspnea. Ultrasound imaging can be used to determine the amount of ascites and guide the site of needle insertion. Ultrasound can also help rule out the underlying etiology of abdominal distention as opposed to other disease processes that may not require a paracentesis (Fig. 13.6). In addition, using ultrasound allows practitioners to identify and sample smaller volumes of fluid in the abdominal cavity, which traditional paracentesis techniques do not allow [14].

Equipment Recommended equipment for ultrasound-guided paracentesis includes [14–16]:

- Ultrasound machine with curvilinear (2–5 MHz) probe
- Probe cover
- Sterile gloves, mask, cap, and gown
- Fenestrated drape
- Blood culture bottles
- Blood specimen tubes
- Vacuum container

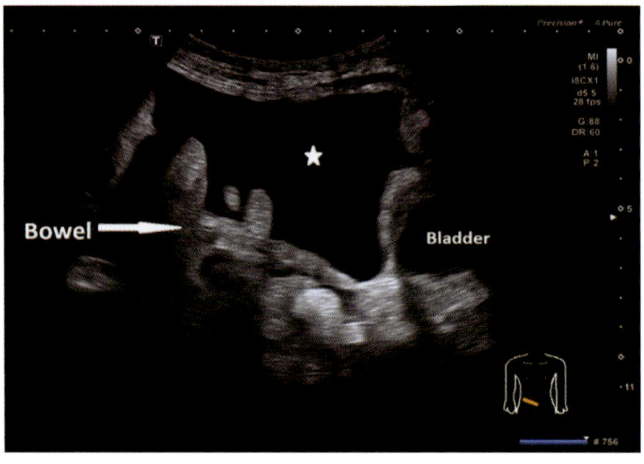

FIGURE 13.6 Image shows a large amount of peritoneal ascites (*). Bowels (white arrow) floating in the ascites can be observed in real-time B-mode ultrasound.

- Sterile gauze
- Sterile syringes
- Chlorhexidine
- Alcohol wipes
- 1% Lidocaine with syringe/needle
- Adhesive bandage
- #11 Scalpel blade
- Paracentesis needle
- 8 Fr catheter over 18-gauge × 7.5-inch needle with 3-way stopcock and self-sealing valve
- Tubing set with roller clamp

Patient Position Patient's head should be elevated to allow for maximal drainage. The patient should be placed in a supine or slight lateral decubitus position. Just prior to starting the procedure, the abdomen ultrasound should be performed, and the patient should then remain in the same position throughout the procedure [14].

Procedure Ultrasound can be used as an adjunct to a paracentesis procedure in two ways. First, a practitioner can utilize ultrasound statically by first scanning the abdomen and marking the entry site prior to inserting the needle. The other option is to use ultrasound dynamically and observe the needle entering the peritoneal cavity under ultrasound guidance in real-time (Fig. 13.7). One advantage of the dynamic approach is that smaller volumes of fluid can be aspirated safely [14].

The ultrasound probe should be set to the "abdominal setting." Ascites fluid will appear anechoic on the screen. In order to select a location for fluid to be drained, locate the area with the thinnest abdominal wall and the largest fluid pocket, with the fluid pocket being at least 3 cm deep, and assess vessels in the abdominal wall by using Doppler to avoid a potential source of bleeding [14]. After the location has been identified, prep the patient with chlorhexidine and sterile draping. Anesthetize the skin, then anesthetize the peritoneum following the catheter tract. Using a scalpel to

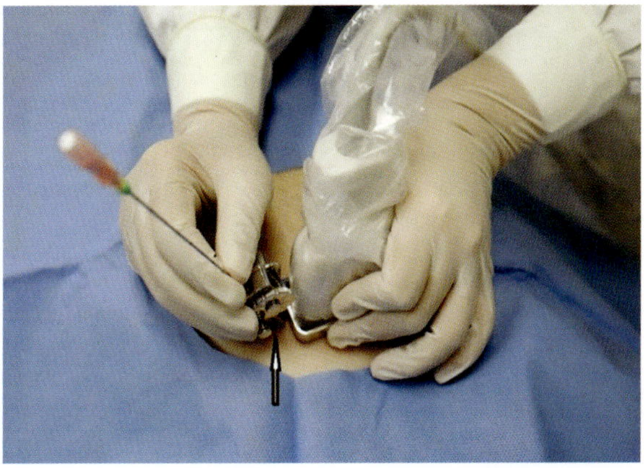

FIGURE 13.7 Image shows the position of the needle and the transducer. An ultrasound guide (arrow) is used in the procedure.

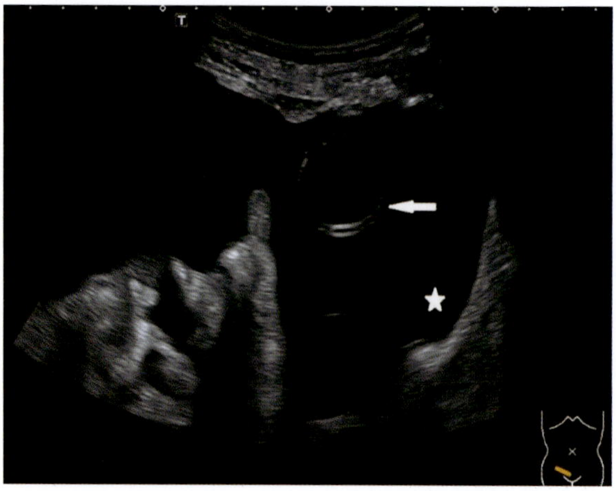

FIGURE 13.8 Image shows the catheter (white arrow) being inserted into the peritoneal ascites (*).

create a small incision in the skin. Traction should be applied to the entry site with the practitioner's nondominant hand. The catheter will be inserted over the needle (Fig. 13.8).

After inserting the needle and catheter, the syringe should fill easily. At that point, the catheter should be inserted over the needle and advanced 3 mm. Withdraw the needle and attach the three-way stopcock to the catheter. If paracentesis is being performed for diagnostic purposes, obtain samples for lab testing. If the paracentesis is for therapeutic purposes, attach tubing and the vacuum container for fluid aspiration. After adequate fluid has been removed, remove the catheter. Firm pressure and an adhesive bandage should be applied to the entry site [14–16].

Thoracentesis

A thoracentesis is used to remove pleural fluid from a patient's chest cavity. Like paracentesis, thoracentesis can be diagnostic or therapeutic. Patients with newly diagnosed pleural effusions should undergo diagnostic thoracentesis to determine the underlying etiology of fluid collection. Therapeutic thoracenteses are beneficial for patients with symptomatic pleural effusions, which usually cause dyspnea. B-mode ultrasound shows a pleural effusion (Fig. 13.9). Using ultrasound to guide thoracentesis allows for better visualization of the underlying anatomy, which leads to higher success rates, lower complication rates, and decreased complications, including hemorrhage and pneumothorax [17].

Equipment Recommended equipment for ultrasound-guided thoracentesis includes [17, 18]:

- Ultrasound machine with a curvilinear array (3.5–5 MHz) probe with probe cover
- Sterile gloves, mask, cap, gown, and drape
- Vacuum container
- Sterile gauze

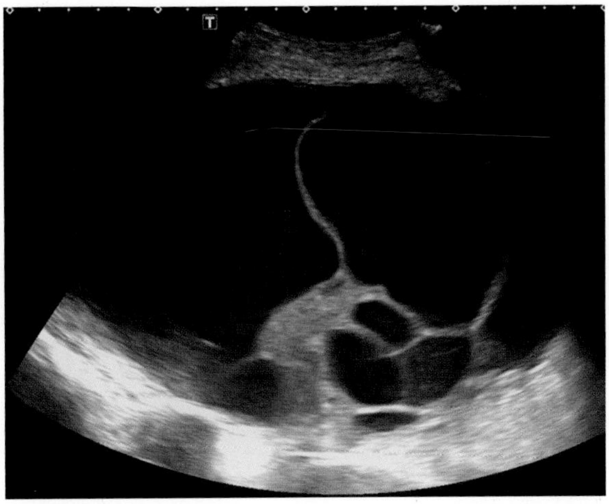

FIGURE 13.9 Pleural effusion with septation and internal echoes on B-mode ultrasound.

- Sterile syringes
- Chlorhexidine and alcohol wipes
- 1% Lidocaine with syringe/needle
- Adhesive bandage
- #11 Scalpel blade
- Thoracentesis needle
- 8 Fr catheter over 18-gauge × 7.5-in. needle with three-way stopcock and self-sealing valve
- Tubing set and specimen vials

Patient Position Positioning depends on the ability of the patient. If able, the patient should sit upright with his or her arms resting on a bedside table just below shoulder level. Having the patient sit upright keeps the ribs aligned in a way that minimizes the risk of the aspiration needle hitting the superior intercostal bundle (Fig. 13.10a). If the patient is critically ill or unable to sit upright, he or she should be placed in the lateral recumbent position (Fig. 13.10b), with the pleural effusion facing upright. The patient's arm should be placed over the head in order to access the chest wall, if possible [19].

Procedure The patient should first be properly positioned. The ultrasound probe should be placed perpendicularly between the seventh and ninth ribs, and between the posterior axillary line and the patient's midline if the patient has a large amount of pleural effusion. On ultrasound, pleural fluid will appear anechoic against hyperechoic atelectatic lung. Be sure to avoid the diaphragm, which appears as curvilinear/linear echogenic structure inferiorly, when selecting a puncture site. Practitioners can use B-mode ultrasound to evaluate the thickness of the chest wall, depth of the lung, and the amount of fluid (Fig. 13.11a), which helps determine the depth that the needle and/or catheter can be introduced safely [20]. Once the appropriate site has been marked, the patient should be prepped with chlorhexidine and draped using sterile technique [19].

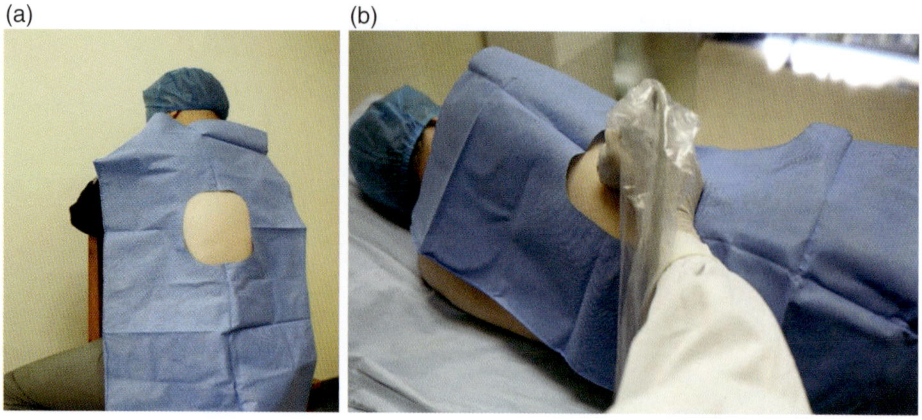

FIGURE 13.10 (a, b) To perform thoracentesis, patient is in the upright position (a) or lateral recumbent position (b).

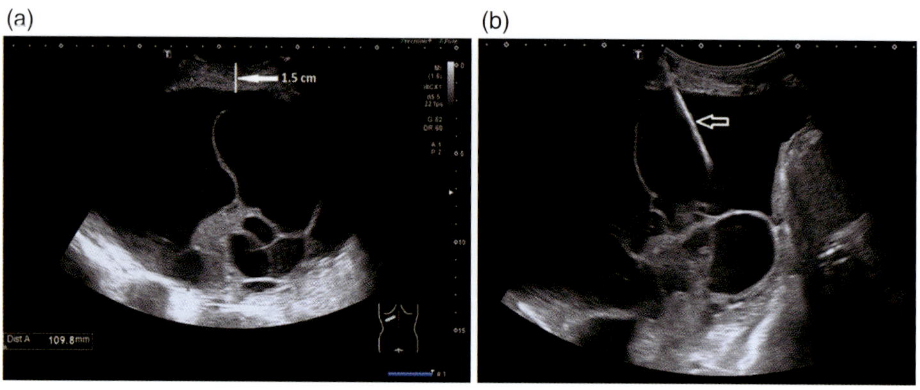

FIGURE 13.11 (a, b) (a) Ultrasound image of pleural effusion. The distance from the skin to pleural space measures 1.5 cm (arrow). The largest amount of pleural effusion measures 109.8 mm (Dist. A, distance between two electronic clippers). (b) B-mode image shows the needle (arrow) and guidewire in pleural effusion space for thoracentesis.

Administer 1% lidocaine in the skin. Then, anesthetize the upper margin of the lower rib and "walk" over the superior margin of the rib, being careful to avoid the neurovascular bundle. Be sure to utilize ultrasound to provide real-time guidance of the needle insertion (Fig. 13.11b). A large volume syringe is then used through the anesthetized tract, and fluid should then be aspirated [19].

If performing diagnostic thoracentesis, remove approximately 20–70 mL for analysis. If performing a therapeutic thoracentesis, advance a catheter through the anesthetized tract to access the fluid pocket. The needle should be stabilized by hand or puncture guide rack, followed by advancing the over-the-needle catheter into the pleural fluid. Drainage tubing is then attached to the stopcock to limit air entrapment. Fluid can be drained by a syringe or aspirated using a vacuum container [19].

At the end of the procedure, whether diagnostic or therapeutic, the catheter should be removed as the patient holds his/her breath in expiration. The procedure site should be covered with sterile dressing after removal of the needle and catheter. A chest X-ray is commonly requested to assess the presence of pneumothorax after thoracentesis [19].

Abscess and Cyst Aspirations

A cyst is a collection of fluid that is typically benign, as opposed to an abscess, which is a fluid collection caused by an infection [21]. Both can be treated with aspiration to remove tissue, air, or local body fluids from a specific area of the body and can be sent to the lab for definitive analysis. Before the advent of ultrasound, diagnostic and therapeutic interventions associated with the care of abscesses, cysts, and aspirations were complex, often requiring open surgery. With ultrasound guidance, practitioners can easily identify pathology and limit the need for invasive procedures to improve patient outcomes and decrease procedural-related complications [22].

Equipment Recommended equipment for ultrasound-guided abscesses, cysts, and aspirations includes [23, 24]:

- Ultrasound machine with a high-frequency linear (5–12 MHz) probe.
- Probe cover
- Ultrasound gel
- Appropriate needle(s) for the procedure
- 1% lidocaine with syringe/needle
- Sterile gloves, drapes, and gauze
- Chlorhexidine
- Appropriate needle and syringe for desired procedure
- Scalpel
- Forceps
- Scissors
- Wound dressings
- Culture swabs (if necessary)

Patient Position The patient is placed in supine position with proper exposure of the area in need of intervention. The practitioner should hold the ultrasound probe in his or her nondominant hand to ensure comfort so that the procedure can be performed with his or her dominant hand.

Procedure The patient should first be properly positioned. Sterile techniques should be followed throughout the procedure. The area is anesthetized with local anesthetic. Sterile ultrasound gel is placed on the patient's skin. The ultrasound transducer is then used to carefully locate an abscess, cyst, or another tissue area in need of aspiration (Fig. 13.12a,b). Once identified, a needle is inserted into the appropriate area under ultrasound guidance. If drainage of a fluid collection is indicated, exchange the needle with a guidewire, through which a drainage catheter is placed. If performing a diagnostic aspiration procedure, tissue or fluid samples will

(a) (b)

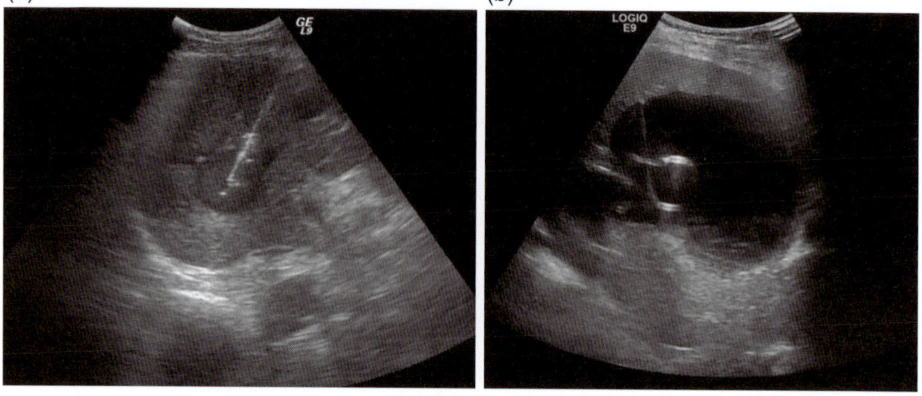

FIGURE 13.12 (a, b) B-mode images of abscess drainage (a) and liver cyst aspiration (b).

be obtained as needed. Once the procedure is over, the needle or catheter is removed, and the area is dressed [22].

Peripheral Nerve Blocks

Equipment The equipment needed for peripheral nerve blocks (interscalene brachial plexus, femoral nerve, and popliteal sciatic nerve) includes the following [25].

Ultrasound machine with a linear transducer (8–14 MHz), sterile sleeve, and gel

- Standard nerve block tray
- A 20-mL syringe containing the local anesthetic
- A 5-cm, 22-gauge needle
- Sterile gloves

Brachial Plexus

The ultrasound-guided brachial plexus block can provide rapid and definitive pain relief caused by traumatic injuries to the upper extremity. The brachial plexus can be blocked at several locations: the neck with an interscalene block, above the clavicle with a supraclavicular block, below the clavicle with an infraclavicular block, or in the axilla region with an axillary block (Fig. 13.13). The most common one is the interscalene block.

While the interscalene block is most known for its use in surgery of the shoulder and proximal upper extremity, this nerve block is also indicated for clavicular fractures, proximal and mid-humeral fractures, reduction of shoulder dislocations, drainage of deltoid abscesses, and laceration repairs of the lateral arm. This approach anesthetizes the C5–C7 nerve roots, as well as the superficial cervical plexus (clavicle, shoulder, and lateral arm above the elbow). Depending on the volume of local anesthetic injected, the interscalene block may not anesthetize the lower trunk (roots C8–T1) and may not provide analgesia for medial (ulnar distribution) hand surgery [26].

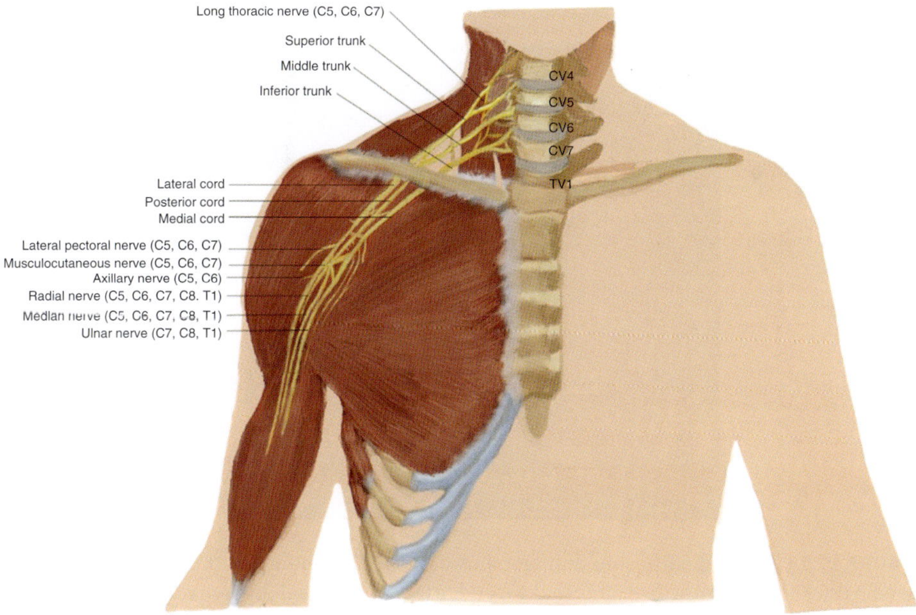

FIGURE 13.13 Illustration of brachial plexus.

Patient Position The patient is positioned supine, with the head turned away from the side being anesthetized. The physician then palpates and identifies the sternal notch, the sternal and clavicular heads of the sternocleidomastoid muscle, the clavicle, and the anterior and middle scalene muscles lying just posterior to the clavicular head of the sternocleidomastoid muscle [26].

Procedure The physician places the transducer in the transverse plane, just above the clavicle. Next, the pulsation of the subclavian artery is identified by directing the beam of the transducer toward the first rib. In this position, the trunks of the brachial plexus appear as a bundle lateral to the subclavian artery, overlying the first rib.

The brachial plexus is traced superiorly, with the transducer maintained in an axial position. At about the C6 level, the nerve roots of the brachial plexus are visualized in a vertical "stoplight" orientation within the interscalene groove. Insert the needle using an in-plane approach directed toward these nerves from lateral to medial. The needle tip is placed next to the nerve roots (Fig. 13.14). After negative aspiration for blood, a total of 12–30 mL of local anesthetic is injected, in 5-mL increments, with aspiration in-between injections. Stop if the patient experiences pain or paresthesia at any time during the injection. Spread of anesthetic should be visualized surrounding the roots. Remove the needle and discard safely in the appropriate sharps container. Clean the patient from excess ultrasound gel and then dress the injection site with the appropriate dressings [26].

Femoral Nerve Block

The femoral nerve block is utilized to anesthetize or provide analgesia to the anterior thigh and knee, often for treatment of a hip fracture, femur fracture, knee injury, including patellar fracture, incision and drainage of abscess, laceration repair, or postoperative

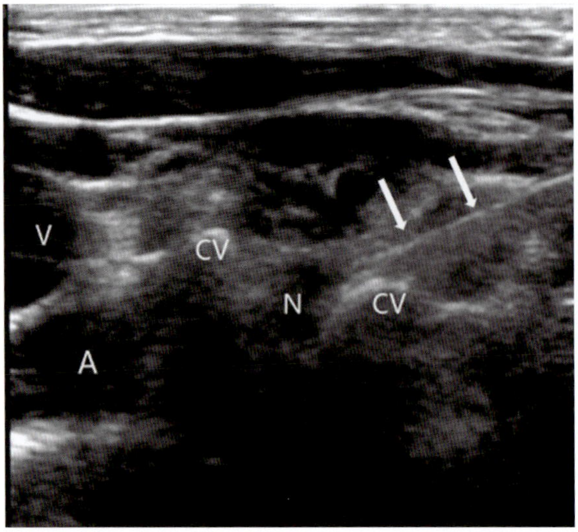

FIGURE 13.14 B-mode ultrasound image shows the needle tip next to the nerve root and needle track (white arrows). A, internal carotid artery; V, internal jugular vein; N, brachial plexus; CV, cervical vertebrae.

care. The ultrasound-guided technique allows the practitioner to monitor the distribution of local anesthetic, as well as provide extra precision during needle placement. Ultrasound guidance may also reduce the risk of femoral artery puncture [27].

Patient Position The patient is placed in the supine position. Drapes are placed so that sensitive areas are covered, while exposing the inguinal region.

Procedure The ultrasound transducer is placed at the inguinal crease. Locate the hyperechoic femoral nerve, which can be seen lateral to the hypoechoic, pulsating common femoral artery, superficial to the iliopsoas, and deep to the fascia lata and fascia iliaca (Figs. 13.15 and 13.16). In-plane or out-of-plane approaches may be

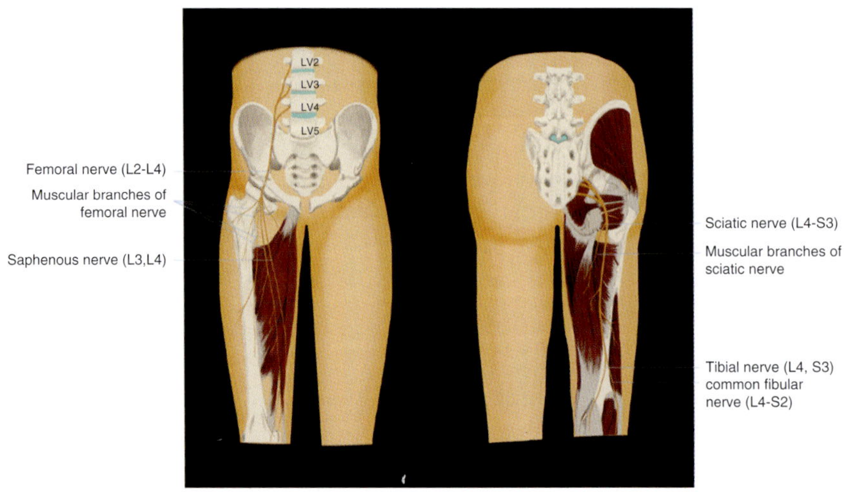

FIGURE 13.15 Illustration of the femoral nerve.

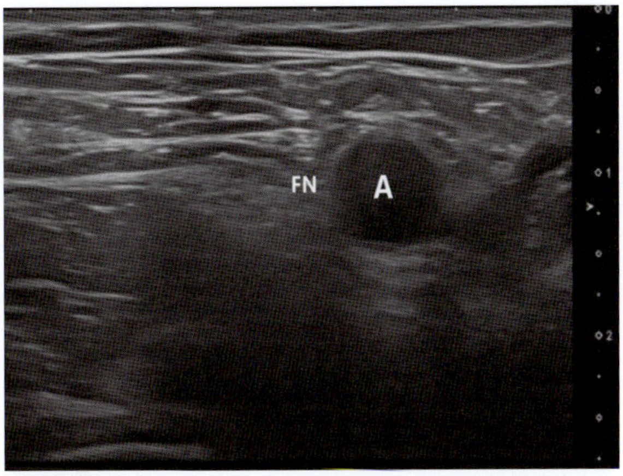

FIGURE 13.16 B-mode ultrasound image shows the right femoral nerve when the ultrasound transducer is placed at the inguinal crease. A, femoral artery; FN, femoral nerve.

used. Insert the needle with the tip adjacent to the nerve. After negative aspiration, 20–40 mL of local anesthetic is injected in 5 mL increments, with gentle aspiration between each injection. Anesthetic should be visualized spreading above, below, or circumferentially around the nerve. Remove the needle and discard it in the sharp container. Clean the patient from excess ultrasound gel [27].

Popliteal Sciatic Nerve Block

The sciatic nerve block provides complete anesthesia of the leg below the knee. Sciatic nerve block can be used to provide analgesia for surgery, fractures, laceration repairs, and abscess laceration and drainage [27].

Patient Position There are three common patient positions for a popliteal sciatic nerve block, determined by patient mobility:

Prone: the patient is prone with a pillow under the foot to slightly flex the knee.

Lateral decubitus: the patient is placed in the lateral decubitus position, operative side up.

Supine: the patient is supine, with the calf and foot elevated with the hip flexed to approximately 45° with knee flexed 90° as well for access to the popliteal fossa [27].

Procedure The popliteal fossa and crease are identified. The ultrasound transducer is placed over the popliteal crease transversely. Visualize the pulsation of the popliteal artery as an initial landmark (Fig. 13.17). The tibial nerve is then identified superficial to the popliteal artery. The popliteal vein lies between the popliteal artery and the tibial nerve but is very easily compressed. Follow the tibial nerve superiorly to the bifurcation of the sciatic nerve: the common fibular nerve laterally and the tibial nerve medially. This branch point is generally 7 cm above the popliteal crease in adults but is widely variable. The nerve block can be performed at proximal

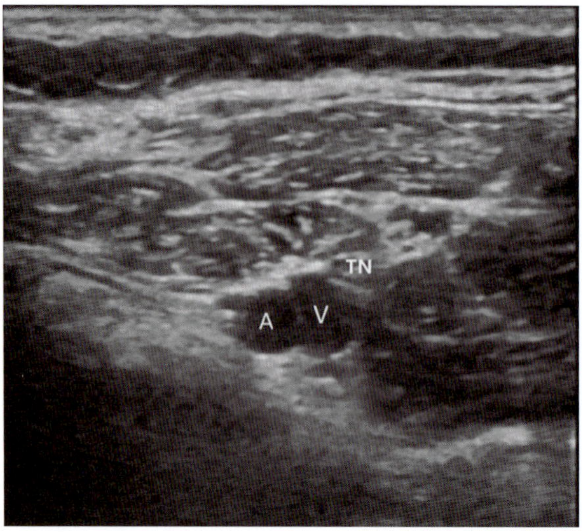

FIGURE 13.17 B-mode ultrasound image shows the left tibial nerve when the ultrasound transducer is placed over the popliteal crease in a transverse plane. A, popliteal artery; V, popliteal vein; TN, tibial nerve.

or distal to the branch point. The needle is inserted in the lateral thigh parallel to the transducer, directed toward the hyperechoic nerve. After negative aspiration, 20–30 mL of local anesthetic is injected in 5 mL increments, with confirmatory negative aspirations between each injection.

Local spread of anesthetic should be visualized around the entire sciatic nerve or around each of the two branches. Remove the needle and discard it in a sharp container. Clean the patient from excess ultrasound gel [27].

Summary

Ultrasound plays an important role in interventional procedures. The guidance with real-time ultrasound can improve the success rate and reduce complications. Physicians require all knowledge of anatomy, ultrasound physics, instrumentation, standard protocol for specific procedures, and experience in performing successful ultrasound-guided procedures.

Review Questions

1. Which transducer type would provide the highest resolution for superficial structures?
   - **a.** 5 MHz phased array
   - **b.** 10 MHz linear array
   - **c.** 5 MHz curvilinear
   - **d.** 3 MHz linear array

2. Which of the following describes an "acoustic" imaging artifact?
   a. Error in presentation of ultrasound information
   b. Error in interpretation
   c. Error in perception
   d. Electrical noise
3. In what direction is the ultrasound probe placed when accurately measuring the transverse plane of the artery?
   a. Perpendicular to the artery
   b. Parallel to the artery
   c. Adjacent to the artery
   d. Using beam steering techniques
4. Where is the ultrasound probe placed when performing thoracentesis?
   a. Between ribs 7 and 9, between the anterior axillary line and midline
   b. Between ribs 7 and 9, between the posterior axillary line and midline
   c. Between ribs 4 and 6, between the posterior axillary line and midline
   d. Between ribs 4 and 6, between the anterior axillary line and midline
5. In what position should a patient be placed for an ultrasound-guided thoracentesis procedure?
   a. Supine
   b. Prone
   c. Lateral recumbent with the pleural effusion facing down
   d. Sitting upright position
6. What ultrasound probe should you use to perform an interscalene nerve block?
   a. Phased array
   b. Endocavity
   c. Curvilinear
   d. Linear array
7. What structure should be identified just medial to the femoral nerve when performing a femoral nerve block?
   a. Femoral artery
   b. Lateral cutaneous femoral nerve
   c. Lymphatic channel
   d. Adductor canal
8. What patient position is ideal for the performance of an internal jugular vein cannulation?
   a. Prone trendelenburg
   b. Supine trendelenburg
   c. Left lateral decubitus
   d. Supine with drape used to cover sensitive areas

Correct answers: 1. b; 2. a; 3. a; 4. b; 5. d; 6. d; 7. a; 8. b.

References

1. Rippey J. Ultrasound guidance should be the standard of care for most invasive procedures performed by clinicians. Australas J Ultrasound Med. 2015; 15(4):116–120. https://doi.org/10.1002/j.2205-0140.2012.tb00194.x.
2. AIUM. AIUM practice parameters for documentation of an ultrasound examination. *J Ultrasound Med* 2020; 39: E1–E4. https://doi.org/10.1002/jum.15187.
3. Tirado A, Nagdev A, Henningsen C, et al. Ultrasound-guided procedures in the emergency department: needle guidance and localization. *Emerg Med Clin North Am* 2013; 31: 87–115.
4. AIUM.org. AIUM practice parameter for the performance of selected ultrasound-guided procedures. https://www.aium.org/resources/practice-parameters. Published 2016.
5. Cervini P, Hesley GK, Thompson RL, et al. Incidence of infectious complications after an ultrasound-guided intervention. *AJR* 2010; 195: 846–850.
6. Centers for Disease Control and Prevention. Disinfection and sterilization guidelines. https://www.cdc.gov/infection-control/hcp/disinfection-and-sterilization. Published 2019.
7. Sites BD, Brull R, Chan VW, et al. Artifacts and pitfall errors associated with ultrasound-guided regional anesthesia: Part II: A pictorial approach to understanding and avoidance. *Reg Anesth Pain Med* 2010; 35(2 Suppl): S81–S92.
8. Butcher C, Aziz S. CHAPTER 18, Ultrasound guidance for common procedures. In: Levitov A, Dallas P, Slonim A (eds). Bedside ultrasonography in clinical medicine. New York: McGraw-Hill Professional, 2010 https://studylib.net/doc/8385439/ultrasound-guidance-for-common-procedures.
9. Bushberg JT. The essential physics of medical imaging. Google Books, 2011 https://books.google.com/books/about/The_Essential_Physics_of_Medical_Imaging.htm.Published.
10. Miller AG, Bardin AJ. Review of ultrasound-guided radial artery catheter placement. *Respir Care* 2016; 61: 383–388. doi.org/10.4187/respcare.04190.
11. Theodore A, Clermont G, Dalton A. Intra-arterial catheterization for invasive monitoring: Indications, insertion techniques, and interpretation. Up to Date. https://www.uptodate.cn/contents/intra-arterial-catheterization-for-invasive-monitoring-indications-insertion-techniques-and-interpretation. Published 2019.
12. Weiner R, Ryan E, Yohannes-Tomicich J. CHAPTER 89, Arterial line monitoring and placement. In: Oropello JM, Pastores SM, Kvetan V (eds). Critical care. New York, NY, McGrawHill; New York 1–7 https://accessmedicine.mhmedical.com/content.aspx?sectionid=143522170&bookid=1944&Resultclick=2.
13. AIUM.org. AIUM practice parameter for the use of ultrasound to guide vascular access procedures. https://www.aium.org/resources/practice-parameters. Published 2019.
14. ACEP. Ultrasound-guided paracentesis. ACEP Now. https://www.acepnow.com/article/ultrasound-guided-paracentesis. Published 2012.
15. Shlamovitz G. What equipment is used in paracentesis? Medscape. https://www.medscape.com/answers/80944–32458/what-equipment-is-used-in-paracentesis#qna. Published 2019.
16. Verma S. Diagnostic and large-volume abdominal paracentesis. Up to Date. https://www.uptodate.cn/contents/diagnostic-and-large-volume-abdominal-paracentesis. Published 2025.
17. Heffner J, Mayo P. Ultrasound-guided thoracentesis. Up to Date. https://www.uptodate.cn/contents/ultrasound-guided-thoracentesis. Published 2019.
18. Brauner M. What equipment is needed to perform thoracentesis? Medscape. https://www.medscape.com/answers/80640–94896/. Published 2019.
19. Schweickert W, Puchalski J. Thoracentesis, pleural biopsy, and thoracic ultrasound. Pulmonology Advisor. www.pulmonologyadvisor.com. Published 2019.
20. ACEP. Ultrasound for thoracentesis. ACEP Now. https://www.acepnow.com/article/ultrasound-thoracentesis. Published 2013.

21. Adhikari S and Blaivas M. The ultimate guide to point-of-care ultrasound-guided procedures. Situ-LaCasse E, Javedani P, Devis P, Arif-Tiwari H. Ultrasound-guided percutaneous drainage procedures. 2019. 205–223. Springer, New York.
22. Image-guided drainage. *Interventional Radiol* https://muschealth.org/medical-services/digestive/tests/interventional-radiology/image-guided-drainage.
23. Becker T. Technique for skin abscess drainage. Uptodate.com. https://www.uptodate.cn/contents/techniques-for-skin-abscess-drainage. Published 2019.
24. Meer J, Taylor T, Beck S. Emergency medicine. Emergency ultrasound: soft-tissue assessment. MDedge Emergency Medicine. https://www.mdedge.com/content/emergency-ultrasound-soft-tissue-assessment. Published 2015.
25. NYSORA. Ultrasound-guided interscalene brachial plexus block. NYSORA. https://www.nysora.com/techniques/upper-extremity/intescalene/ultrasound-guided-interscalene-brachial-plexus-block. Published 2020.
26. Jeng C, Rosenblatt M. Upper extremity nerve blocks: techniques. Uptodate.com. https://www.uptodate.cn/contents/upper-extremity-nerve-blocks-techniques. Published 2020.
27. Jeng C, Rosenblatt M. Lower extremity nerve blocks: techniques. Uptodate.com. https://www.uptodate.cn/contents/lower-extremity-nerve-blocks-techniques. Published 2020. www.uptodate.com/contents/overview-of-peripheral-nerve-blocks. Updated: Jul 30, 2025.

CHAPTER 14

Ultrasound in Resuscitation

Robert Russell[1], Austin Page[1], and Xiang Fei[2]

[1] Rocky Vista University, College of Osteopathic Medicine, Ivins, Utah, USA

[2] Department of Ultrasound, The First Medical Center, General Hospital of PLA, Beijing, China

Introduction

Ultrasound is a standard imaging tool used in the assistance of resuscitation according to the American College of Emergency Physicians [1]. To help physicians effectively and efficiently determine diagnoses and treatment plans, several resuscitative ultrasound protocols have been developed. One of the most widely implemented point-of-care protocols is the Rapid Ultrasound for Shock and Hypotension (RUSH) exam [2]. This protocol outlines a standardized sequence of ultrasound scans that distinguish different causes, various states, and the underlying pathologies of shock. The mnemonic HI-MAP, which stands for heart, inferior vena cava (IVC), Morison's pouch, aorta, and pneumothorax, has been used to help physicians follow standard sequence while performing ultrasound scans [2]. The whole concept of ultrasound examination is to assess organs and vessels that exhibit dysfunction of the pump, the tank, and the pipes in the circulation system. The RUSH protocol sequences a standard order of scanning; however, various scanning protocols include, but are not limited to, the FEEL-resuscitation [3], the ACES exam [4], FALLS protocol [5], and FATE [6], which may be appropriate depending on the physician's diagnostic acumen. These protocols can be especially helpful with patients who present shock without a clear medical history to explain their current critical condition [7]. In this chapter, we will explore HI-MAP RUSH protocol, one of the commonly used ultrasound techniques in our institution. We will also present a conglomeration of techniques that assist in determining a patient's fluid status in a critical care scenario.

Anatomy

Aorta

The aorta originates from the left ventricle, initially ascending approximately 2 in. From there, it loops left and descends along the left side of the vertebral column as the thoracic aorta. Once through the opening of the diaphragm, it becomes the abdominal aorta. At the level of the 4th lumbar vertebra, the aorta will bifurcate into the common iliac arteries [8].

Inferior Vena Cava

The IVC returns blood to the heart from all areas of the body below the diaphragm. The IVC is formed at the junction of the two common iliac veins on the right side at the level of the 5th lumbar vertebra. The left and right renal veins also connect to the IVC at the level of the 1st lumbar vertebra (Fig. 14.1). The IVC then travels upwards along the right side of the aorta and through the central tendon of the diaphragm, ultimately arriving at the right atrium [8].

Morison's pouch (hepatorenal recess) is the space between the liver and the right kidney. It is located in the right upper quadrant (RUQ) between the 8th and 11th ribs (Fig. 14.2). In normal conditions, there is no free fluid between the liver and right kidney [1].

Lungs

The apex of both lungs, the top of lungs is located approximately 1–1.5 in. above the first rib, while the bases of the lungs rest on the diaphragm. The right lung is broader,

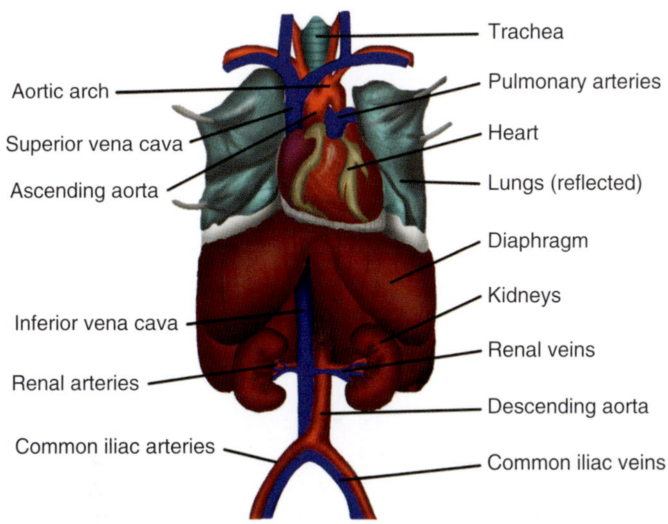

FIGURE 14.1 Anatomy illustration of Aorta and IVC.

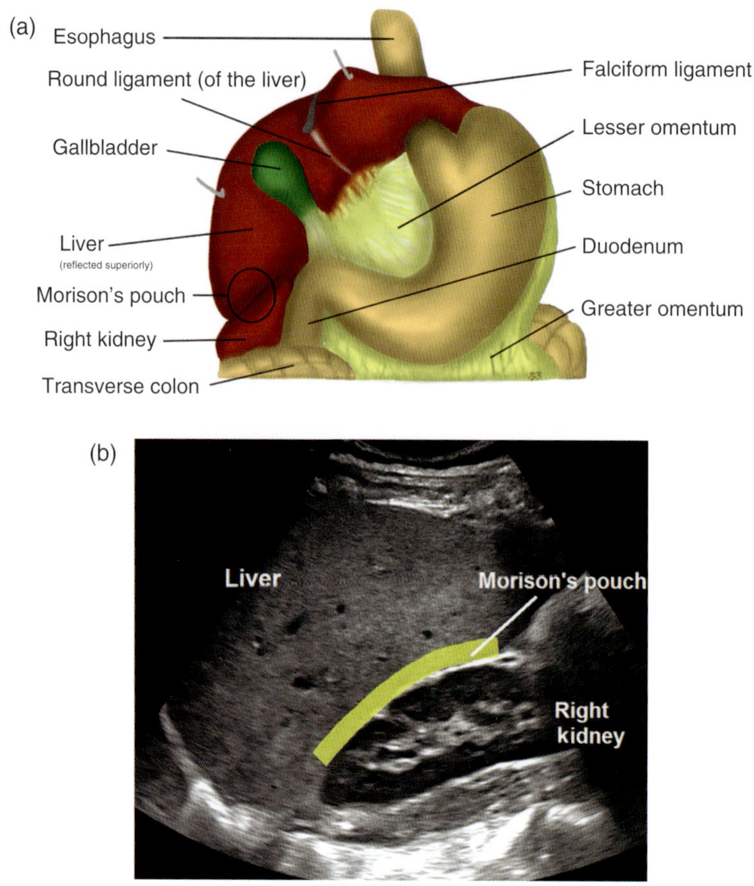

FIGURE 14.2 (a, b) Illustration (a) and ultrasound image (b) of Morison's pouch (highlighted yellow) with the liver and superior border of the kidney visible. There is no fluid in this space under normal conditions.

heavier, and shorter than the left lung and sits higher due to its position above the liver. The lungs are encased in a visceral pleura and a parietal pleura that also envelope the roots of the lungs, which contain the bronchial tube, the pulmonary artery and veins, the bronchial arteries and veins, the pulmonary plexus, the bronchial glands, and lymphatics [8].

Anatomy of the chest and heart is introduced in Chapter 3 and Chapter 4 of this book.

Ultrasound Techniques

Ultrasound is typically performed when the patient is lying in a supine position unless otherwise specified [9]. The physician can use a phased array probe (2–5 MHz) for visualizing the heart and IVC. This exam is designed to be performed quickly, transitioning from one view to the next without interruption [2].

Abdominal Aorta

To find the transverse view of the aorta, the probe is placed directly midline and angled posteriorly, with the indicator pointed laterally to the patient's right. The aorta is located directly anterior to the vertebral bodies, with the IVC on the right. All four portions of the aorta should be imaged by ultrasound in both transverse and longitudinal planes: (1) just below the heart; (2) superior to the renal arteries (Fig. 14.3); (3) inferior to the renal arteries; and (4) proximal and distal to the common iliac artery bifurcation (Fig. 14.4) [2]. Scans should be carefully performed from the proximal abdominal aorta below the diaphragm to the aortic bifurcation due to the possible development of an abdominal aortic aneurysm (AAA) at any one of these portions. The normal diameter of the aortic lumen should be less than 3 cm, measured transversely from the outer wall on one side to the outer wall on the other side.

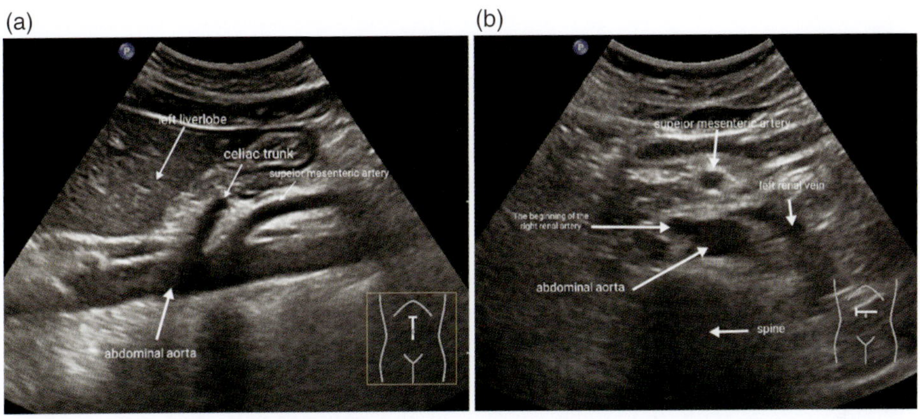

FIGURE 14.3 (a, b) Longitudinal proximal abdominal aorta (a) and transverse mid abdominal aorta at the level of renal arteries (b).

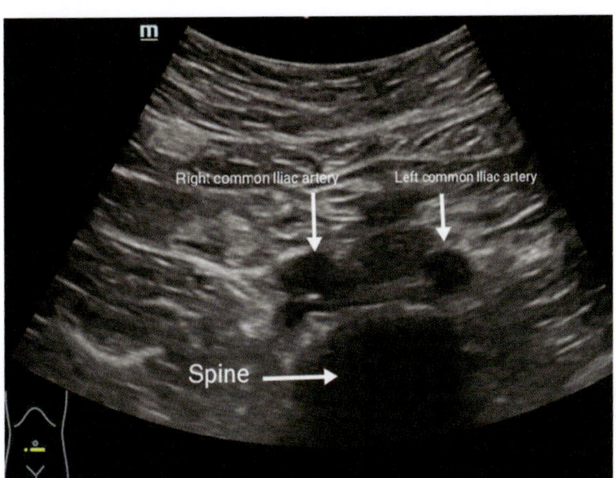

FIGURE 14.4 Transverse B-mode ultrasound image of the common iliac arteries.

Heart

The heart is a muscular organ that resides between the lungs, encased within the pericardium. The heart is divided into four chambers: the right atrium, right ventricle, left atrium, and left ventricle, and functions with four valves: the tricuspid valve, pulmonary valve, mitral (bicuspid) valve, and aortic valve [8].

The heart's position in the chest is oblique, with the base of the heart toward the right shoulder, and the apex toward the left pelvis. Due to the heart's oblique position and its obstructed location behind the inferior portion of the sternum, ultrasound image of the heart relies on the use of four different views: parasternal long axis, parasternal short axis, apical four-chamber, and subxiphoid [8].

Parasternal Long Axis and Short Axis To find the parasternal long-axis view, position the probe in the third or fourth intercostal space just left of the sternum. The sound beam should be pointed toward the patient's right shoulder. If positioned properly, the left ventricle and mitral valve should be clearly seen in the middle of the screen [10]. The left atrium, right ventricle, mitral valve, aortic valve, and interventricular septum should also be visible simultaneously. The details of performing parasternal short axis of the heart can be found in Chapter 4 of this book.

Apical Four-Chamber To find the apical four-chamber view, position the probe at the apex of the heart with the probe marker pointing to the patient's left. The apex is generally located just inferior and medial to the left midclavicular line in the fourth or fifth intercostal space. Once in position, tilt the probe so that the transducer is angled toward the patient's right shoulder [11]. If positioned correctly, all four chambers, the mitral valve, and the tricuspid valve should be visible.

Subxiphoid To find the subxiphoid view, position the probe inferior to the xiphoid process, with the probe marker to the patient's left, and point superiorly toward the head and slightly toward the patient's left shoulder [11]. Adjust the scanning direction of the probe anteriorly and posteriorly until a view of the four chambers of the heart is visible (Fig. 14.5). A part of the left hepatic lobe as an acoustic window may also be seen in the subxiphoid view of the heart.

Inferior Vena Cava

Ultrasound of the IVC can be used to help predict the patient's intravascular volume levels and identify a patient in hypovolemic shock [12].

To image the IVC, begin by obtaining a subxiphoid view of the heart as described in the previous section. The IVC should be visible longitudinally and transversely (Fig. 14.6). It is best to view the IVC superior to the insertion of the hepatic veins and inferior to the junction with the right atrium [13].

Morison's Pouch and FAST Exam

The focused assessment of sonography for trauma (FAST) exam (see Chapter 12) is a widely accepted protocol for identifying free fluid in the abdominal cavity during emergent situations [14]. A complete FAST exam may be performed for this step of

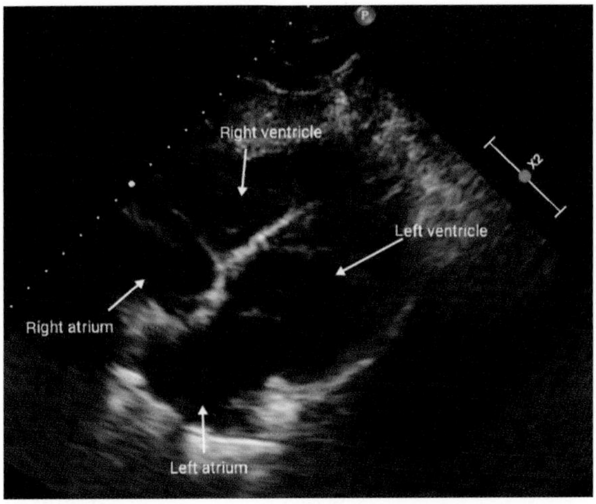

FIGURE 14.5 Subxiphoid view of the heart.

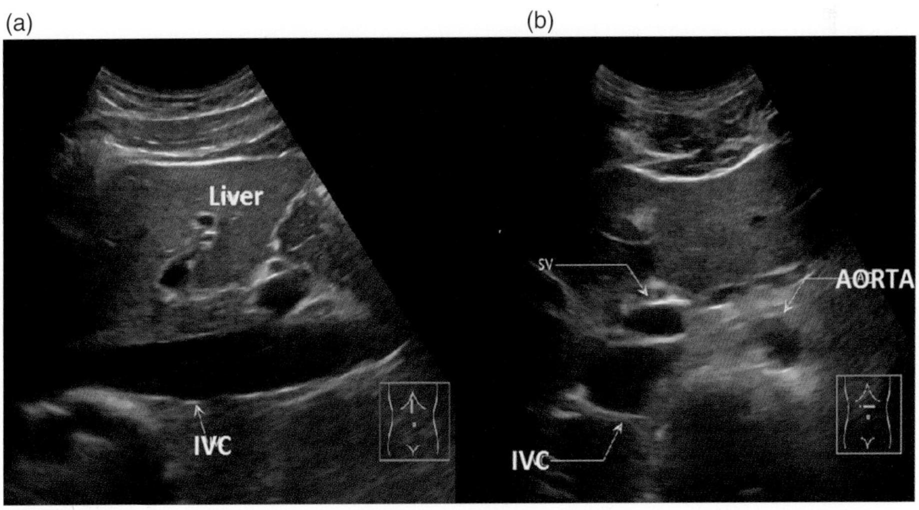

FIGURE 14.6 Longitudinal (a) and transverse (b) B-mode ultrasound images of inferior vena cava (IVC).

the RUSH protocol. If time does not allow for a complete FAST exam, a quick examination of Morison's pouch, the space between the right kidney and the liver, with the patient in the Trendelenburg position, may be used to examine for intraperitoneal blood or fluid. Since Morison's pouch does not contain any fluid in healthy patients, it is considered a potential space of accumulating free fluid in a patient with blunt trauma [15].

Morisons Pouch To find Morison's pouch, begin by placing the patient in supine position. Then place the probe at the right midaxillary line between the liver and right kidney, with the indicator pointed superiorly [14, 15].

Chest

An ultrasound scan of the chest is used to identify the presence of a pneumothorax. To scan for a pneumothorax, begin by placing the patient in a supine position if the patient is stable. Then place the probe on the patient's anterior chest in a sagittal orientation at the midclavicular line in the 2nd intercostal space [16]. Identify two ribs in the field of view by viewing the posterior shadow that will appear on the image. If two ribs are not present, slide the probe superiorly/inferiorly until two ribs are in the field of view [16]. Normally, a view of the lung will show the pleural layers sliding against one another between the ribs. This dynamic movement of the pleura is a sign of normal lung tissue and occurs during respiration. On M-mode, a normal ultrasound of the lungs will show a grainy image that has been identified as a "sandy beach" appearance (Chapter 3, Fig. 3.2). B-lines less than 3 or Z lines in the lung B-mode image may also be considered normal. B-lines are present due to ultrasound reverberation artifacts [16].

Common Pathologies in Resuscitation

Bedside ultrasonography can be utilized to recognize pre-shock, compensated shock, uncompensated shock, and cardiac arrest. Early recognition of undifferentiated hypotension is important to patient management [17].

Ultrasound may be used to assess the types of shock present in a patient. Hypovolemic shock can be ruled into one's differential based upon the intravascular volume of the patient. Cardiogenic shock can be determined by the location of pump failure: either left or right ventricular (RV) systolic or diastolic failure. Obstructive shock can be assessed by recognizing the presence of a pneumothorax, pulmonary embolism, cardiac tamponade, or other obstruction that can affect the filling of the ventricles. Distributive shock can be indicated by the degree of vascular vasodilation [7].

During cardiopulmonary resuscitation, point-of-care ultrasound can be beneficial for determining the location of tracheal tube placement, assessing cardiac movement of the heart, determining filling status of the heart during the pauses between chest compressions, and while the pulse is being checked [18].

Cardiac Tamponade

Cardiac tamponade is caused by pericardial effusion, the presence of fluid inside the pericardium, which is associated with obstructive shock. Fluid within the pericardium causes increased pressure on the heart, resulting in inhibition of its ability to relax and fill with blood [19]. The first step in scanning for cardiac tamponade is to look for a pericardial effusion. With the parasternal long-axis view in place, look for an anechoic stripe surrounding the heart. The pericardial effusion can exist on one side of the heart or encircle the entire heart [20]. It is important to note that a pericardial effusion and a pleural effusion can appear very similar in the parasternal long-axis view. To differentiate between the two situations, one must look at the aorta posterior to the wall of the pericardium. In a pericardial effusion, the anechoic fluid will be seen anterior to the posterior wall of the pericardium and descending aorta. In a pleural effusion, the anechoic fluid will be seen posterior to the posterior wall of the pericardium and descending aorta [21].

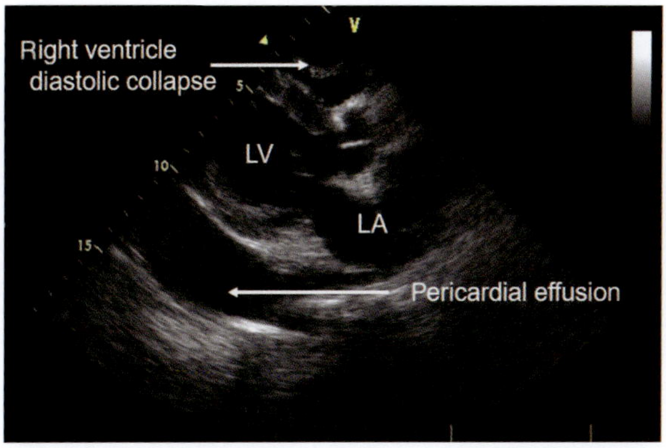

FIGURE 14.7 Severe cardiac tamponade with collapsed right ventricle on B-mode image.

After assessing a pericardial effusion, further investigation is required to evaluate the ability of the heart to relax. Increased pressure caused by the pericardial effusion can impair diastolic filling and cause collapse of the cardiac chambers, which can be assessed by viewing the right atrium and right ventricle during right atrial diastole and right ventricular diastole, respectively. The right atrium's collapse has been recognized as one of the earliest signs indicating the presence of cardiac tamponade but has a low specificity for the condition [22]. In addition to right atrium collapse, right ventricle collapse during diastole can be useful in identifying tamponade [22]. While viewing the cardiac chambers from either a subxiphoid or parasternal axis, one can use M-mode to view the right ventricle during diastole to assess whether the ventricle collapses. The degree of collapse can vary depending on the severity of tamponade. With mild tamponade, there may be a slight decrease in right atrial and ventricular relaxation. In more severe cases, the right atrium will become concave, and the right ventricle (Fig. 14.7) will completely collapse into the septum [23].

Left Ventricular Dysfunction

Evaluation of the left ventricle (LV) can help physicians identify the underlying cause of shock. A hypodynamic LV may indicate a cardiogenic cause of shock, while a hyperdynamic LV may indicate a distributive or hypovolemic cause of shock. The dynamics of the LV are evaluated by calculating fractional shortening of the LV using the following equation: $FS = (LVIDd - LVIDs)/LVIDd \times 100\%$, where FS = fractional shortening, LVIDd is left ventricular internal diameter at the end of diastole and LVIDs is left ventricular internal diameter at the end of systole [24]. M-mode parasternal long-axis view (Fig. 14.8) is used to measure the internal diameter of the left ventricle [24].

Calculating the fractional shortening with the method described is most accurate; however, with adequate training, physicians can estimate the ventricular function simply by observing several cycles of heart movement [25].

A dramatically increased left ventricular contraction can also be problematic. Patients with a ventricular wall diameter change of greater than 90% could be in shock secondary to hypovolemia or sepsis. Extreme cases can show the walls surrounding the ventricle converging and completely closing the chamber [2]. When patients present with undifferentiated, nontraumatic, symptomatic hypotension, the findings of a hyperdynamic left ventricle are specific for sepsis as the etiology of shock [26].

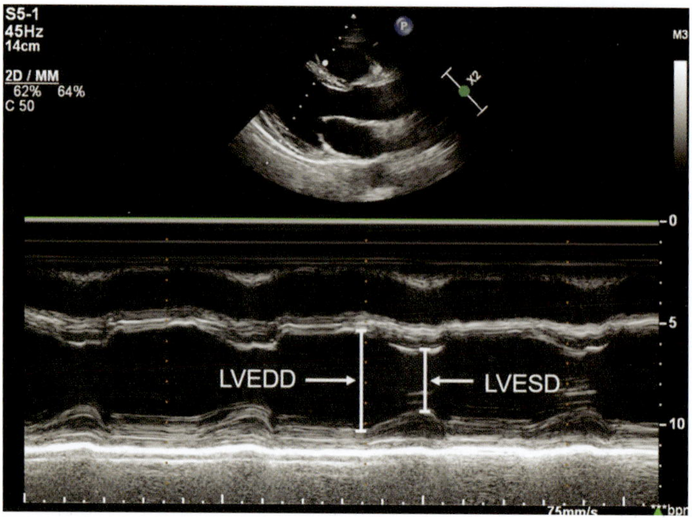

FIGURE 14.8 Parasternal long axis and measuring diameter of the left ventricle in M-mode ultrasound. LVEDD, left ventricle end diastolic diameter; LVESD, left ventricle endsystolic diameter.

Right Ventricular Failure

Signs of right ventricular (RV) dilatation can be identified by ultrasonography in the apical four-chamber view. Determining the presence of RV dilatation can be done by comparing the size of the RV with the LV; the RV should be approximately ⅓ the size of the LV [27]. If the RV is similar in size to the LV, this indicates RV dilatation (Fig. 14.9). Dilatation of the RV indicates fluid overload or increased pulmonary afterload. Other causes of RV dilatation and dysfunction can also be due to pulmonary hypertension, RV infarction, RV outflow obstruction, such as an embolism, or cardiac arrest [28, 29].

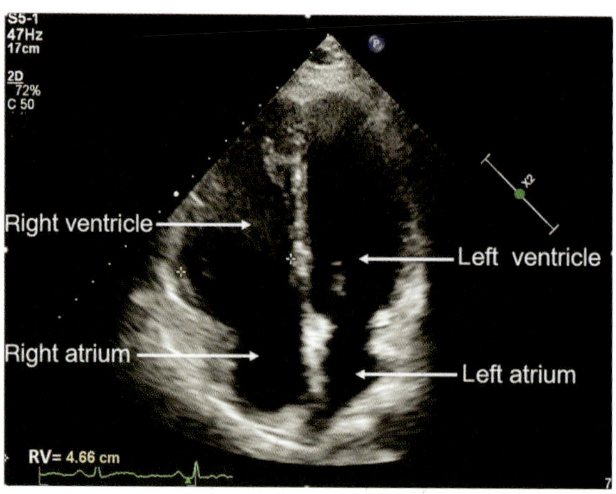

FIGURE 14.9 Four-chamber view of the heart shows right ventricle dilatation (4.66 cm) on B-mode ultrasound image.

Right heart function can be estimated by the displacement of the tricuspid valve during systole or tricuspid annular plane systolic excursion (TAPSE). This measurement determines the displacement of the tricuspid annulus toward the apex of the heart during systole [30]. The greater the displacement of the tricuspid annulus, the better the systolic function of the heart. Using M-mode (color flow imaging to assess blood flow direction may also be used), align the cursor with the right ventricular wall in an apical four-chamber view of the heart. Values less than 17 mm are abnormal. This measurement is widely used and is easily accomplished. It is significantly associated with outcomes of pulmonary hypertension and severity of right ventricular systolic failure [30].

Hypovolemia and Inferior Vena Cava

The volume status and central venous pressure (CVP) can be estimated using ultrasound of the IVC. This measurement can help predict which patients would benefit from fluid administration for correcting hypotension.

One method used to estimate CVP is the caval index. The caval index is the percentage of change in IVC during respiration. The diameter of the IVC reduces during inspiration and expands during expiration [15, 30]. To measure the diameter of the IVC, record the IVC in a longitudinal view using B-mode and M-mode to measure the distance from one wall to the opposite (Fig. 14.10). To calculate the caval index, you will need the diameter during inspiration and expiration. The equation for caval index is: $[(IVCe - IVCi)/IVCe] \times 100$, where IVCe is the diameter of the IVC in expiration and IVCi is the diameter of the IVC during inspiration [31, 32].

The American Society of Echocardiography has established guidelines for estimating the CVP via ultrasound and recommended its use as less invasive than traditional venous catheterization. CVP is measured by the IVC diameter and collapsibility. The site for measuring IVC diameter is 1–2 cm inferior to the junction of the right atrium and IVC. An IVC diameter of less than 2.1 cm along with a collapse of greater than 50% during inspiration indicates a CVP of less than 3 mmHg (range 0–5 mmHg).

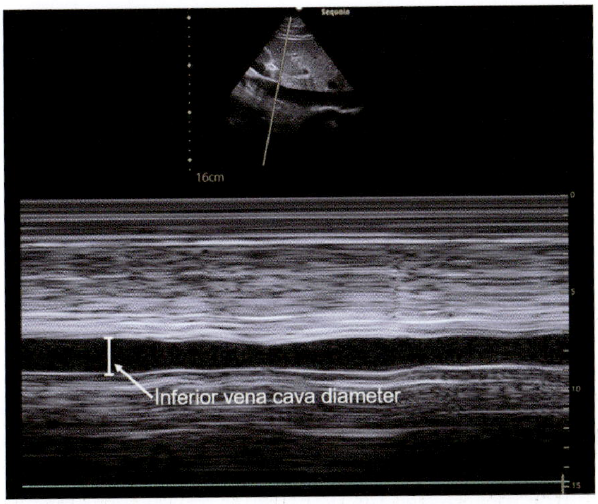

FIGURE 14.10 Change in lumen diameter of the inferior vena cava in expiration and inspiration on M-mode ultrasound.

An IVC diameter of greater than 2.1 cm along with a collapse of less than 50% during inspiration indicates a CVP of greater than 15 mmHg (range 10–20 mmHg) [32]. Low or normal CVP is consistent with hypovolemic or distributive shock. A high CVP is consistent with cardiogenic or obstructive shock.

It is noted that the changes in IVC diameter are reversed in a patient on mechanical ventilation compared to patients having spontaneous breathing [15, 31]. The IVC expands during inspiration and collapses during expiration. While ventilated, during the inspiratory phase of respiration, the pleural pressure increases, leading to an increase in the right atrial pressure (RAP), causing the IVC to remain dilated. The opposite occurs at the IVC during expiration on a ventilated patient [33].

Abdominal Aortic Aneurysm

Risk factors for developing an AAA include age, male, smoking history, atherosclerosis, hypertension, and family history of AAA [34]. The size of the aorta measures from the outer wall of the vessel to the opposite side of the outer wall. AAA is diagnosed if the aorta lumen is greater than 3 cm in diameter and the shape of the aorta is bulging or outpouching [2]. The presence of a thrombus or plaque buildup may occlude the lumen and make it difficult to determine the actual wall. When screening for an AAA, the operator should measure three dimensions (length, width, and anteroposterior) in the upper, middle, and lower portions of the abdominal aorta. It is important to note that most AAAs occur below the renal arteries (infrarenal segment) and may extend into the iliac arteries [2, 35].

There are two different types of aneurysms: fusiform and saccular. With the fusiform aneurysm, the aorta balloons on all sides of the vessel, while the ballooning occurs on only one side of the aorta in the saccular aneurysm. Due to the increased wall stress, it is surmised that saccular aneurysms have a greater risk of rupturing [36]. An aneurysm with dissection (Fig. 14.11), appearing with a thin arterial wall and flap, also has potential for rupture and bleeding, which requires urgent intervention [37]. In addition, AAA greater than 5 cm have an increased risk of rupture and bleeding into the retroperitoneal cavity. Consequently, patients with ruptured AAA may present with hypotension, flank or back pain, or a pulsatile mass [34]. It is difficult to identify retroperitoneal bleeding from a ruptured AAA using ultrasound alone. Unstable patients with a confirmed AAA and consistent clinical symptoms should be considered to have an AAA rupture and treated accordingly [21]. A CT scan is recommended for further evaluation if an aneurysm is present [34].

Intra-Abdominal Bleeding

Intra-abdominal bleeding is a common and severe cause of shock. Such bleeding can present due to many different causes, including, but not limited to, blunt trauma, penetrating trauma, rupture of vessels, and ruptured ectopic pregnancy [38]. A patient's volume status can first be assessed via ultrasound of the IVC and further investigated by performing a FAST exam. In the case of intra-abdominal bleeding or other causes of intra-abdominal fluid, there may be an anechoic accumulation of fluid between the kidney and the liver (Fig. 14.12).

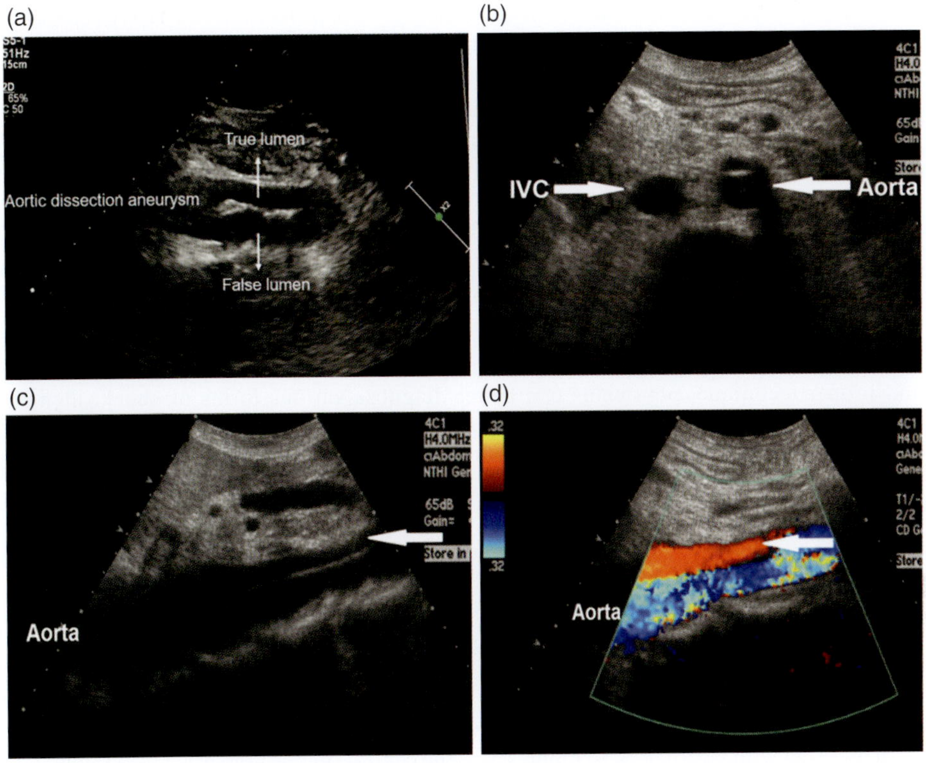

FIGURE 14.11 Ultrasound images of abdominal aorta aneurysm dissection in longitudinal (a) and transverse (b) planes. True lumen (white arrow) and false lumen on B-mode (c) and color flow imaging (d).

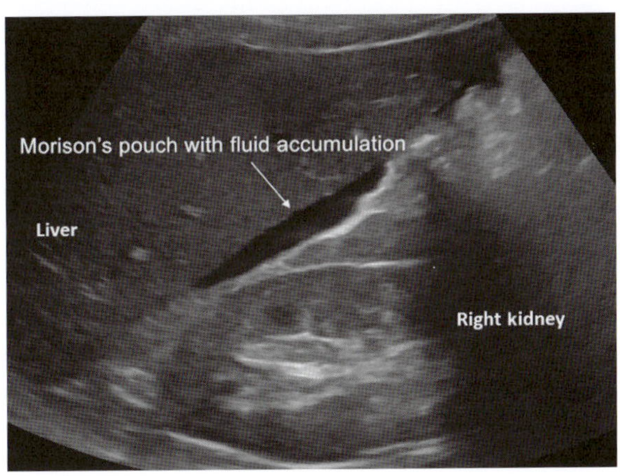

FIGURE 14.12 Image of Morison's pouch with fluid accumulation on B-mode image.

Pneumothorax

In the event of a pneumothorax, absence of the dynamic movement of the pleura is suggestive of a potential pneumothorax [39, 40]. On M-mode lung ultrasound, if there is loss of the dynamic movement of the pleura (absence of "seashore" sign), then lung sliding will appear as a static view as "barcode" sign or the "stratosphere" sign (Chapter 12, Fig. 12.8) [16].

The only movement that can be seen is chest wall movement in the event of a pneumothorax. It is important to distinguish between the normal movement of the pleura against one another and that of the chest wall. The presence of dynamic movement of the pleura rules out a pneumothorax, but the absence of this dynamic sliding of the pleura does not necessarily indicate a pneumothorax. Differentials from pneumothorax include hemothorax and hypercarbic respiratory failure [41, 42].

Summary

Ultrasound is an important tool in the emergency department. With concise protocols and proper technique, physicians can better diagnose various forms of shock, identify underlying causes (or at least narrow differential diagnosis), and guide management to correct hypovolemia. While other, more time-consuming, diagnostic modalities may be more sensitive or specific, ultrasound remains an effective diagnostic tool for assisting resuscitation.

Review Questions

1. True or False: While scanning the inferior vena cava, if the diameter of the vessel is greater than 2.1 cm with less than 50% compression, the central venous pressure (CVP) is low.
2. When viewing the RUQ of a patient, between ribs 8 and 11, what pouch can be filled with fluid between the liver and the right kidney?
   a. Pouch of Douglas
   b. Morison's pouch
   c. Vesicouterine pouch
   d. Paracolic gutter
3. The presence of the "barcode sign" on M-mode ultrasound when viewing the anterior chest wall is potentially indicative of what condition?
   a. Pleural effusion
   b. Atelectasis
   c. Pneumothorax
   d. Mediastinal mass
4. The preferred single probe for viewing all the lung and cardiac images described in this chapter is:
   a. Phased array
   b. Curvilinear probe
   c. Linear probe
   d. Endocavity probe
5. Which of the following views is not always pertinent in a routine focused cardiac ultrasound?
   a. Parasternal long axis
   b. Apical four-chamber
   c. Subxiphoid
   d. Transesophageal

6. To help in determining whether pelvic fluid is present, one may position the patient in:
   a. Reverse Trendelenburg
   b. Trendelenburg
   c. Semi-fowler
   d. Fowler
7. All the following are examples of obstructive shock, EXCEPT:
   a. Tension pneumothorax
   b. Pulmonary embolism
   c. Cardiac tamponade
   d. Heart failure
8. True or False: The size and shape of the abdominal aorta may change following respiratory variation in real-time B-mode ultrasound.
9. When determining the size of the aortic lumen, one should measure from the ____ to the ____.
   a. Inner wall, inner wall
   b. Outer wall, outer wall
   c. Lumen, wall
   d. Wall, lumen
10. True or False: When performing an ultrasound on a patient for suspected cardiac tamponade, the collapsibility of the right atrium during diastole is more specific than the right ventricle collapsing during diastole for tamponade.

Correct answers: 1. False; 2. b; 3. c; 4. a; 5. d; 6. a; 7. d; 8. False; 9. b; 10. False.

References

1. American College of Emergency Medicine. Ultrasound guidelines: emergency, point-of-care and clinical ultrasound guidelines in medicine. *Ann Emerg Med* 2017; 69: e27–e54. https://doi.org/10.1016/j.annemergmed.2016.08.457.
2. Weingart SD, Duque D, Nelson B. Rapid ultrasound for shock and hypotension (RUSH-HIMAPP). http://emedhome.com. Published 2009.
3. Breitkreutz R, Price S, Steiger HV, et al. Focused echocardiographic evaluation in life support and peri-resuscitation of emergency patients: a prospective trail. *Resuscitation* 2010; 81: 1527–1533.
4. Atkinson PRT, McAuley DJ, Kendall RJ, et al. Abdominal and cardiac evaluation with sonography in shock (ACES): an approach by emergency physicians for the use of ultrasound in patients with undifferentiated hypotension. *Emerg Med J* 2009; 26: 87–91.
5. Lichtenstein DA, Karakitsos D. Integrating ultrasound in the hemodynamic evaluation of acute circulatory failure (FALLS-the fluid administration limited by lung sonography protocol). *J Crit Care* 2012; 27: 53.e11–533.e19.
6. Jensen MB, Sloth E, Larsen KM, Schmidt MB. Transthoracic echocardiography for cardiopulmonary monitoring in intensive care. *Eur J Anaesthesiol* 2004; 21: 700–707.
7. Estoos E, Nakitende D. Diagnostic ultrasound use in undifferentiated hypotension. Treasure Island, FL: StatPearls Publishing, 2020. https://www.ncbi.nlm.nih.gov/books/NBK499955.
8. Gray H, Carter HV, Pick TP, Howden R. Anatomy: descriptive and surgical. New York: Fall River Press, 2012; 93–97, 434–442, 450–451, 525–527, 596, 957–962.

9. Gillman LM, Ball CG, Panebianco N, et al. Clinician performed resuscitative ultrasonography for the initial evaluation and resuscitation of trauma. *Scand J Trauma Resusc Emerg Med* 2009; 17: 34. https://doi.org/10.1186/1757-7241-17-34.
10. Aquilina O, Felice H, Fenech A, Grech V. Normal adult echocardiography - apical views. *Images Paediatr Cardiol* 2007; 9: 1–9.
11. Mitchell C, Rahko PS, Blauwet LA, et al. Guidelines for performing a comprehensive transthoracic echocardiographic examination in adults: recommendations from the American Society of Echocardiography. *J Am Soc Echocardiogr* 2019; 32: 1–64. https://doi.org/10.1016/j.echo.2018.06.004.
12. Rahman NH, Ahmad R, Kareem MM, Mohammed MI. Ultrasonographic assessment of inferior vena cava/abdominal aorta diameter index: a new approach of assessing hypovolemic shock class 1. *Int J Emerg Med* 2016; 9: 8. https://doi.org/10.1186/s12245-016-0101-z.
13. Goldflam K, Lewiss R, Saul T, Solomon R. *Inferior* vena cava ultrasound. ACEP Now website. https://www.acepnow.com/article/inferior-vena-cava-ultrasound/?singlepage=1&theme=print-friendly. Published 2011.
14. Franzen D. FAST examination. FAST exam. https://www.saem.org/cdem/education/online-education/m3-curriculum/bedside-ultrasonagraphy/fast-exam. Published 2016.
15. Vincent JL, Rhodes A, Perel A, et al. Clinical review: update on hemodynamic monitoring--a consensus of 16. *Crit Care* 2011; 15: 229. https://doi.org/10.1186/cc10291.
16. Husain LF, Hagopian L, Wayman D, et al. Sonographic diagnosis of pneumothorax. *J Emerg Trauma Shock* 2012; 5: 76–81. https://doi.org/10.4103/0974-2700.93116.
17. Jones AE, Tayal VS, Sullivan DM, Kline JA. Randomized, controlled trial of immediate versus delayed goal-directed ultrasound to identify the cause of nontraumatic hypotension in emergency department patients. *Crit Care Med* 2004; 32: 1703–1708.
18. Volpicelli G. Usefulness of emergency ultrasound in nontraumatic cardiac arrest. *Am J Emerg Med* 2010; 29: 216–223. https://doi.org/10.1016/j.ajem.2009.03.018.
19. Cardiac Tamponade. Clinical key elsevier point of care. https://www-clinicalkey-com.proxy.rvu.edu/#!/content/clinical_overview/67-s2.0-ab580412-524c-4e24-a7b3-e0286a23be90. Published 2019.
20. Goodman A, Phillips P, Mailhot T, Diku M. The role of bedside ultrasound in the diagnosis of pericardial effusion and cardiac tamponade. *J Emerg Trauma Shock* 2012; 5: 72–75. https://doi.org/10.4103/0974-2700.93118.
21. Seif D, Perera P, Mailhot T, et al. Bedside ultrasound in resuscitation and the rapid ultrasound in shock protocol. *Crit Care Res Prac* 2012; 2012: 1–14. https://doi.org/10.1155/2012/503254.
22. Nagdev A, Stone MB. Point-of-care ultrasound evaluation of pericardial effusions: does this patient have cardiac tamponade? *Resuscitation* 2011; 82: 671–673. https://doi.org/10.1016/j.resuscitation.2011.02.004.
23. Shabetai R. Pericardial effusion: haemodynamic spectrum. *Heart* 2004; 90(3): 255–256. https://doi.org/10.1136/hrt.2003.024810.
24. Chengode S. Left ventricular global systolic function assessment by echocardiography. *Ann Card Anaesth* 2016; 19: 26–34. https://doi.org/10.4103/0971-9784.192617.
25. Moore CL, Rose GA, Tayal VS, et al. Determination of left ventricular function by emergency physician echocardiography of hypotensive patients. *Acad Emerg Med* 2002; 9: 186–193. https://doi.org/10.1111/j.1553-2712.2002.tb00242.x.
26. Jones AE, Craddock PA, Tayal VS, Kline JA. Diagnostic accuracy of left ventricular function for identifying sepsis among emergency department patients with nontraumatic symptomatic undifferentiated hypotension. *Shock* 2005; 24: 513–517.
27. Ho SY, Nihoyannopoulos P. Anatomy, echocardiography, and normal right ventricular dimensions. *Heart* 2006; 92: i2–i13. https://doi.org/10.1136/hrt.2005.077875.
28. Rudski LG, Wyman WL, Afilalo J, et al. Guidelines for the echocardiographic assessment of the right heart in adults: a report from the American Society of Echocardiography. *J Am Soc Echocardiogr* 2010; 23: 685–713.

29. Pinsky MR. The right ventricle: interaction with pulmonary circulation. *Crit Care* 2016; 20: 266. https://doi.org/10.1186/s13054-016-1440-0.
30. Mangion JR. Assessment of right ventricular structure and function. In: Felker GM, Mann DL (eds). Essential echocardiography: a companion to Braunwalds heart disease. Philadelphia, PA: Elsevier, 2019; 180–189.
31. Mok KL. Make it SIMPLE: enhanced shock management by focused cardiac ultrasound. *J Intensive Care* 2016; 4: 51. https://doi.org/10.1186/s40560-016-0176-x.
32. Rudski LG, Lai WW, Afilalo J, et al. CME exam for guidelines for the echocardiographic assessment of the right heart in adults: a report from the American Society of Echocardiography. *J Am Soc Echocardiogr* 2010; 23: 786–788.
33. Jardin F, Vieillard-Baron A. Ultrasonographic examination of the venae cavae. *Intensive Care Med* 2006; 32: 203–206. https://doi.org/10.1007/s00134-005-0013-5.
34. Dalman R, Mell M. Overview of abdominal aortic aneurysm. https://www-uptodate-com.proxy.rvu.edu/contents/overview-of-abdominal-aortic-aneurysm. Published 2019.
35. Guideline Developed in Collaboration with the American College of Radiology; Society of Radiologists in Ultrasound. AIUM practice guideline for the performance of diagnostic and screening ultrasound examinations of the abdominal aorta in adults. *J Ultrasound Med* 2015; 34: 1–6. https://doi.org/10.7863/ultra.34.8.15.13.0003.
36. Nathan DP, Xu C, Pouch AM, et al. Increased wall stress of saccular versus fusi form aneurysms of the descending thoracic aorta. *Ann Vasc Surg* 2011; 25: 1129–1137. https://www.ncbi.nlm.nih.gov/pubmed/22023944.
37. Kiru G, Bicknell C, Falaschetti E, et al. An evaluation of the effect of an angiotensin-converting enzyme inhibitor on the growth rate of small abdominal aortic aneurysms: a randomised placebo-controlled trial (AARDVARK). Southampton (UK): NIHR Journals Library; 2016 Jul. (Health Technology Assessment, No. 20.59.) Chapter 3, Ultrasound measurements and quality assurance. Available from: https://www.ncbi.nlm.nih.gov/books/NBK378857
38. Pariyadith M, Snead G. Emergency ultrasound in adults with abdominal and thoracic trauma. https://www-uptodate-com.proxy.rvu.edu/contents/emergency-ultrasound-in-adults-with-abdominal-and-thoracic-trauma. Published 2019.
39. Ball CG, Ranson K, Dente CJ, et al. Clinical predictors of occult pneumothoraces in severely injured blunt polytrauma patients: a prospective observational study. *Injury* 2009; 40: 44–47.
40. Lichtenstein DA, Menu Y. A bedside ultrasound sign ruling out pneumothorax in the critically ill. Lung sliding. *Chest* 1995; 108: 1345–1348.
41. De Luca C, Valentino M, Rimondi MR, et al. Use of chest sonography in acute-care radiology. *J Ultrasound* 2008; 11: 125–134. https://doi.org/10.1016/j.jus.2008.09.006.
42. Mallow C, Isakow W. Risk factors for loss of lung sliding in a medical intensive care population with acute respiratory failure. *J Bronchology Interv Pulmonol* 2019; 26: 102–107. https://doi.org/10.1097/LBR.0000000000000525.

CHAPTER 15

Ultrasound of the Breast

Rachel McCann[1], Christine Kai[1], Andy Nigh[1], and Han-Xue Zhao[2]

[1]Rocky Vista University, College of Osteopathic Medicine, Ivins, Utah, USA

[2]Department of Ultrasound, Beijing Tongren Hospital, Capital Medical University, Beijing, China

Introduction

Ultrasonography of the breast has proven to be a noninvasive diagnostic tool that physicians and professionals can utilize in office settings and breast imaging centers to investigate breast pathologies. Breast ultrasound is often scheduled when a lump is felt during a clinical breast examination [1]. No preparation is required prior to the ultrasound scan. Physicians and ultrasound operators who perform breast ultrasound scans and image interpretation should undergo appropriate and accredited training. Knowledge of breast anatomy, common breast pathologies, patient's position, transducer placement, and ultrasound machine settings is critical to acquire high quality of breast ultrasound images. Mammography is the standard method of breast cancer screening; supplemental ultrasound of the breast can be useful in the detection of early-stage breast cancers, especially in dense breast tissue [2]. Early detection of breast cancers can yield a better prognosis, as treatment in early stages is most effective [1]. Ultrasound of the breast can determine the difference between cystic lesions and solid masses, which is typically difficult to make with mammography. Many other symptoms can also be evaluated using ultrasonography, including new lumps, skin changes, skin thickening, nipple discharge, and unexplained pain [1]. The diagnostic capabilities, along with the ease of use and low cost, make ultrasound an accessible and powerful tool for assessing breast pathologies.

Anatomy

The breast is an anatomical structure that lies on the anterior surface of the thorax. It is composed of the mammary gland, fat, connective tissue, vessels, nerves, and lymphatics (Fig. 15.1). This organ matures as a modified sweat gland that is a highly specialized cutaneous structure involved in the ejection and secretion of milk for the nourishment of offspring. It is specific to mammals and very similar throughout

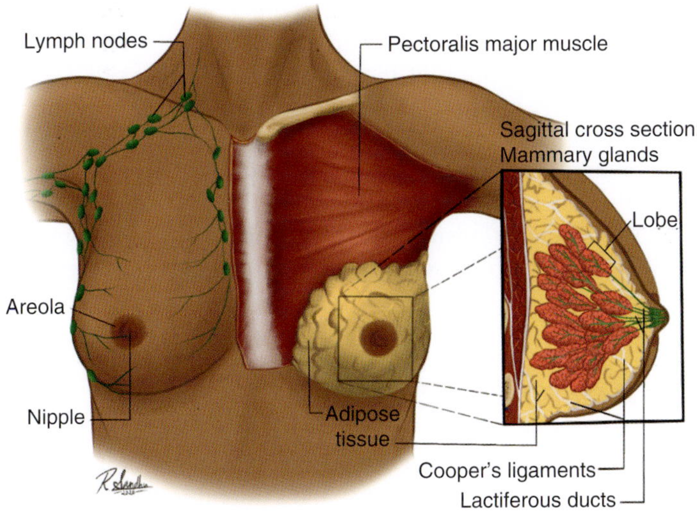

FIGURE 15.1 Illustration of breast anatomy.

various species. In humans, the mammary gland is composed of 15–20 lobes that originate from the areola and nipple and diffuse along the anterior and lateral thoracic wall as they further subdivide into lobules [3]. Around age 20, women have fully developed breasts following puberty; however, as women near the age of 40, breast tissue begins to atrophy due to menopausal hormonal changes. Pregnancy and lactation also induce striking growth and functional changes to the breast tissue. Various changes also occur during a woman's menstrual cycle due to the fluctuation of hormone levels [3].

The breast spans from the second to the sixth rib and from the sternum to the midaxillary line, bilaterally. The tissue of the breast can expand beyond these borders, superolateral into the axilla (axillary tail), superiorly to the clavicle, and inferiorly to the epigastric space. The organ is invested by the superficial fascia and the thoracic wall. The posterior border of the breast is the deep layer of the superficial fascia, which lies on top of the pectoralis major, serratus anterior, and external oblique muscles (Fig. 15.1). Between the deep layer of the superficial fascia and the deep investing fascia of the pectoralis major muscle is the retromammary bursa, which contributes to the mobility of the breast [3, 4].

The glandular portion of the breast has a protuberant, conical shape. Generally, around the apex of the breast, the dermis becomes more pigmented, keratinized, and wrinkled. This more pigmented area is the areola that contains sebaceous and sweat glands. In the center of the areola is the nipple. The nipple contains numerous free nerve endings and muscular tissue that enable the suckling of an infant. The lobes that comprise the mammary gland end in a lactiferous duct that opens through an orifice onto the nipple. These lobes are suspended by fibrous connective tissue, which forms a lattice framework of ligaments, called Cooper's ligaments, to support the lobes, maintain breast shape, and contribute to mobility. This framework is surrounded by the subcutaneous adipose tissue [3].

The blood supply of the breast includes branches of the internal mammary artery, posterior intercostal arteries, and axillary artery. Venae comitantes of the breast closely follow the path of the arterial supply and drain toward the axilla. Anastomoses of the intercostal veins with the vertebral plexus allow for metastasis.

The sensory innervation of the breast is provided mainly by branches of the second to sixth intercostal nerves, with a few contributions from the supraclavicular nerve of the cervical plexus. The lymph of the breast drains principally into the axillary lymph nodes. The axillary lymph nodes are divided into six groups: lateral, external mammary, subscapular, central, subclavicular, and interpectoral lymph nodes [4]. The internal mammary and axillary nodes also play a role in lymph drainage of the breast; however, they do not drain to the axilla [5]. Understanding the anatomy of the breast is imperative when performing an ultrasound scan, yet this procedure is only useful when proper examination technique is also implemented (Fig. 15.1).

Indications for Breast Ultrasound

Ultrasonography has proven to be a successful imaging technique in diagnosing breast abnormalities, assisting in cyst aspirations, and evaluating tissue density, implants, and masses [1]. Although mammography has been instrumental in increasing the diagnosis of breast cancer, it is limited in detecting or interpreting all incidences of breast pathologies due to issues such as dense breast tissue and the resulting low-resolution image. Thus, it is recommended that abnormalities that are discovered upon a mammogram or palpated in a breast exam be further investigated using ultrasonography [1]. This procedure can be particularly useful in distinguishing a fluid-filled cyst from a solid mass detected upon palpation (Fig. 15.2).

Ultrasound of the breast is commonly indicated in women under the age of 35, who typically have relatively dense breast tissue that can be difficult to thoroughly examine with mammography alone [2]. Women who may be pregnant or have breast implants should also avoid exposure to the radiation from a mammogram, and therefore, ultrasonography is recommended for evaluation of the breast and the implant, if applicable.

Procedures such as cyst aspirations, surgical breast biopsies, and other interventional procedures can benefit from guidance with ultrasound [2]. Preoperative

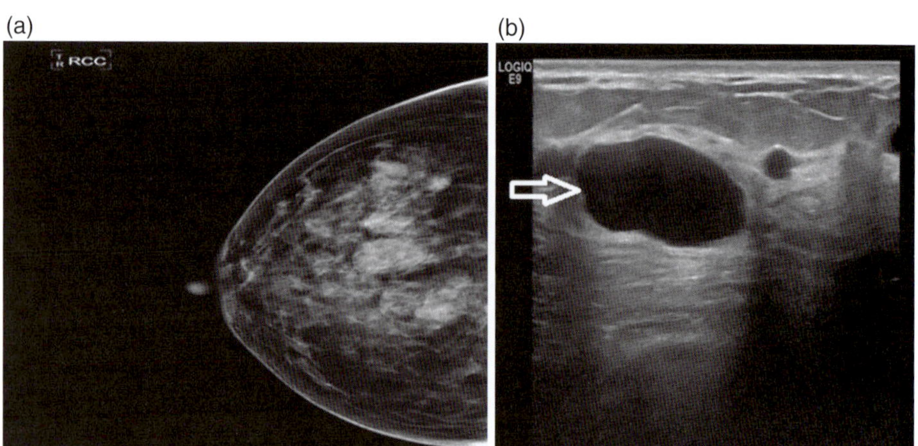

FIGURE 15.2 (a, b) Mammogram (a) and transverse plane B-mode ultrasound image (b) of fluid-filled cyst (arrow) correlated with the lesion in mammogram.

ultrasound-guided breast biopsy can provide histopathological information of the breast lesion and localization to mark the site of the breast tumor. Breast ultrasound is an integral part of designing a successful breast surgery [2].

In women that have previously diagnosed malignant masses or any findings that are highly suggestive of malignancy, ultrasound can be used to help identify axillary lymphadenopathy. Such identifications can help to recognize and monitor breast cancer metastasis [1, 2]. When indicated and in conjunction with knowledge of proper examination technique and anatomy of the breast, ultrasound is an invaluable tool to help identify a wide range of breast conditions, benign or malignant.

Ultrasound Techniques

When performing a high-resolution breast ultrasound, a linear-array, broad-bandwidth transducer with a center frequency of at least 12 MHz or higher should be used [1]. This would allow for 5–6 cm of penetration into the tissue with high image resolution. Variable frequencies may be required, depending on the depth and characteristics of the area of interest, to obtain optimal images. However, the depth of the focus should be greater than 3 cm, and gain should be set so that the subcutaneous fat is completely gray. Pectoral muscles along the chest wall should be visible to demonstrate that the entire breast is in view (Fig. 15.3). Color and spectral Doppler imaging can also be used to assess blood flow in the area scanned [6]. High-frequency transducer, a gel pad, or a thick layer of gel may facilitate imaging of superficial lesions.

Imaging is best acquired after placing the patient in a supine position with the ipsilateral arm above the head. This positioning allows the skin over the breast to be spread thinner. Proper draping techniques should be applied for covering any portion of the breasts that are not being scanned. While performing the scan, the transducer should be kept parallel to the breast surface so that the beam is perpendicular to the tissue. Failure to keep this position can result in reflective and refractive attenuation. Pressure needs to be applied on B-mode to flatten out the Cooper's ligaments to avoid artifacts. The pressure then needs to be lessened when performing color flow imaging and elastography [7].

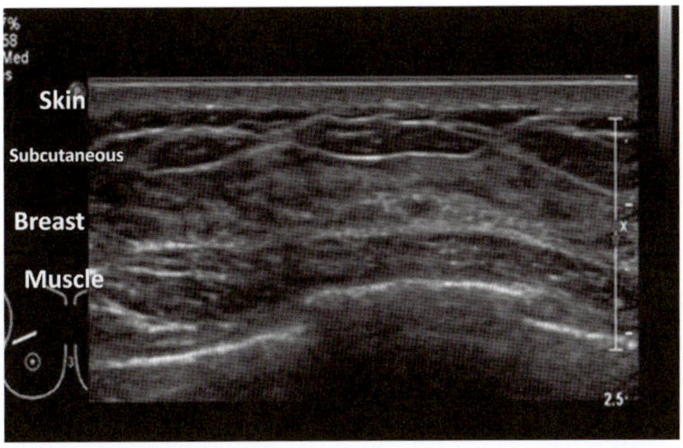

FIGURE 15.3 Longitudinal B-mode ultrasound image of normal breast tissues.

If scanning the entire breast, it is imperative to have multiple different planes of scanning, including sagittal, transverse, radial, and tangential, as well as scanning the axillary region. Radial scanning is used to detect masses in the ducts, which would otherwise be overlooked. The scan should be done in a systematic fashion so as to not to neglect any portion of the breast. For example measurements for a breast lesion should include longitudinal, transverse, and anteroposterior dimensions. To better localize and identify a potential lesion, the medical professional should palpate the mass in the breast directly to guide ultrasound scan [7].

Ultrasound-guided interventional procedures involving needle placement should be set up so that the entire needle can be observed inside the breast. The most important aspect of this is ensuring proper placement of the transducer. If ultrasonography is being used as a supplement to mammographic or other imaging studies, the images should be directly compared. When documenting a lesion in a scan, it should be labeled with breast laterality, distance from the nipple itself (not the areola), clock-face notation, and orientation of the transducer during the scan [2]. Knowledge of proper examination technique will not only help identify pathologies accurately, but more importantly, will allow professionals to rule out such conditions and reassure patients with normal tissue [1].

Ultrasound of Normal Breast

When beginning ultrasound examination of the breast tissue, visualize the pectoral muscles, ribs, and chest wall at the bottom of the screen to ensure that the entire breast is in plane. Starting from the top of the image, the skin will appear as a bright, linear echo. Directly under the skin is an echo-poor region of subcutaneous fat. The pectoral muscle is visualized at the bottom of the image, appearing as echo-poor linear striations along the long axis of the muscle (Fig. 15.3). Under the pectoral muscle are ribs, often round or oval in cross-section. As ultrasound cannot penetrate the bone, the image behind the ribs will often show an acoustic shadow [1, 8].

The parenchyma, or breast tissue, lies underneath the subcutaneous fat and consists of tissues with varying echogenicity. The adipose tissue appears more hypoechoic, while the connective tissue appears more hyperechoic. Glandular tissue density varies based on age, parity, and hormonal status. Younger women commonly have dense glandular tissue, while the makeup of the breast tissue in older women transitions into fat over time [1].

The fibrous connections responsible for maintaining the shape of the breast are called Cooper's ligaments. As connective tissue of the breast, Cooper's ligaments are visualized as linear, echogenic structures. Attenuation, the loss of intensity due to absorption, reflection, or scattering, can occur around Cooper's ligaments (Fig. 15.4) and appear as a lesion [1]. Varying the angle of the transducer and reading in multiple planes is recommended to rule out lesions.

Leading from the breast lobules to the nipple are mammary ducts, anatomically tubular structures present throughout the breast but best visualized in the subareolar area. Ducts can be visualized as echo-free tubes that lead to the nipple. The nipples are echo-poor, oval structures made of dense connective tissue.

Lymph nodes can be visualized most easily in the axillary region, though some may be detected within the breast. Lymph nodes appear as solid, echo-poor, oval shapes with a hyperechoic hilum. Larger arteries and their corresponding veins may

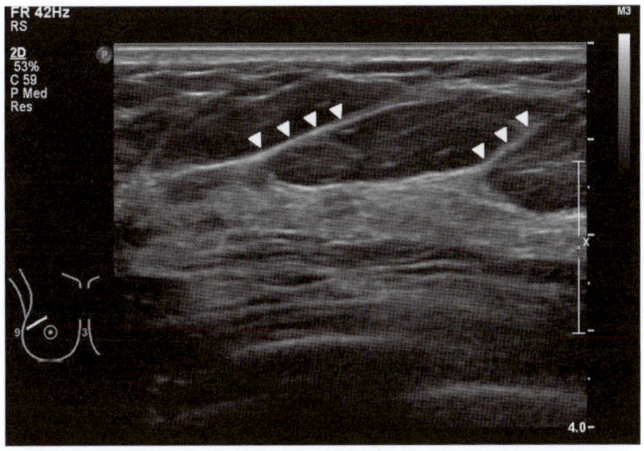

FIGURE 15.4 Transverse plane of Cooper's ligaments on B-mode ultrasound image (white arrow heads).

be visualized along their course of perfusion of the breast tissue. Veins are oval in cross-section and may collapse with pressure or respiration, while arteries are generally rounder and have stronger wall echoes [1, 8]. When using ultrasound, it is important to be able to identify normal tissue in the breast in order to compare the differences when faced with pathology.

Common Pathologies of the Breast

Detection of potential lesions depends on the operator and their assessment of the characteristics of the lesion. Using the lexicon of descriptors set forth by the American College of Radiology promotes less variation and more clinical efficacy in reporting lesions found by breast ultrasound [7].

Breast Cyst

The most commonly found benign disease of the breast via ultrasound is a cyst [1]. Ultrasound can differentiate with high accuracy between fluid-filled cysts and solid lesions, and under ideal conditions can visualize small 2–3 mm cysts. Characteristics of a simple cyst are defined precisely as echo-free, round or oval shaped with a smooth border, well-defined margins, and posterior enhancement. The posterior enhancement appears as a brighter zone behind the cyst caused by echo enhancement and is often seen with fluid-filled structures (Fig. 15.5). Calcification of cysts can also lead to a loss of visualization of posterior enhancement. Sebaceous cysts within the skin of the breast often appear with well-defined margins, uniform low-level echoes throughout, and posterior enhancement [1].

Complex cysts filled with hemorrhagic or inflammatory debris and proteins appear as lesions with inner echoes, septations, well-defined margins, and posterior enhancement. Indicators of a malignant lesion may include markedly thick walls and papillary lesions vegetating within the lumen. Color flow imaging can also be used to find vascular areas in intracystic cancers [9].

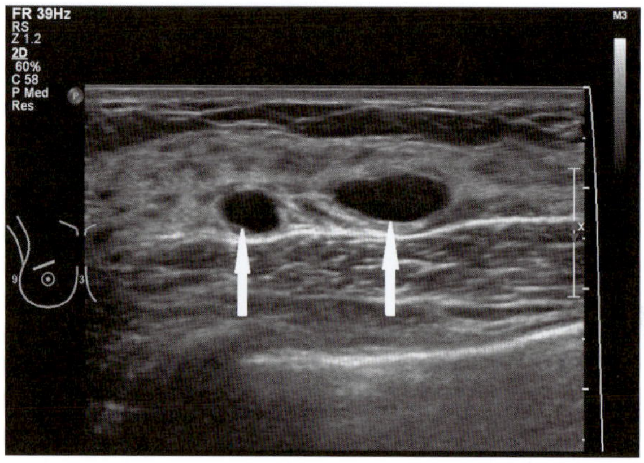

FIGURE 15.5 Simple breast cysts (white arrows) in B-mode ultrasound image.

Breast Fibroadenoma

Fibroadenomas are the most common type of benign, solid breast tumors, occurring most frequently in younger, premenopausal women [1]. Fibroadenomas are painless, unilateral, marble-like masses that are comprised of both epithelial and stromal fibrocyte tissues. They vary in size but stop growing as they reach a maximum diameter of 2–3 cm unless they are inappropriately stimulated by a hormone. Fibroadenomas shrink in size postmenopause. Under ultrasound, fibroadenomas are oval or roundish lesions with echo-poor centers, consisting of either regular or multilobular margins and no posterior enhancement (Fig. 15.6). There are exceptions to these rules, and in a small percentage of cases, fibroadenomas can have irregular margins, inhomogeneous distribution of the lesions, and posterior enhancement [1].

Inflammation

Mastitis, inflammation of breast tissue, can also be visualized via ultrasound. Acute mastitis is common in breastfeeding women but can also affect other women and may involve an infection. Mastitis can appear as either an echo-rich or echo-poor

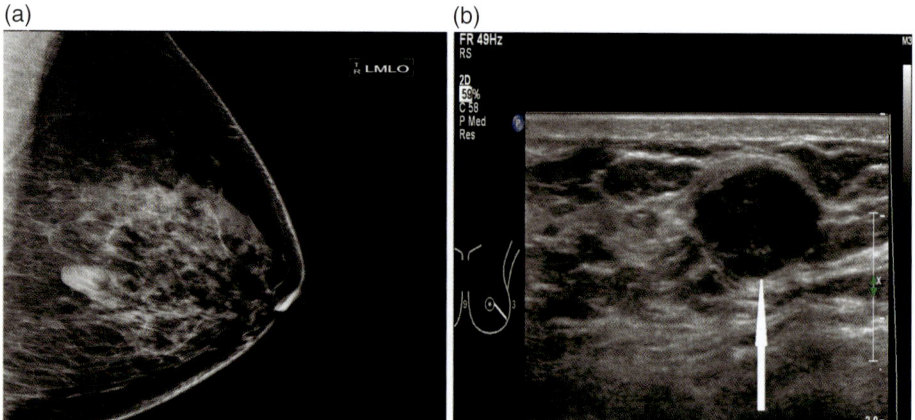

FIGURE 15.6 (a, b) Breast fibroadenoma on mammogram and B-mode ultrasound (arrow).

area with blurred margins and a mixed echoic internal structure. Abscesses have varying inner echoes depending on their fluid and debris levels, inner sedimentations, and posterior enhancement. Inflammatory carcinomas are not always possible to differentiate from mastitis or abscess on ultrasound; therefore, ultrasound-guided aspiration for histology analysis is recommended [10].

Breast Cancer

The most common types of malignant breast neoplasms are ductal carcinoma in situ, invasive ductal carcinoma, and invasive lobular carcinoma [11]. Ultrasound can show limited qualities of these epithelial cancers with the use of high-frequency ultrasound transducers and color flow imaging.

Ductal carcinoma *in situ* are noninvasive group of neoplastic cells that do not disrupt the basal membrane [11]. Microcalcifications are present in some breast lesions, although it can be difficult to visualize [1]. Under ultrasound examination, microcalcifications can be seen in isolated clusters, though the morphology may be unclear. Ductal carcinoma in situ can also appear as an echo-poor lesion, with or without internal calcification. Use of a high-frequency ultrasound transducer can be used to aid in visualizing the distribution of microcalcifications more clearly (Fig. 15.7).

Invasive ductal carcinoma is breast cancer that has spread into surrounding tissue and is the most common type of breast cancer [11]. Beginning in the milk duct of the breast, neoplastic cells break through the wall of the duct and continue to grow into the surrounding breast tissues. It may also metastasize to other parts of the body via nearby lymphatic structures and vasculature. Ultrasound can be used to estimate the size of the lesion. Lesions appear as hypoechoic, irregular in shape, and without clear margins. Shadowing from the fibrous tissue within invasive ductal carcinoma can be seen in 30–40% of cases [1]. An echogenic halo surrounding the lesion distinguishes the lesion from the desmoplastic reaction occurring in the tissues the tumor has invaded. Spiculated margin is a diagnostic feature of malignancy, as strands of tissue can be seen radiating out from the irregularly shaped lesion.

However, spiculated margins are not specific to invasive ductal carcinomas. Fibroadenomas, radial scars, and fat necrosis can also be associated with the stellate

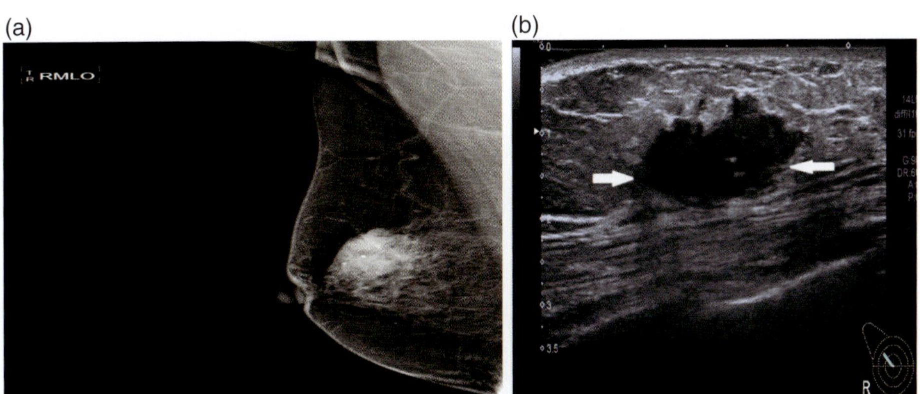

FIGURE 15.7 (a, b) Breast cancer with calcification on mammogram and B-mode ultrasound (arrows) images.

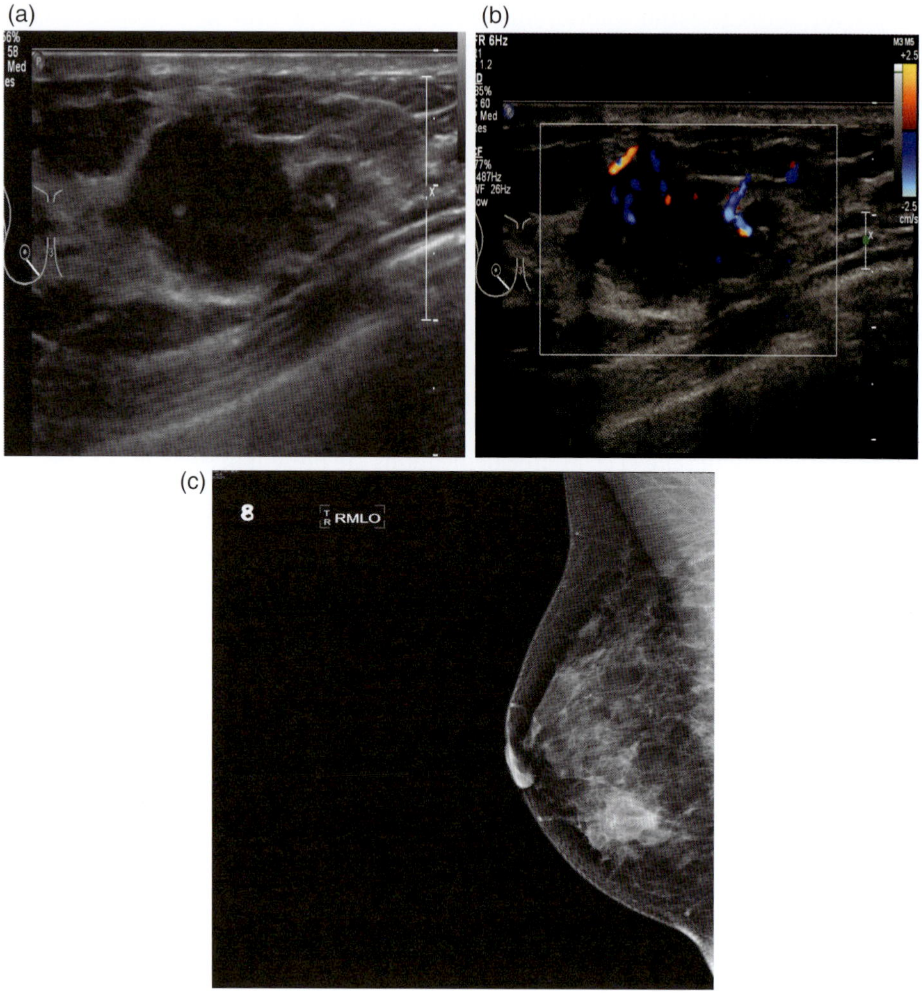

FIGURE 15.8 (a–c) A lesion of invasive ductal carcinoma on B-mode image (a), color flow imaging (b), and mammogram (c).

shape of spiculated margins. Biopsy is necessary to confirm the diagnosis of invasive ductal carcinoma. In smaller neoplasms, margins are more defined, and the echoic halo from desmoplastic reactions may not be present. High-frequency transducers can be used to analyze the thickening of skin, subcutaneous tissue, and Cooper's ligaments due to tumor infiltration. Color flow imaging (Fig. 15.8) can show increases in vascular supply due to invasive ductal carcinomas [12].

Lobular carcinoma in situ is neoplasia inside the milk-producing glands of the breast that do not grow through the lobule [11]. Lobular carcinoma in situ is typically diagnosed histologically after biopsy for a lesion seen on mammography and/or ultrasonography. Invasive lobular carcinoma, like invasive ductal carcinoma, can metastasize to other parts of the body. Ultrasound imaging of invasive lobular carcinoma is characterized by a hypoechoic lesion with ill-defined borders and minimal or no shadowing (Fig. 15.9). Vascular supply to the lesion can sometimes be seen [1].

Characteristics of ultrasound imaging of malignant breast neoplasms may include irregular shape and orientation, spiculated margins, echogenic halo boundaries,

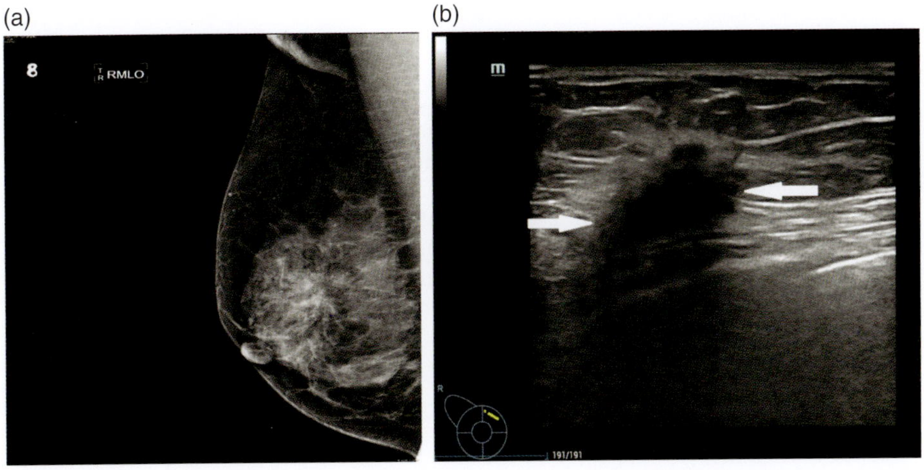

FIGURE 15.9 (a, b) Lobular carcinoma of the breast in mammogram (a) and B-mode ultrasound (b). The lesion appears hypoechoic and ill-defined borders in B-mode ultrasound image (b).

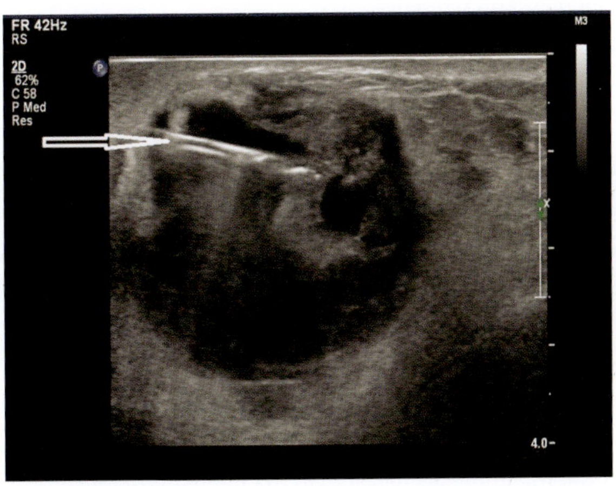

FIGURE 15.10 Ultrasound-guided breast lesion biopsy (arrow: biopsy needle).

hypoechoic lesions, microcalcifications, or the presence of hypervascularity. The finding of these features warrants a biopsy (Fig. 15.10).

Reporting of Results and Quality Control

Reporting of results of diagnostic images should follow accepted guidelines, including a BI-RADS score with documentation of appropriate recommendations and follow-up. A vigorous quality control program should be in place with documentation of sensitivity and specificity of results mapped against BI-RADS classifications, patient education, and infection rates [12, 13].

Summary

Breast ultrasound can be used to investigate the normal anatomy of breast tissue, along with any suspected palpable mass. When used as a complement to mammography, ultrasound can detect breast lesions or abnormalities that are not easily visible on mammography and can lead to early detection of neoplasms. Ultrasound can also aid procedures such as biopsies, aspirations, and preoperative localization. It is important to consult with breast imaging specialist when a breast lesion is palpated and identified. Further assessment for breast lesions with BI-RADS score is recommended in clinical patient care [13].

Review Questions

1. Which patient would not need a breast ultrasonography?
   - a. A 50-year-old woman with normal breast exam and normal screening mammogram. The breasts are not dense.
   - b. A 25-year-old pregnant woman
   - c. A 37-year-old woman with dense breast tissue
   - d. A 29-year-old woman with breast implants
2. Which of the following are true statements regarding transducer and imaging technique?
   - a. Low-frequency transducers always provide ideal breast images
   - b. High-frequency transducers always provide ideal breast images
   - c. Wide-bandwidth transducers are useful in providing ideal breast images
   - d. Acoustic standoffs are not needed in breast imaging due to the normal fatty breast tissue providing an adequate acoustic interface
3. Where is the common transducer placement for the breast ultrasound?
   - a. 3–8th ribs from the sternum to the midaxillary line
   - b. 5–10th ribs from the midclavicular line to the midaxillary line
   - c. 2–6th ribs from the midclavicular line to the midaxillary line
   - d. 2–6th ribs from the sternum to the midaxillary line
4. What should you do if a breast mass is detected during an ultrasound scan?
   - a. Stop the ultrasound immediately and consult an oncologist
   - b. Obtain scans of the mass in at least two planes, with and without caliper measurements
   - c. Obtain scans of the mass in all planes possible with caliper measurements
   - d. Obtain one clear scan of the mass without caliper measurements
5. Which muscle lies directly below the breast?
   - a. Serratus anterior
   - b. Transversus abdominis
   - c. External oblique
   - d. Pectoralis major

6. What is an anechoic focal lesion with posterior acoustic enhancement on B-mode image?
   a. Subcutaneous tissue edema
   b. Ductal carcinoma
   c. Benign cyst
   d. Solid mass
7. Which of the following ultrasound findings suggests malignancy?
   a. Uniform increased echogenicity
   b. Spiculated margins and internal microcalcifications
   c. Hypoechoic lesion with ill-defined margins
   d. Echo-poor lesion without internal calcification
8. Which of the following displays a hypoechoic lesion with no posterior enhancement?
   a. Subcutaneous tissue edema
   b. Liquidated abscess
   c. Simple cyst
   d. Fibroadenoma
9. Which of the following is NOT true reason for breast ultrasound?
   a. It replaces mammography in breast cancer screening
   b. Noninvasive in-office appointments with no preparation required
   c. Visualization of dense breast tissue
   d. Distinguishing a fluid-filled cyst from a solid mass
10. A lesion appears hypoechoic, irregular in shape, with spiculated margins on B-mode ultrasound. What is the next step to diagnose invasive ductal carcinoma?
    a. No further work-up is necessary; a diagnosis can be made from ultrasound alone
    b. Chest CT scan
    c. Biopsy
    d. Repeat ultrasound scan by another technician

Correct answers: 1. a; 2. c; 3. d; 4. b; 5. d; 6. c; 7. b; 8. d; 9. a; 10. c.

References

1. Buscarini E, Lutz H, Mirk P. Manual of diagnostic ultrasound. Vol 2. 2nd ed. Geneva,: World Health Organization, 2013.
2. Bark L, D'Orsi C, Paltiel H (eds). ARC practice parameter for the breast ultrasound examination. American College of Radiology, 2016.
3. Pillary J, Davis T. Physiology, lactation. Treasure Island: StatPearls Publishing, 2019.
4. Bland K, Copeland E, Klimberg S, et al. The breast: comprehensive management of benign and malignant diseases. 5th ed. Elsevier, 2017.
5. Suami H, Pan WR, Mann GB, Taylor GI. The lymphatic anatomy of the breast and its implications for sentinel lymph node biopsy: a human cadaver study. *Ann Surg Oncol* 2008; 15: 863–871.
6. Skaane P, Engedal K. Analysis of sonographic features in the differentiation of fibroadenomas and invasive ductal carcinoma. *AJR Am J Roentgenol.* 1998; 170: 109–114. https://doi.org/10.2214/ajr.170.1.9423610.

7. Mendelson EB, Berg WA. Training and standards for performance, interpretation, and structured reporting for supplemental breast cancer screening. *AJR* 2015; 204: 265–268.
8. Lutz H, Buscarini E. Manual of diagnostic ultrasound. Vol Vol 1. 2nd ed. Geneva, Switzerland: World Health Organization, 2011.
9. Rodríguez MC, Secades AL, Angulo JM. Best cases from the AFIP: intracystic papillary carcinoma of the breast. *Radiographics* 2010; 30: 2021–2027.
10. Yeh ED, Jacene HA, Bellon JB, et al. What radiologists need to know about diagnosis and treatment of inflammatory breast cancer: a multidisciplinary approach. *Radiographics* 2013; 33: 2003–2017.
11. American Cancer Society. invasive breast cancer (IDC/ILC): types of invasive breast carcinoma. https://www.cancer.org/cancer/breast-cancer/understanding-a-breast-cancer-diagnosis/types-of-breast-cancer/invasive-breast-cancer.html. Published 2017.
12. Popli MB. Pictorial essay: mammographic features of breast cancer. *Indian J Radiol Imaging* 2001; 11: 175–179.
13. ACR practice parameter for the performance of a diagnostic breast ultrasound. https://www.acr.org/–/media/ACR/Files/Practice-Parameters/US-Breast.pdf

CHAPTER 16

Ultrasound in Global Medicine

Richard Rodriguez-Brizuela, Andrew Wojtanowski, Tyler Burke, and Camille Z. Bentley
Rocky Vista University, College of Osteopathic Medicine, Parker, Colorado, USA

Introduction

According to the World Health Organization (WHO), approximately 3–4 billion people are at risk for preventable widespread loss and death due to a lack of access to radiologic assessments. Potential imaging modalities, such as ultrasound, have been recommended for improving access to radiologic assessments in developing countries by specialists, including Palmer, Mets, Weber, and Mindel in the late 20th century [1].

Since its first appearance in the mid-20th century, ultrasound imaging has gained even greater recognition because of its diverse diagnostic capabilities. For "underserved populations" in the developing world, it has opened a new dimension in healthcare for those living in remote areas, because of its accuracy, user-friendly interface, cost-efficiency, and portability. Furthermore, ultrasound imaging is relatively inexpensive and safe when compared to other imaging modalities such as computed tomography (CT) and magnetic resonance imaging (MRI) [2]. CT scans carry the risk of exposing patients to ionizing radiation, while MRI scans are relatively contraindicated in individuals with cardiac pacemakers and defibrillators, and neither is widely available [3, 4].

Ultrasound has demonstrated remarkable versatility in various clinical settings such as cardiology, internal medicine, obstetrics/gynecology (OB-GYN), surgery, and emergency medicine. This is especially true in areas such as Latin America, the Middle East, Africa, and Asia Pacific, where quality improvement and availability of basic medical imaging are relied heavily on [1]. Although ultrasound technology is widely used for diagnosis, one review article indicates that many healthcare providers in developing countries lack adequate training and do not meet the minimum standards set by the WHO [5]. Despite these limitations, further research is needed, as ultrasound remains a valuable, noninvasive tool for evaluating thousands of patients [6].

In this chapter, we will discuss pathologies commonly seen in the developing world and the importance of ultrasound in the diagnosis of these conditions. This chapter should be used in conjunction with the review of ultrasound techniques and the understanding of normal images of systems from other chapters in this book.

Cardiovascular Disorders

Rheumatic Heart Disease

Rheumatic heart disease (RHD) is one of the most significant acquired forms of heart disease (HD) in children and young adults. RHD remains a significant global burden of disease [7]. It is the consequence of unchecked exposure or poorly treated group A *streptococcus pyogenes* [8]. Although the disease is rare in the developed world, RHD currently leads to 250,000 premature deaths worldwide annually [9]. RHD is usually present in young children in the form of shortness of breath and fatigue. Upon physical examination, an apical holosystolic murmur (mitral valve regurgitation, MR), an apical mid-diastolic murmur (Carey Coombs murmur), and/or a basal early systolic murmur (aortic valve regurgitation) may be detected. However, MR is the most common early manifestation. Transient pericarditis occurs in 15% of cases of Acute Rheumatic Fever (ARF) and may present with precordial chest pain and pericardial friction rub. As the disease progresses, heart failure (HF) and left ventricular dilation (LVD) result from the severe valvular disease (aortic valve and/or mitral valve) [10]. Any child suspected of ARF should be evaluated for murmurs associated with rheumatic carditis. Likewise, any child with a new or worsening pathologic cardiac murmur should be suspected of exposure to a group A streptococcal infection.

The use of ultrasonography enables the assessment of valve morphology and the severity of valve dysfunction. RHD is associated with mitral valve findings consistent with mitral stenosis such as valve leaflet doming into the left ventricle, increased leaflet thickening (>2 mm), and valve calcinosis (evident by relative hyperechogenic foci). These findings may occur independently or in combination. Left atrial dilation may be found in response to mitral valve stenosis [11]. Echocardiography can also be used to assess left and right ventricular size and function and may provide an accurate estimation of pulmonary artery systolic pressure and monitor disease progression.

Chagas' Disease

Chagas' disease, also called American Trypanosomiasis, is a potentially life-threatening illness caused by the protozoan parasite *Trypanosoma cruzi*. The protozoan is transmitted by an insect vector called the triatomine bug, also known as the "kissing bug," which is endemic to the tropics of Latin America [12].

Chagas' disease manifests in three phases: acute, intermediate, and chronic. The acute phase is typically asymptomatic, lasting weeks to months. Physical examination of an infected patient may reveal signs of edema at the bite site called a "chagoma," enlarged lymph nodes on palpation, skin rash, and fever [12]. In the intermediate phase, the patient may remain asymptomatic for more than 20 years. By the chronic phase, the patient may present significant signs and symptoms of the disease, including cardiac and gastrointestinal complications. The acute phase of Chagas' disease may be confirmed by microscopic examination of a blood smear, while later stages of the disease may be confirmed by testing for *T. cruzi* antibodies [12].

Ultrasound visualization of Chagas' disease is an incredibly valuable tool in viewing the acute phase. Acute Chagas' myocarditis manifests in ultrasound imaging with pericardial effusion (Chapter 3), evident by anechoic fluid in the pericardial space. In late-stage Chagas' disease, approximately half of symptomatic patients demonstrate left ventricular dilation [13]. Treatment for bloodborne *T. cruzi* consists of benznidazole and nifurtimox in addition to supportive care [12]. Antiparasitic treatment is effective regardless of the disease stage; however, long-term care management should be followed by appropriate specialists. Disease prevention includes disinfecting fomites, utilizing insecticide-treated bed nets, using personal protective equipment (PPE), and applying insect repellent to exposed skin [13].

Respiratory Disorders

Pulmonary Tuberculosis (TB)

Pulmonary tuberculosis (TB) is a highly communicable disease caused by *Mycobacterium tuberculosis* infection. The WHO estimated up to 10.8 million infections and 1.25 million deaths from TB in 2023 [14]. Patients infected with TB may present with a cough, lymphadenopathy, fevers, night sweats, and weight loss. Despite nonspecific signs and symptoms, people should take precautionary measures when working in endemic regions where the TB burden is high [14].

TB can be diagnosed through a positive nucleic acid amplification (NAA) test or acid-fast bacilli (AFB) smear. Other confirmatory tests to further support the diagnosis of TB include positive tuberculin skin test (TST) or interferon-gamma release assay (IGRA) and chest X-rays (or CT). Unfortunately, these tests may not be available in developing countries endemic to TB, suggesting possible undetected cases leading to new incidences. In rural settings, the management of clinically diagnosed cases of TB is to quarantine and use appropriate PPE such as face masks to prevent the spread of disease. Local health departments are encouraged to actively contain TB, while healthcare providers are instructed on precautionary guidelines for airborne diseases in TB-prevalent areas [14].

Ultrasound imaging can provide a noninvasive workup of TB in medically scarce regions of the world [15, 16]. Suspected tuberculosis infections may show adjunct evidence of pulmonary effusion, which can be assessed with ultrasound, potentially detecting effusions as small as 5 mL [17]. In TB, pleural effusion is due to an exudative process along the costophrenic angle and will likely be hypoechoic [16, 18]. For pleural effusions within the lowest part of the chest cavity (dependent areas), a longitudinal, transthoracic ultrasound study may be performed with the patient in a seated or lateral recumbent position.

Pneumothorax

Pneumothorax is an abnormal collection of air in the pleural space of the thoracic cavity, which can either be spontaneous or acquired in the setting of blunt or penetrating trauma. Many cases of the former can go undiagnosed. Primary spontaneous pneumothorax (PSP) is a significant global health burden with an annual incident rate of 7.4–18 cases per 100,000 population for men and 1.2–6/100,000 women [19]. Although there are limits to quantifying the global cases of traumatic pneumothorax, the WHO estimates road injury as one of the leading causes of mortality worldwide [20]. Furthermore, it has been found that 25% of deaths due to trauma are associated with thoracic trauma [21]. Therefore, being able to recognize and quickly diagnose pneumothorax in the context of thoracic trauma is paramount in patient management, considering the possible sequelae [22].

Patients with a pneumothorax usually present with acute mild to severe dyspnea and pleuritic chest pain. With increasing severity of the condition, pain is usually unilateral with decreased chest excursion on the affected side. On physical examination of the affected side, the physician will note diminished breath sounds and hyperresonant percussion. Some associated signs may include neck vein distension and contralateral tracheal deviation [22]. However, pain and discomfort can be very mild or even absent in those with existing lung diseases complicated by a chronic pneumothorax.

Laboratory findings are typically nonspecific and may reveal mild leukocytosis with the absence of a left shift. An additional finding also includes normal to low peripheral oxygen saturation [23]. Traditionally, the radiologic diagnostic test for a pneumothorax is either X-ray and/or CT. However, portable bedside ultrasound has been increasingly popular for rapid imaging and diagnosis of pneumothorax [23].

Sonography of a pneumothorax is often visualized over the anterior chest, at the midclavicular lines between ribs 2–4 with the patient supine [24]. A high-frequency, low-penetrating view is appropriate for this visualization. Pneumothorax can be assessed in either a B-mode (standard) or M-mode. From the B-mode, a qualitative absence of movement along the hyperechoic pleural interface will be noted. If the observer is unsure of the qualitative difference, assessment of the unaffected contralateral side may be used for comparison and standardization of the image. The M-mode can provide an objective assessment of pneumothorax. Setting the motion detection at the intercostal space with M-mode in a healthy, unaffected patient will demonstrate horizontal lines above the pleural interface and a granular, speckled appearance devoid of lines below the pleural interface. In the affected patient with a pneumothorax, the entire image (above and below the pleural interface) will demonstrate horizontal lines as the characteristic "barcode" sign [24]. Details regarding ultrasound in the assessment of pneumothorax can be found in Chapter 3 of this book. Treatment for pneumothorax is urgent and includes bed rest, oxygen therapy, observation, simple aspiration, closed intercostal tube drainage, and tube thoracostomy [22, 25].

Hepatobiliary Disorders

Amebic Liver Abscess

Amebic liver abscess is the most common extraintestinal manifestation of amoebiasis, caused by the protozoan *Entamoeba histolytica*. It is transmitted through the fecal-oral route with the ingestion of contaminated food and water, as well as from poor hand hygiene between individuals [26]. Amebiasis poses a major global burden in endemic areas of developing countries, despite most infections being asymptomatic. Developing countries with limited resources and inadequate sanitation face a higher risk of distribution of this protozoan [27].

Amebiasis primarily affects middle-aged adults, especially men. These individuals may present with ongoing right upper quadrant pain and fever over the course of several weeks. The pain may range from dull to sharp and may refer to the epigastrium, the right chest, or the shoulder. Other associated symptoms may include cough, sweating, malaise, weight loss, and anorexia. Patients may also present with concurrent diarrhea and jaundice. In 50% of amoebiasis cases, hepatomegaly and tenderness are noted on the physical exam. Possible life-threatening conditions that may occur include hepatic vein thrombosis, inferior vena cava thrombosis, or liver abscess rupture into either the chest or abdominal cavity [28]. The diagnosis of amebic liver abscess is usually confirmed through proper serological and antigenic testing with supplemental stool microscopy or stool antigenic testing [29]. However, serology testing is not available in many developing regions of the world. In the case of limited serologic testing and high clinical suspicion, ultrasound imaging may be used to assist in diagnosing liver amebiasis. Liver abscesses can have a variable appearance depending on the etiology and the case. Whereas bacterial and fungal causes tend to have multiple foci, amebic abscesses are more often present as a single focus. Echogenicity can range from an anechoic center to hyperechoic. The abscess itself may be simple or complex with septations. Considering the variable appearance, it is important for the interpreter of the ultrasound to be able to distinguish these foci from the generally homogenous liver tissue. Using color Doppler can help distinguish an abscess (negative for flow) from a vascular mass (positive for flow) [30].

Identification and evaluation of the severity of an abscess is the first step toward treating this condition. With serious complications such as a possible abscess rupture, a referral to surgery is warranted. Otherwise, the standard treatment consists of a combination of metronidazole or tinidazole to resolve parasitic infections within the tissues, followed by a course of paromomycin to eliminate intramural cysts [26].

Cholecystitis/Ascending Cholangitis

Cholelithiasis (gallstones) are deposits of hardened digestive material within the gallbladder. Gallstones typically form when bile becomes oversaturated with cholesterol, when the biliary tract is not draining properly, or when the liver excretes too much bilirubin. Cholelithiasis has a relatively high incidence worldwide and often leads to cholecystitis [31].

Cholecystitis refers to acute or chronic inflammation of the gallbladder. Frequently, it occurs when the cystic duct is obstructed by a gallstone, leading to inflammation or impaired emptying of the gallbladder [32]. Similarly, ascending cholangitis occurs when gallstones obstruct the common bile duct and leads to inflammation. Both conditions can become life-threatening if not addressed promptly. When clinical suspicion is high, patients may benefit from having accessible, safe, noninvasive screening methods offered by their providers [31].

Patients with acute cholecystitis typically present with complaints of steady, severe, and prolonged postprandial right upper quadrant and/or epigastric abdominal pain. Cholecystic pain may radiate to the neck, right shoulder, or back. Associated complaints may include fever, nausea, vomiting, and anorexia [32]. On physical examinations, patients usually appear ill, tachycardic, and physically motionless due to peritoneal inflammation causing worsening of pain with movement. Further examination of the abdomen may reveal voluntary guarding and a positive Murphy's sign. Some patients may present with a classic complication of acute cholangitis known as Charcot's triad, which consists of fever, abdominal pain, and jaundice.

Symptoms of acute cholangitis are secondary to the lodging of a biliary stone in the common bile duct, which requires immediate medical attention [31].

When clinical suspicion is high, ultrasound is often the first radiographic study used in the diagnosis of gallstones in the gallbladder. A right upper quadrant scan of the gallbladder and biliary system will aid in identifying these pathologies. Gallstones located in the intra-cystic duct of the gallbladder may appear as hyperechoic focus with or without shadowing. Gallstones may not be visible if they are well embedded in the neck of the gallbladder or they are too small in size.

Cholecystitis will likely present with secondary findings of peri-cholecystic fluid (anechoic fluid around the gallbladder capsule) and thickening of the gallbladder wall greater than 3 mm; however, gallstones may not be necessary to diagnose cholecystitis (see Figures in Chapter 5). A "sonographic" Murphy sign may support the diagnosis of cholecystitis through the reproduction of the right upper quadrant pain when pressure is applied over the gallbladder with the ultrasound probe.

When evaluating ascending cholangitis, the bile duct system is assessed for bile duct dilation (suggestive of stasis and/or obstruction), bile duct wall thickening (suggestive of local inflammation), and heterogeneity of hypoechoic substances in the intraductal space (which may represent exudate). After the ultrasound analysis, patients can be referred to a hospital for further evaluation and treatment [33].

Genitourinary Disorders

Placenta Previa

Placenta previa refers to the presence of placental tissue that extends over the uterine internal cervical os during pregnancy. This can result in complications during the last two trimesters of pregnancy such as vaginal bleeding or hemorrhage, preterm birth, and/or the need for a cesarean delivery. Although 90% of confirmed placenta previa in the developed world with <20 weeks of gestation resolve before delivery, the remaining 10% of placenta previa cases can result in major complications for the mother and fetus [34].

In developed countries, the majority of placenta previa cases are discovered with routine transabdominal ultrasounds at 16–20 weeks of gestation. Transabdominal ultrasounds are utilized to screen for placenta previa prior to digital vaginal exams to prevent possible severe hemorrhage secondary to the palpation of a placenta previa. However, only 50% of women worldwide receive the recommended antenatal care, and nearly 50% of all births in the developing world occur in nonhospital settings. The use of transabdominal ultrasound in these cases would assist in the early detection of high-risk pregnancies such as those with placenta previa and multiple gestations [35].

Pregnant women in their second or third trimesters who present with painless vaginal bleeding are strongly encouraged to be evaluated for possible placenta previa with ultrasound imaging, given its safety for use in pregnancy. Due to the dynamic migration of the placenta in the earlier stages of gestation, assessment for placenta previa is generally completed after 20 weeks. While assessing for placenta previa with a transabdominal view, it is imperative that the study be done with an empty bladder, as an overdistended bladder may produce a false positive on a sonographic exam [36]. The placenta will appear as an echogenic structure lining the anechoic gestational sac. The vascular nature of the placenta allows color Doppler sonography to confirm flow and aids in the identification of the placenta [37]. A reading showing thickness of the placental tissue between 2.8 and 4.2 cm maximizes the specificity and the sensitivity of the exam [35]. If placenta previa or vasa previa is suspected, an additional transvaginal ultrasound may be used to confirm and monitor the location of the placenta. More information on the ultrasound assessment of placenta previa can be found in Chapter 6 in this book.

Nephrolithiasis and Staghorn Calculi

Nephrolithiasis (kidney stones) are crystal deposits typically formed in the kidneys but can also develop in the walls of the urinary bladder. Kidney stones may accumulate from many sources, as mentioned in earlier chapters (Chapter 7), but staghorn calculi tend to be one of the rarest and most problematic kinds of nephrolithiasis. Staghorn calculi are large, branching stones often composed of ammonium phosphate that occur with increased ammonia production and elevated urine pH. They are typically seen in individuals who develop an upper urinary tract infection with urease-producing organisms like *Proteus mirabilis* and *Klebsiella* [38]. Staghorn calculi are more common in women than men, with a ratio of 3:1, respectively [39]. These calcified masses can grow to fill the entire renal pelvis and calyces over a period of weeks to months.

Patients with staghorn calculi may present symptoms similar to a urinary tract infection, which can include flank pain, lower abdominal pain, dysuria, and hematuria. A urinalysis of a patient with staghorn calculi may indicate elevated nitrites, leukocyte esterase, and trace blood. However, an alkaline strip (pH >8) should raise concerns for calculus formation [37, 38].

The standard for confirming any renal stone is a non-contrast CT scan of the abdomen and pelvis. However, in the rural setting, ultrasound devices in the B-mode can localize a stone. A longitudinal kidney study may demonstrate a hyperechoic stone with accompanying posterior acoustic shadowing. The size of the stone can be more accurately measured by obtaining the width of the shadow instead of the width of the stone [40]. In addition, twinkling artifacts below the stone can often be seen using color flow imaging, which can be useful for the detection of smaller stones. For optimal results, it is suggested that the patient drink 8–24 ounces of clear fluid and have a full bladder before the procedure.

Conservative measures have been shown to be ineffective in the management of staghorn calculi. If left untreated, a staghorn calculus may increase the risk of kidney damage secondary to obstruction and infection. Monitoring staghorn calculi recurrences with a kidney ultrasound is highly recommended for patients following treatment [41].

Benign Prostatic Hyperplasia with Hydronephrosis

Benign prostatic hyperplasia (BPH) is a common global condition among older men due to progressive cellular enlargement of the prostate gland with age. BPH is partially due to the increased production of dihydrotestosterone (DHT) by the enzyme 5α-reductase. The smooth muscle of the prostate may also be under the influence of increased α1-adrenergic receptor activity, which may lead to increased muscle tone when stressed. Both these factors can lead to urinary outflow tract obstruction [42].

Patients suspected of BPH will often present with urinary frequency, decreased force of urinary stream, nocturia, strained voiding, and urgency. BPH is characterized by a non-tender, relatively enlarged prostate with a regular, smooth surface on digital rectal exam. A urinalysis should be conducted to rule out a urinary tract infection. Individuals with chronic urinary retention should be evaluated for hydronephrosis with ultrasound.

A longitudinal view of the kidneys may show an enhanced-anechoic fluid-filled space within the renal sinus as well as dilation of the renal pelvis (>20 mm anteroposterior diameter) and calyces [40]. Hydronephrosis may also show dilation of the proximal ureters and distal regions adjacent to the ostium, which is not usually seen under normal conditions. Urinary tract obstruction may lead to significant impairment of renal function. Additional imaging may show diffuse bladder wall thickness (>5 mm) and diffuse prostatic hyperplasia on a transverse view of the lower abdomen and pelvis [43]. An ultrasound image with hydronephrosis is presented in Chapter 7 of this book.

Soft Tissues

Skin and Soft Tissue Infections (Cellulitis and Abscesses)

Skin and soft tissue infections, including abscesses and cellulitis, are common medical conditions that pose a major global health burden of more than 650,000 hospital admissions per year in the United States [44]. In resource-limited communities, efficient recognition and diagnosis of these infections are paramount to a complete resolution.

Skin and soft tissue infections are the result of a breach of the epidermal layer of the skin through bites, minor scratches, or abrasions. These infections are particularly prominent in the setting of poor hygiene [45]. Cellulitis is an infection of the deep dermis and subcutaneous tissue distinguished by expanding erythema, warmth, tenderness, and swelling. In contrast to cellulitis, a skin abscess is a collection of pus within the dermis or subcutaneous space and often manifests as a painful, fluctuant, and erythematous nodule [46].

Patients with soft tissue infections typically present with localized symptoms; however, these infections may also present with a fever, which is indicative of a systemic infection in a minority of cases [45]. Though differentiating soft tissue infections is difficult, ultrasound imaging can enhance distinctions for a more accurate diagnosis. Cellulitis may appear outwardly nonspecific, but skin changes may be visibly detected by ultrasound. The most common cellulitis finding seen on ultrasound is cobblestoning, which is an area of hypoechoic fluid that separates subcutaneous tissue and fat in a reticular pattern [47]. Other signs visible on ultrasound include hyperechoic skin and increased echogenicity of the underlying subcutaneous tissue.

Abscesses present as anechoic or hypoechoic cavities on ultrasound due to the accumulation of purulent material and blood. They also exhibit posterior acoustic enhancement from decreased attenuation of the ultrasound beam as it passes through the liquid center of the abscess, creating a hyperechoic shadow along its posterior wall [47]. In addition to these findings, cobblestoning may surround the abscess, as most abscesses will also show signs of cellulitis. In rare cases, abscesses may appear hyperechoic from a collection of loculations or very dense fluid. Gentle pressure with the probe, also known as ultrasonic fluctuance, can be applied over the imaged region to improve visualization of the abscess collection [47]. Ultrasound images of superficial soft tissue structures are optimized by using a high-frequency linear probe (8 MHz). If made available, an acoustic standoff pad may be used to assist the clinician with the imaging of extremely superficial structures by increasing the distance between the transducer and the area of interest. Otherwise, the use of a water bath may provide similar benefits. If a patient has a drainable abscess, it is highly recommended that they undergo ultrasound-guided drainage (see Chapter 13).

Foreign Body

A common cause of soft tissue injuries are open wounds with lodged foreign bodies. One study noted that lacerations and puncture wounds from foreign material are the most common mechanisms of injury involving a foreign body, accounting for 66.1% of all documented cases [48]. Other less common forms of reported injuries include falling onto an object, injuries from operating machinery, needle punctures, staples, and retained piercings. From the possible lacerable foreign material, wood laceration injuries account for the majority of cases at 34% [48]. A small fragment of wood may not be seen using an X-ray; however, the foreign body may be visualized through ultrasound [48].

Patients with foreign bodies often have a recent history of trauma. The most common sites of injuries include the hands and feet, especially in areas of the world where walking barefoot is common practice [49]. In culturally diverse countries where protective foot coverings are less common, ultrasound may be used to assess foreign bodies. Important aspects of a physical examination for foreign bodies include an examination of the wound for signs of infection, visualization of the foreign body, and assessment of damage to nearby structures such as vessels, nerves, muscles, or tendons. Ultrasound imaging can be used when the exact location of the foreign body cannot be visualized [50]. It can also be used to assess the size, shape, and depth of the foreign body. A linear high-frequency transducer (7.5–13 MHz) is typically the preferred method for viewing soft tissue on ultrasound, but in some instances, an acoustic standoff pad or a water bath may be utilized to better visualize superficial structures.

On ultrasound, foreign bodies may present as hyperechoic structures with posterior acoustic shadowing. This shadowing artifact advances visualization of small foreign bodies in complex tissues and can be used as a guide for removal when possible [49, 51].

Sparganosis

Human sparganosis is a foodborne infection caused by the larvae of various *Diphyllobothrium* tapeworms of the genus *Spirometra*. These tapeworms are endemic to South-East Asia, but cases have been reported worldwide [52]. In humans, larval invasion of the brain, eyes, breasts, spinal cord, and subcutaneous tissues may result in local tissue damage, paralysis, blindness, and death [53].

Clinical features of human sparganosis are often nonspecific; however, taking a thorough patient travel history by asking about recent travel to endemic areas may help point towards a diagnosis of sparganosis.

A clinical presentation of sparganosis may include migratory pain and subcutaneous nodules [51]. Preliminary tests such as eosinophil count may reveal eosinophilia. Identification of sparganum antibodies is often not available in the developing world.

A soft tissue study using high-resolution ultrasound (7.5–12 MHz) can be used to identify subcutaneous nodular lesions produced by the larvae. Ultrasonographic findings of sparganosis may show elongated tubular hypoechoic structures with a serpentine-like appearance [54]. Assistance with ultrasound helps ensure the removal of the entire cestode, including possible remnants. The majority of human sparganosis cases are treated with surgical removal of the helminth. In cases where surgical removal is not recommended, the infection can be treated pharmacologically with antihelminthic drugs such as praziquantel or albendazole [53].

Musculoskeletal Disorders

Septic Arthritis

Septic arthritis is the inflammation of a joint from pathological microbial invasion. It most often occurs from infection with *Staphylococcus* spp. secondary to direct trauma to the joint or hematogenous spread from a distant site, such as the lungs from a recent respiratory illness. Most cases are monoarticular, involving primarily the hip or knee joints, but can occasionally affect multiple and smaller joints [54]. Several risk factors for septic arthritis have been identified in children and must be taken into consideration when working in impoverished areas of the developing world. Some of these include malnutrition, prematurity/low birth weight, sickle cell disease, hemophilia, and HIV [55].

Acute septic arthritis typically presents with an inflamed, painful joint, restricted motion, antalgic gait, or diminished weight-bearing on the joint, especially the femoroacetabular joint. Associated symptoms can include sudden onset of high fever, pain, and irritability. The diagnosis of septic arthritis is supported by appropriate laboratory and imaging studies. In a complete blood count (CBC), the peripheral blood white cell count (WBC) is frequently elevated with a predominance of polymorphonuclear cells. In addition to an increased leukocyte count, acute phase reactants such as c-reactive protein (CRP) and erythrocyte sedimentation rate (ESR) are often markedly raised [54].

Ultrasound imaging has become a reliable method for assisting with the diagnosis of septic arthritis. A high-frequency B-mode study can be used to evaluate for joint effusion, particularly in areas where fluid buildup is not visually evident such as the femoroacetabular joint. An ultrasound scan may reveal an anechoic area or zone with low echogenicity, which may be displaceable or affected by compression. Depending on the joint of interest, the ultrasound probe may be positioned in either a longitudinal or transverse view. A transducer is placed longitudinally over the suprapatellar region, while a transverse view will help visualize the medial and lateral compartments of the knee. Ultrasound-guided joint effusion aspiration can be used to assess the type of inflammation and reduce fluid collection in the joint, which aids in diagnosis and guides selection of appropriate treatment with antimicrobial agents [56].

Osteomyelitis

Osteomyelitis is the pathological invasion of bone by microorganisms with subsequent inflammation that may involve either the trabecular or cortical bone, bone marrow, and periosteum [57]. *Staphylococcus aureus* and *S. epidermidis* are the most common pathogens in normal skin flora and significantly contribute to the increased risk of deep tissue or bone infections in penetrating injuries. Other precipitating events may include open fractures, puncture injuries, foreign bodies, local infections, recent surgery, or hematogenous spread [58]. Severe manifestations of osteomyelitis have been noted to occur more frequently in the developing world than in industrialized nations. The increased incidence of chronic osteomyelitis and associated complications is often attributed to insufficient medical care and malnutrition.

Local and systemic symptoms of osteomyelitis include pain, swelling, erythema, fever, and chills. Since these findings are similar to those of septic arthritis, it is imperative to find a method to differentiate osteomyelitis from septic arthritis [57]. One method to detect infection is with laboratory values that may show an elevated white blood count, CRP, and ESR. However, additional procedures such as a needle-biopsy and cultures from the aspirate will be used to confirm the diagnosis.

Ultrasound imaging can aid in the diagnosis of osteomyelitis in two ways. First, a high-frequency B-mode study can be used to localize the area of necrotic bone. If available, an acoustic standoff pad or a water bath may be used to assist with the imaging of extremely superficial structures by increasing the distance between the transducer and the area of interest. Ultrasound findings of osteomyelitis vary depending on the duration of the disease. Early in the disease, soft tissue swelling may show up as cobblestoning, while periosteal thickening may show up as a zone that appears hyperechoic. Later findings will show increased periosteal thickening, subperiosteal exudate or abscess formation, and cortical bone erosions [56]. Since the needle used for biopsy must be placed within the infected area with liquefaction, a high-frequency ultrasound transducer should be used to guide the needle aspiration to the appropriate site. After confirming the diagnosis, antibiotics and/or surgical intervention may be utilized for the management of osteomyelitis [57].

Summary

Ultrasound has proven to be an invaluable tool in global medicine. The convenience and economical nature of ultrasound compared to CT and MRI have contributed to its increasing usage in developing countries. By using portable ultrasound and hand-held scanners, ultrasound imaging can assess a variety of conditions in adults and pediatric populations that may otherwise be left untreated. However, it is vital that the establishment of a standard protocol and technical training is enforced to improve the proper application of ultrasound in global medicine. Below is a limited list of other applications of ultrasound in the developing world:

- **Long bone fracture**: Long bone fracture is one of the most common trauma-associated pathologies worldwide. Ultrasound has been shown to have good accuracy for diagnosing long bone fractures and assessing the success of reduction attempts [59].
- **Schistosomiasis infection**: Among the multiple uses of ultrasound to detect and characterize different liver pathologies, ultrasound has been shown to assist in the diagnosis and monitoring of hepatosplenic involvement of *Schistosomiasis mansoni* in endemic areas [60].
- **Ocular infections**: B-mode ultrasound can be used for suspected intraocular infections for imaging of the posterior segment. This can be useful when the view becomes obscured by small pupillary size or poor view of the fundus due to the opacity of the media [61].
- **Ocular trauma**: Timely evaluation of ocular trauma can be done with point-of-care ultrasound, including vitreous hemorrhage and retinal detachment [62].
- **Facial and odontogenic infections**: Ultrasound has shown to be effective in localizing soft tissue infections in the face, neck, and oral cavity. It also has high predictability in determining the stages of infections [61].
- **Pregnancy monitoring**: Ultrasound is commonly used in the developing world for general first-, second-, and third-trimester screening obstetrical ultrasound to look for fetal viability, fetal presentation and number, cause of vaginal bleeding during pregnancy, among other things. For more details, please refer to the earlier chapter of the text (see Chapter 6).
- **Other clinical applications**: Ultrasound is useful in the assessment of ascites, hepatomegaly, and splenomegaly with variable etiologies and testicular pathologies (torsion, malignancy, hydrocele), which are described in early chapters.

Review Questions

1. What is the most advantageous quality of ultrasound in global medicine?
   - **a.** Portability
   - **b.** Informative
   - **c.** Radiation free
   - **d.** Cost-effectiveness
   - **e.** All above
2. Ultrasound is able to depict a solid lesion deep in the lungs.

   True

   False
3. Which image modality listed below is considered the first line of study in the diagnosis of gallstones in rural areas?
   - **a.** CT
   - **b.** MRI

   c. Ultrasound
   d. Nuclear imaging
   e. MRE

4. In the third trimester of pregnancy, ultrasound is commonly used to assess vaginal bleeding caused by:
   a. Placenta previa
   b. Uterine myoma
   c. Ovarian cyst
   d. Uterine prolapse
   e. Intrauterine growth retardation

5. How to distinguish the lesion of soft tissue abscess from vascular malformation with ultrasound imaging?
   a. Based on echogenicity of the lesion
   b. Based on internal vascularity of the lesion
   c. Based on the size of the lesion
   d. Based on the location of the lesion
   e. Based on the palpability of the lesion

Correct answers: 1. e; 2. False; 3. c; 4. a; 5. b.

References

1. Conlon R. Teaching ultrasound in tropical countries. *J Ultrasound* 2012; 15: 144–150.
2. Sippel S, Muruganandan K, Levine A, Shah S. Review article: use of ultrasound in the developing world. *Int J Emerg Med* 2011; 4: 72. https://doi.org/10.1186/1865-1380-4-72.
3. Wiest PW, Locke JA, Heintz PH, Mettler FA Jr. CT scanning: a major source of radiation exposure. *Semin Ultrasound CT MR* 2002; 23: 402–410.
4. Nordbeck P, Ertl G, Ritter O. Magnetic resonance imaging safety in pacemaker and implantable cardioverter defibrillator patients: how far have we come? *Eur Heart J* 2015; 36: 1505–1511. https://doi.org/10.1093/eurheartj/ehv086.
5. LaGrone LN, Sadasivam V, Kushner AL, Groen RS. A review of training opportunities for ultrasonography in low and middleincome countries. *Trop Med Int Health* 2012; 17(7): 808–819.
6. Shah SN, Sharma S. Mitral Stenosis. Treasure Island (FL): StatPearls Publishing, 2025.
7. Watkins DA, Johnson CO, Colquhoun SM, et al. Global, regional and national burden of rheumatic heart disease, 1990-2015. *N Engl J Med* 2017; 377: 713–722.
8. Sliwa K, Carrington M, Mayosi BM, et al. Incidence and characteristics of newly diagnosed rheumatic heart disease in urban African adults: insights from the heart of Soweto study. *Eur Heart J* 2010; 31: 719–727.
9. Kelly MC, Jennings R, Heron M. Treatment of trivalvular rheumatic heart disease: why it matters where we live. *BMJ Case Rep* 2014; 2014: bcr2013202006. https://doi.org/10.1136/bcr-2013-202006.
10. Rocha Araujo FD, Brandao KN, Araujo FA, et al. Cardiac tamponade as a rare form of presentation of rheumatic carditis. *Am Heart Hosp J* 2010; 8: 55.
11. Sani MU, Karaye KM, Borodo MM. Prevalence and pattern of rheumatic heart disease in the Nigerian savannah: an echocardiographic study. *Cardiovasc J Afr* 2007; 18: 295–299.

12. Chagas Disease. Centers for disease control and prevention, 2019. http://www.cdc.gov/parasites/chagas.
13. Acquatella H. Echocardiography in Chagas heart disease. *Circulation* 2007; 115: 1124–1131.
14. World Health Organization. Tuberculosis (TB) [Internet], 2025. https://www.who.int/news-room/fact-sheets/detail/tuberculosis.
15. Di Gennaro F, Pisano L, Veronese N, et al. Potential diagnostic properties of chest ultrasound in thoracic tuberculosis – a systematic review. *Int J Res Public Health* 2018; 15(10): 2235. https://doi.org/10.3390/ijerph15102235.
16. Gulati M, Ventkataramu N, Gupta S, et al. Ultrasound guided fine needle aspiration biopsy in mediastinal tuberculous. *Int J Tuberc Lung Dis* 2000; 4: 1164–1168.
17. Zhai K, Lu Y, Shi HZ. Tuberculous pleural effusion. *J Thorac Dis* 2016; 8: E486–E494.
18. Soni NJ, Franco R, Velez MI, et al. Ultrasound in the diagnosis and management of pleural effusions. *J Hosp Med* 2015; 10: 811–816.
19. Onuki T, Ueda S, Yamaoka M, et al. Primary and secondary spontaneous pneumothorax: prevalence, clinical features and in hospital mortality. *Can Respir J* 2017. https://doi.org/10.1155/2017/6014967.
20. World Health Organization. Top 10 causes of death, 2018. https://www.who.int/news-room/fact-sheets/detail/the-top-10-causes-of-death.
21. Ali N, Gali BM. Pattern and management of chest injuries in Maiduguri, Nigeria. *Ann Afr Med* 2004; 3: 181–184.
22. Sharma A, Jindal P. Principles of diagnosis and management of traumatic pneumothorax. *J Emerg Trauma Shock* 2008; 1: 34–41. https://doi.org/10.4103/0974-2700.41789.
23. Kanne JP, Rother MDM. Pneumothorax: imaging diagnosis and etiology. *Sem Roentgenol* 2023; 58: 440–453. https://doi.org/10.1053/j.ro.2023.06.004.
24. Husain LF, Hagopian L, Wayman D, et al. Sonographic diagnosis of pneumothorax. *J Emerg Trauma Shock* 2012; 5: 76–81.
25. Iqbal B, Hallfax R, Rahman NM. Pneumothorax: an update on clinical spectrum, diagnosis, and management. *Clin Med (Lond)* 2025; 25(3): 10037. https://doi.org/10.1016/j.clinme.2025.100327.
26. Prakash V, Bhimji SS. Amebic liver. StatPearls Publishing, 2017. https://www.ncbi.nlm.nih.gov/books/NBK430832.
27. Kannathasan S, Murugananthan A, Kumanan T, et al. Epidemiology and factors associ ated with amoebic liver abscess in northern Sri Lanka. *BMC Public Health* 2018; 18(1): 118.
28. Nath J, Ghosh SK, Singa B, et al. Molecular epidemiology of amebiasis: a cross sectional study among N.E. Indian population. *PLoS Negl Trop Dis* 2015; 9: e0004225.
29. Pritt SB, Clark CG. Amebiasis. *Mayo Clin Proc* 2008; 83: 1154–1159.
30. Bélard S, Tamarozzi F, Bustinduy AL, et al. Point-of-care ultrasound assessment of tropical infectious diseases- a review of applications and perspectives. *Am J Trop Med Hyg* 2015; 94(1): 8–21. https://doi.org/10.4269/ajtmh.15-0421.
31. Stinton LM, Shaffer EA. Epidemiology of gallbladder disease: cholelithiasis and cancer. *Gut Liver* 2012; 6(2): 172–187. https://doi.org/10.5009/gnl.2.12.6.2.172.
32. Indar AA, Beckingham IJ. Acute cholecystitis. *BMJ* 2002; 325(7365): 639–643.
33. Pinto A, Reginelli A, Cagini L, et al. Accuracy of ultrasonography in the diagnosis of acute calculous cholecystitis: review of the literature. *Crit Ultrasound J* 2013; 5(Suppl 1): S11. https://doi.org/10.1186/2036-7902-5-S1-S11.
34. Cresswall JA, Ronsmans C, et al. Prevalence of placenta previa by world region: a systemic review and meta-analysis. *Trop Med Int Health* 2013; 18: 712–724.
35. Quant HS, Friedman AM, Wang E, et al. Transabdominal ultrasonography as a screening test for second-trimester placenta previa. *Obstet Gynecol* 2014; 123: 628–633.
36. Fadl S, Moshiri M, Fligner CL, et al. Placental imaging: normal appearance with review of pathologic findings. *Radiographics* 2017; 37: 979–998.
37. Harvey HB, Ahn R, Price DD, Burke TF. Innovating for the developing world: meeting the affordability challenge. *AJR* 2014; 203: 835–837.
38. Horuz R, Sarica K. The management of staghorn calculi in children. *Arab J Urol* 2012; 10: 330–335.

39. Flannigan R, Choy WH, Chew B, Lange D. Renal struvite stones - pathogenesis, microbiology, and management strategies. *Nat Rev Urol.* 2014; 11: 333–341. https://doi.org/10.1038/nrurol.2014.99.
40. Hansen KL, Nielsen MB, Ewertsen C. Ultrasonography of the kidney: a pictorial review. *Diagnostics (Basel)* 2015; 6: 2. https://doi.org/10.3390/diagnostics6010002.
41. Diri A, Diri B. Management of staghorn renal stones. *Ren Fail* 2018; 40: 357–362.
42. Moul JW, Whitley B. Benign prostatic hyperplasia. In: Chapple CR, McConnell JD, Tubaro A (eds). Conn's current therapy. Elsevier, 2019; 1088–1091.
43. Tyloch JF, Wieczorek AP. The standards of an ultrasound examination of the prostate gland. Part 2. *J Ultrason* 2017; 17: 43–58. https://doi.org/10.15557/JoU.2017.0007.
44. Raff AB, Kroshinsky D. Cellulitis: a review. *JAMA* 2016; 316: 325–337.
45. Wanat K, Norton S. Travelers health: posttravel evaluation - skin and soft tissue infections. CDC website. https://wwwnc.cdc.gov/travel/yellowbook/2020/posttravel-evaluation/skin-and-soft-tissue-infections. Accessed June 24, 2019.
46. Weaver JS, Omar I, Epstein K, et al. High-resolution ultrasound in the evaluation of musculoskeletal infections. *J Ultrason* 2023; 23(95): e272–e284. https://doi/org/10.15557/jou.2023.0034.
47. O'Rourke K, Kibbee N, Stubbs A. Ultrasound for the evaluation of skin and soft tissue infections. *Mo Med* 2015; 112: 202–205.
48. Levine MR, Gorman SM, Young CF, Courtney DM. Clinical characteristics and management of wound foreign bodies in the ED. *Am J Emerg Med* 2008; 26: 918–922.
49. Hiremath R, Reddy H, Ibrahim J, et al. Soft tissue foreign body: utility of high resolution ultrasonography. *J Clin Diagn Res* 2017; 11: TC14–TC16.
50. Rubin G, Chezar A, Raz R, Rozen N. Nail puncture wound through a rubber-soled shoe: a retrospective study of 96 adult patients. *J Foot Ankle Surg* 2010; 49: 421–425.
51. Liu Q, Li MW, Wang ZD, et al. Human sparganosis, a neglected food borne zoonosis. *Lancet Infect Dis* 2015; 15: 1226–1235.
52. Kim SM, Amponsah EK, Eo MY, et al. Clinical manifestation of a patient with forehead sparganosis. *J Craniofac Surg* 2017; 28: 1081–1083.
53. Agarwal A, Aggarwal A. Bone and joint infections in children: septic arthritis. *Indian J Pediatr* 2016; 83: 825–833.
54. Kang SN, Sanghera T, Mangwani J, et al. The management of septic arthritis in children: systematic review of the English language literature. *J Bone Joint Surg (Br)* 2009; 91: 1127–1133.
55. Gaigneux E, Cormier G, Varin S, et al. Ultrasound abnormalities in septic arthritis are associated with functional outcomes. *Joint Bone Spine* 2017; 84: 599–604.
56. Maffulli N, Papalia R, Zampogna B, et al. The management of osteomyelitis in the adult. *Surgeon* 2016; 14: 345–360. https://doi.org/10.1016/j.surge.2015.12.005.
57. Sheedy CA, Snyder SB. Clinician-performed ultrasound in identifying osteomyelitis of the hand. *J Emerg Med* 2014; 47: e121–e123.
58. Chartier LB, Bosco L, Lapointe-Shaw L, Chenkin J. Use of point-of-care ultrasound in long bone fractures: a systematic review and meta-analysis. *CJEM* 2017; 19: 131–142. https://doi.org/10.1017/cem.2016.397.
59. Strahan R, Chiyesu KO, Schneider-Kolsky ME. Ultrasound study of liver disease caused by *Schistosoma mansoni* in rural Zambian schoolchildren. *J Med Imaging Radiat Oncol* 2012; 56(4): 390–397. https://doi.org/10.1111/j.1754-9485.2012.02371.x.
60. Geetha R, Tripathy K. Chorioretinitis. In: StatPearls [Internet]. Treasure Island, FL: StatPearls Publishing, 2022. https://www.ncbi.nlm.nih.gov/books/NBK551705.
61. Skidmore C, Saurey T, Ferre RM, et al. A narrative review of common uses of ophthalmic ultrasound in emergency medicine. *J Emerg Med* 2021; 60: 80–89. https://doi.org/10.1016/j.jemermed.2020.08.003.
62. Ghali S, Katti G, Shahbaz S, et al. Fascial space odontogenic infections: ultrasonography as an alternative to magnetic resonance imaging. *World J Clin Cases* 2021; 9(3): 573–580. https://doi.org/10.12998/wjcc.v9.i3.573.

CHAPTER 17

Ultrasound in Medical Education

Thomas Chandy, Kevin Brighton, Michael Stephens, Jennifer Frazee, and Jill Pitcher
Rocky Vista University, College of Osteopathic Medicine, Parker, Colorado, Ivins, Utah, USA

Introduction

The future for ultrasound is promising. Ultrasound technology has outpaced traditional education, necessitating an early introduction to the technology within the medical education system [1]. This chapter reviews the current state of ultrasound in medical school and postgraduate training and identifies the key methodologies in teaching ultrasound. This chapter discusses the importance of early medical ultrasound training that can assist students in their medical education and prepare them to provide high-quality patient care in the future.

Medical School Training

Year I: Learning Anatomy/Basic Ultrasound Techniques

The first-year of medical school typically focuses on the basic medical sciences, physiology, and anatomy. These courses help establish a foundational framework that prepares medical students for the transition to clinical practice during hospital rotations. However, ultrasound is often not included in the first-year medical school curriculum despite evidence suggesting that early ultrasound training enhances anatomical understanding, spatial orientation, procedural skills, and active learning [2].

Ultrasound education during the first year of medical school has been shown to help students' understanding of normal anatomy and physiology, support the application of basic diagnostic techniques, and improve recognition of pathology [3]. These findings align with reports from students enrolled in gross anatomy courses. [4]. While gross anatomy labs allow students to directly visualize and handle human tissue, ultrasound training complements this experience by demonstrating how these human anatomical structures would appear *in vivo* on imaging. This skill is essential in clinical medicine, where anatomy is frequently assessed with imaging modalities. Ultrasound instruction also enables students to observe real-time physiologic processes such as cardiac function, and helps recognize changes to these physiologic processes associated with disease. As a result, medical students report that ultrasound-integrated curricula strengthen clinical correlations and enhance learning from didactic coursework. [2].

Ultrasound education for first-year medical students may begin with students learning ultrasound basics such as the physics of ultrasound, limitations and advantages of medical ultrasound, proper use of ultrasound instruments, adjustment of settings to acquire optimal visual images, and appropriate probe selection for viewing various anatomical structures based on the location of the targeted structure and organ. Students can learn to differentiate imaging modes, identify common artifacts, and determine which anatomical structures are best visualized with ultrasound versus those requiring other imaging modalities. It has even been suggested to introduce ultrasound use during the first week of medical school (orientation week) to help first-year students become more familiar with the ultrasound equipment and be better prepared to use ultrasound imaging once classes begin [2].

In summary, first-year ultrasound education provides foundational knowledge and skills that integrate within broader medical curricula and serve as a platform for continued development throughout training and into specialty practice. [5]. Many first- and second-year medical students have expressed a desire to greater incorporate ultrasound into their curriculum to support their learning of anatomy, physiology, and pathology [2]. In addition, those who participate in ultrasound training rate themselves as having an increased interest in the clinical use of ultrasound [4]. Compared with other imaging techniques, such as magnetic resonance imaging (MRI), X-ray, and computed tomography, ultrasound offers a unique hands-on learning approach that enhances anatomical learning [1]. Recent advances in ultrasound technology including quality handheld devices have made this instruction scalable and cost effective [5].

Year II: Integrating Ultrasound into Clinical Medicine

During the second year of medical school, students are often transitioning into clinical medicine, developing physical exam skills, and preparing for third- and fourth-year clinical rotations. Ultrasound training during this time is perhaps even more valuable to help prepare medical students for ultrasound application in the clinical world.

As medical students transition from basic medical sciences to clinical medicine, ultrasound education can help improve their understanding of how foundational concepts are applied in clinical practice [2]. This is achieved in part by focusing on pathology visualized through ultrasound. For example, at the University of South Carolina School of Medicine, second-year medical students incorporated ultrasound into their curriculum through comparisons of normal and pathologic images, group-based problem solving cases, and examinations assessing ultrasound knowledge. After completing this training, students reported that the ultrasound-integrated curriculum "increased clinical correlation with basic science instruction" [2]. This improved understanding and confidence may help explain the association between ultrasound education and improved performance on clinical examinations [6].

Studies have demonstrated that implementing a point-of-care ultrasound (POCUS) program can improve students' overall understanding and performance of the physical examination, even when ultrasound skills are not being directly tested [6]. These findings suggest that ultrasound education plays a important role in developing and applying strong physical exam skills [6]. This training will not only help medical students become more competent in patient care, but also help them prepare for test questions focused on physical assessment. As physical exam skills are taught throughout all four years of medical school, ultrasound education represents a valuable addition to the curriculum that strengthens physician training [7].

Ultrasound education in the second year can be a terrific way to prepare medical students for third- and fourth-year rotations. By learning a variety of ultrasound techniques and procedures, medical students may become more engaged, knowledgeable, and competent during clinical rotations [5]. For example, learning how to perform a FAST exam may help prepare students for an emergency medicine (EM) rotation [8, 9]. Likewise, familiarity with echocardiogram acquisition and interpretation is another valuable skill, as it applies across multiple rotations, especially in cardiology [10]. Additionally, understanding Doppler ultrasound findings in conditions such as aortic valve stenosis allows students to identify abnormal blood flow patterns and communicate effectively with their attending physicians while on clinical rotations [11]. Although these ultrasound exams and associated skills are most frequently used during third- and fourth-year rotations, introducing them in the second year allows students sufficient time to develop proficiency and supports a smoother transition to clinical medicine [2]. Early training also enables students to participate more actively in patient care during later rotations, enriching their overall learning experience.

Years III and IV: Ultrasound in Clinical Rotations

Once a medical student completes the first two years of medical school and starts clinical rotations, they can begin to apply the ultrasound skills they developed in a clinical setting. Clinical rotations provide an opportunity to broaden their ultrasound skills and gain insight from different specialties on the diverse applications of ultrasound in medical practice. For instance, third-year students may be taught to recognize the general indications for specific focused ultrasound examinations, determine the appropriate timing for their use in clinical scenarios, and develop a deeper understanding of ultrasound as a tool for procedural guidance [1]. During fourth year, students will then be able to recognize the sensitivity and specificity of various ultrasound procedures and attain insight into the limitations, risks, and benefits of ultrasound use [1]. While students in their first- and second-year medical school training primarily focus on obtaining appropriate ultrasound images, third- and fourth-year students emphasize image interpretation for diagnosis and potential differentials [12]. Furthermore, some curricula also include an objective structured clinical examination (OSCE) at the end of a rotation to evaluate the ultrasound skills and knowledge gained by students during that period [2]. Implementation of online ultrasound lectures congruent with the student's clinical rotation training may assist in improving their ultrasound knowledge while on clinical rotations [1].

Ultrasound training at this stage of medical education often varies depending on the rotation site and the supervising physician's expertise in the use of ultrasound. In many cases, opportunities for students to apply ultrasound in clinical settings remain limited, due to a lack of faculty familiarity with focused ultrasound [1]. For example, radiologists may be particularly interested in teaching medical students the appropriate use of ultrasound in clinical settings, whereas specialties that use ultrasound less frequently may not have such an interest.

While ultrasound training during rotation years is dependent on the attending physician's knowledge and experience of ultrasound, rotations can provide a great opportunity for medical students to practice their ultrasound skills in a variety of settings. Medical students who receive ultrasound training during clinical rotations are more likely to seek additional training in their residency programs and are more likely to use ultrasound in their clinical practice [13]. Using ultrasound during the third and fourth year can help medical students feel more confident in their ultrasound skills and ultimately prepare them to apply ultrasound in their chosen specialty.

Third- and fourth-year medical students can further their ultrasound education by attending the annual American Institute of Ultrasound in Medicine (AIUM) convention. The convention brings together multidisciplinary experts to share cutting-edge ultrasound research and improved clinical guidelines and provides an inclusive space for continued hands-on ultrasound training. The convention hosts lectures and seminars that aim to expand attendees' knowledge and use of ultrasound. The AIUM convention also hosts an event, SonoSlam, that encourages medical students to team up and participate in various ultrasound scanning challenges. It is a great way for students to network, develop new ultrasound skills, and showcase the skills they gained throughout their medical school training. While there are many things to do and learn at this convention, as both emerging and established providers, the conference itself testifies to the growing importance of ultrasound education in medical schools. As shown at this conference, the versatility of ultrasound substantiates its use as the new standard of care in many areas of medicine [14].

Ultrasound in Residency Training

Ultrasound training is becoming more common in residency programs' curricula because of its affordability, accessibility, and accuracy. The American Academy of Family Physicians (AAFP) states that POCUS is the biggest advance in bedside diagnosis since the advent of the stethoscope 200 years ago [14]. For several decades, ultrasound training has been an integral part of several specialty practices, including emergency medicine, obstetrics, cardiology, and radiology. Due to advances in ultrasound technology as well as its affordability, primary care physicians are more frequently using ultrasound as a bedside diagnostic tool. Bedside (portable) ultrasound examinations can be performed in the clinic and in the hospital, and are less costly and time-consuming than CT scan or MRI performed by the radiology department. This section will discuss the current adoption of ultrasound in residency education and will review expected competencies and outcomes after completing training.

A growing number of physicians are using ultrasound at the bedside because of its cost-effectiveness, timeliness, and accuracy. POCUS is noninvasive and does not require ionizing radiation, making it an ideal instrument for physicians [15]. As a result, major academic societies have endorsed POCUS and begun to establish clinical guidelines for their respective clinical fields and training programs. The American College of Emergency Physicians (ACEP) has made ultrasound a universal requirement for emergency medicine (EM) residency training per the Accreditation Council for Graduate Medical Education guidelines [16]. Consequently, POCUS has become the standard for rapid diagnosis in emergency medicine. Other major medical societies have recognized the value of ultrasound and are working to establish guidelines and best practices for ultrasound training during residency. The American College of Physicians (ACP) has formally acknowledged the important role of POCUS in internal medicine [17]. In a written statement of support for ultrasound, ACP emphasized the need to expand ACP's POCUS training programs to enable more internists to attain competency in POCUS [17]. The AAFP stated that a large body of evidence clearly demonstrates that using POCUS improves clinical outcomes, reduces failure and complication rates during procedures, rapidly narrows differential diagnoses, shortens times to definitive treatment, lowers costs, and reduces the use of ionizing radiation of computed tomography imaging [1]. The recent acknowledgment and adoption of ultrasound by major academic medical societies demonstrates the growing importance of ultrasound in clinical practice.

Despite the broad acceptance of ultrasound, residency ultrasound training requirements vary by specialty. Emergency medicine has taken a leadership role in the establishment and education of bedside, clinical, and POCUS by clinicians in the United States and around the world [16]. ACEP states that emergency physicians should have a basic education in ultrasound physics, instrumentation, procedural guidance, and focused assessment with sonography in trauma (FAST) as part of their EM practice [16]. While emergency medicine has made ultrasound a requirement for board certification, other specialties have only recommended guidelines for ultrasound residency curriculum without requiring ultrasound training for board certification. Recently, the AAFP developed ultrasound residency curriculum guidelines with specific knowledge requirements and competencies. The AAFP has yet to make ultrasound a requirement in family medicine training. Subsequently, only a small number of family medicine programs have an established curriculum [15]. In the field of internal medicine, many hospitalists are already incorporating POCUS into their daily practice because it adds value to their bedside evaluation of patients [18]. Although there has been acknowledgment, endorsement, and acceptance of ultrasound as a standard in clinical practice in primary care, many residency programs are only just beginning to provide ultrasound training. As reported in a national survey of internal medicine program directors and assistant program directors in 2012, only 25% of internal medicine programs had a formal ultrasound curriculum, and only 25% planned to start one within the next year [15].

Each year, an increasing number of medical schools are integrating POCUS into their curricula [13]. Multiple studies have shown that the current generation of medical students and residents have increased exposure to POCUS and desire more POCUS training during residency [14]. Ultrasound has become a key tool employed by physicians in clinical practice, and the adoption of ultrasound will continue to increase as more medical schools and residency programs integrate ultrasound training into their core curriculum.

As more residency programs incorporate ultrasound training into their curriculum, new standards to assess physician knowledge of ultrasound are being established. Several academic medical societies are making specific recommendations for the skill sets and competencies that each resident should be able to independently perform or appropriately refer to other specialists. Basic knowledge of ultrasound includes fundamentals of ultrasound physics, safety, anatomy, physiology, and device operation. Basic knowledge can be taught by multiple methods, including live or recorded lectures, online modules, or readings [18]. The AAFP has recommended specific ultrasound skill requirements in the following basic core applications: (1) obstetrics and gynecology (OB/GYN), (2) cardiac, (3) trauma, (4) aorta, (5) biliary, (6) urinary tract, (7) deep venous thrombosis (DVT), (8) soft tissue/musculoskeletal, (9) thoracic/pulmonary, (10) ocular, (11) procedural guidance, and (12) clinical protocols [14]. Each of these core applications in the AAFP guideline includes competencies that are recommended for training programs to assess a resident's ability. For example the AAFP recommends that a resident should be able to perform skills in OB/GYN ultrasound, including transabdominal and transvaginal scanning techniques, detect fetal heart activity, and longitudinally assess fetal and maternal health throughout each trimester of pregnancy. In a recent position statement, the Society of Hospital Medicine recommends that residents develop specific skills in image acquisition, image interpretation, and clinical integration. The Society of Hospital Medicine recommends that assessments of competency include knowledge-based questions, image acquisition using task-specific checklists on human or simulation models, image interpretation using a series of videos or still images with normal and abnormal findings, and clinical integration using "next best step" in a multiple-choice format with POCUS images and simulation-based clinical scenarios. It also encourages a final assessment at the end of training that includes an evaluation of a resident's knowledge and hands-on skills. Hospital medicine residency programs are recommended to use formative assessments for evaluation. These programs assess a resident's knowledge using quantitative scoring systems derived from structured checklists [18]. As an early adopter of required ultrasound training in medicine, the ACEP recommends that "training exams need to include patients with different conditions and body types in different settings including clinical and educational" [16]. The ACEP also states that "abnormal or positive scans should be included in a significant number of training exams used to meet credentialing requirements and trainees should complete a benchmark of 150–300 emergency ultrasound exams depending on the number of applications being utilized" [16]. The growth of ultrasound as a bedside diagnostic tool has been a catalyst for the development of initial ultrasound guidelines for use. As these guidelines develop, competency standards should be developed to assess a trainee's knowledge and skills, which will help to standardize both training and practice expectations.

Ultrasound in Continuing Medical Education

Ongoing ultrasound training is recommended because ultrasound skills can decay with lack of use. Several medical societies recommend that POCUS users should continue using POCUS regularly in clinical practice and participate in POCUS continuing medical education (CME) activities, with ongoing assessment [18]. CME is a requirement for physicians in all medical specialties. Physicians use CME to maintain competence in current skill sets and advance knowledge of new and developing areas in their field. Ultrasound CME activities include conference attendance, online educational activities, research, hands-on training, textbook and journal reading, program administration, and in-service examinations [16]. As previously mentioned, the AIUM, is a multi-disciplinary professional association that provides high-quality education, encourages lifelong learning, and promotes the importance and value of medical ultrasound. The AIUM offers a number of CME activities, including webinars, lecture series, journal articles, and specialty courses focused on ultrasound for students and clinicians. In the AIUM's POCUS and general medicine courses materials are designed to cover POCUS for generalists. Live demonstrations, simulations, and didactic lectures are used to provide a comprehensive and in-depth look at how and where medical ultrasound can effectively be used in point-of-care and general medicine settings [19]. Several other organizations, including nonprofit academic institutions and societies, offer ongoing ultrasound CME activities. For example, the International Society of Professionals in Ultrasound for Obstetrics and Gynecology offers ongoing training in assessing fetal anomalies in the heart and central nervous system (CNS). Weill Cornell has a CME training course, Hospital Medicine Point-of-Care Ultrasonography, which is intended to give physicians the skills to integrate POCUS into their everyday practice [20]. The Society of Ultrasound in Medical Education (SUSME) is an organization with a specific focus on ultrasound education on a global scale. It partners with other organizations such as the World Interactive Network Focused on Critical Ultrasound (WINFOCUS) and the AIUM to support this global education goal [21]. In addition to ongoing training courses, some organizations such as the Society of Hospital Medicine promote quality assurance programs run by a committee within hospital groups to help physicians maintain their ultrasound skills. Quality assurance is aimed at ensuring that physicians maintain basic competency in using POCUS to appropriately influence bedside decisions. Oversight of POCUS includes ensuring that providers using POCUS are adequately trained, can use the equipment correctly, and can document images properly [18]. ACEP has launched the quality improvement process to evaluate images for technical competence, interpretations for clinical accuracy, and provide feedback to improve physician performance [16]. As more physicians adopt ultrasound into their clinical practices, ongoing ultrasound education and quality assurance programs are critical to help physicians maintain their skills and stay up to date with the current ultrasound technology.

Summary

This chapter highlighted the role of ultrasound in medical education and explored how various teaching methods across different training settings can influence a student's future career. The items covered provide a resource that can be used for standard ultrasound training and help prepare doctors for the future.

Review Questions

1. What ultrasound skills are developed during the first year of medical school?
   a. Understanding ultrasound physics
   b. Probe selection for viewing various anatomical structures

c. Adjusting ultrasound settings
d. Transducer and image orientations
e. All the above

2. Ultrasound education in the second year of medical school has proven to:
 a. Decrease clinical correlation with basic science instruction
 b. Be best studied in isolation and quiet
 c. Improve test scores
 d. Limit preparation of second-year students for third- and fourth-year rotations
 e. Only enhance study on anatomy
3. Ultrasound training in the third- and fourth-year of medical school is dependent on:
 a. The attending physician's knowledge and experience in ultrasound
 b. Access to high-end ultrasound equipment
 c. Lowering the cost of medical student training
 d. Access to radiology faculty
 e. The number of clinical patients
4. What is true about "Point-of-Care Ultrasound?"
 a. It is extremely expensive, and thus not applicable in most clinical settings
 b. POCUS takes longer than traditional imaging to obtain quality diagnostic results
 c. It requires ionizing radiation before and after use
 d. POCUS is accurate, timely, and cost-effective
 e. It is easy to perform with no training requirement
5. Quality assurance in ultrasound training is useful for:
 a. Determining which patients are most vulnerable to an infectious disease
 b. Assessing clinical accuracy, technical competency, and providing feedback
 c. Evaluating small and rural clinics' ability to manage trauma
 d. Determining whether a patient needs image studies
 e. Determining the profit of ultrasound service in clinics

Correct answers: 1. e; 2. c; 3. a; 4. d; 5. b.

References

1. Bahner DP, Adkins EJ, Hughes D, et al. Integrated medical school ultrasound: development of an ultrasound vertical curriculum. *Crit Ultrasound J* 2013; 5(1): 6. https://doi.org/10.1186/2036-7902-5-6.
2. Hoppmann RA, Rao VV, Bell F, et al. The evolution of an integrated ultrasound curriculum (iUSC) for medical students: 9-year experience. *Crit Ultrasound J* 2015; 7(1): 18. https://doi.org/10.1186/s13089-015-0035-3.
3. Baltarowich OH, Di Salvo DN, Scoutt LM, et al. National ultrasound curriculum for medical students. *Ultrasound Q* 2014; 30: 13–19.
4. Dreher SM, Dephilip R, Bahner DP. Ultrasound exposure during gross anatomy. *J Emerg Med* 2013; 1: 10. https://doi.org/10.1016/j.jemermed.2013.08.028.
5. Arger PH, Schultz SM, Sehgal CM, et al. Teaching medical students diagnostic sonography. *J Ultrasound Med* 2005; 24: 1365–1369.

6. Liu RB, Suwondo DN, Donroe JH, et al. Point-of-care ultrasound: does it affect scores on standardized assessment tests used within the preclinical curriculum? *J Ultrasound Med* 2019; 38: 433–440.
7. Steinmetz P, Oleskevich S, Dyachenko A, et al. Accuracy of medical students in detecting pleural effusion using lung ultrasound as an adjunct to the physical examination. *J Ultrasound Med* 2018; 37: 2545–2552. https://doi.org/10.1002/jum.14612.
8. Arafat R, Golea A, Dărămuş I, Badea R. Medical education for emergency physician focused on basic competence (focused assessment with sonography in trauma). Evaluation of the Romanian national program: "regional emergency medical services systems." *Med Ultrason* 2011; 13: 283–291.
9. Lee SH, Yun SJ. Diagnostic performance of ultrasonography for detection of pediatric elbow fracture: a meta-analysis. *Ann Emerg Med* 2019; 74: 493–502.
10. Berthelot E, Jourdain P, Bailly MT, et al. Echocardiographic evaluation of left ventricular filling pressure in patients with heart failure with preserved ejection fraction: usefulness of inferior vena cava measurements and 2016 EACVI/ASE recommendations. *J Card Fail* 2020; 26(6): 507–514. https://doi.org/10.1016/j.cardfail.2020.01.018.
11. Hansen KL, Møller-Sørensen H, Kjaergaard J, et al. Aortic valve stenosis increases helical flow and flow complexity: a study of intra-operative cardiac vector flow imaging. *Ultrasound Med Biol* 2017; 43: 1607–1617.
12. Bahner DP, Royall NA. Advanced ultrasound training for fourth-year medical students: a novel training program at the Ohio State University College of medicine. *Acad Med* 2013; 88: 206–213. https://doi.org/10.1097/ACM.0b013e31827c562d.
13. Prats MI, Royall NA, Panchal AR, et al. Outcomes of an advanced ultrasound selective: preparing medical students for residency and practice. *J Ultrasound Med* 2016; 35(5): 975–982.
14. American Academy of Family Physicians. 2016. Recommended curriculum guidelines for family medicine residents: point of care ultrasound. http://www.aafp.org/dam/AAFP/documents/medical_education_residency/program_director.
15. Reaume M, Siuba M, Wagner M, et al. Prevalence and scope of point-of-care ultrasound education in internal medicine, pediatric, and medicine-pediatric residency programs in the United States. *J Ultrasound Med* 2019; 38: 1433–1439.
16 American College of Emergency Physicians. Ultrasound guidelines: emergency, point-of-care, and clinical ultrasound guidelines in medicine, 2016. https://www.acep.org/siteassets/sites/acep/media/ultrasound/ pointofcareultrasound-guidelines.pdf.
17. Schnobrich DJ, Gladding S, Olson APJ, Duran-Nelson A. Point-of-care ultrasound in internal medicine: a national survey of educational leadership. *J Grad Med Educ* 2013; 5(3): 498–502. https://doi.org/10.4300/JGME-D-12-00215.1.
18. Soni NJ, Schnobrich D, Mathews BK, et al. Point-of-care ultrasound for hospitalists: a position statement of the Society of Hospital Medicine. *J Hosp Med* 2019; 14: E1–E6. https://doi.org/10.12788/jhm.3079.
19. AIUM. AIUM practice parameter for the performance of point-of-care ultrasound examinations. *J Ultrasound Med* 2019; 38: 833–849. https://doi.org/10.1002/jum.14972.
20. Weill Cornell Medicine. Introduction to HM-POCUS course. https://medicine.weill.cornell.edu/divisions-programs/general-internal-medicine/education/point-care-ultrasound-training/hm-pocus-class.
21. Hoffmann B, Blaivas M, Abramowicz J, Bachmann M, Badea R, et al. Medical student ultrasound education, a WFUMB position paper, part II. A consensus statement of ultrasound societies. Med Ultrason 2020; 22(2):220–229. https://doi.org/10.11152/mu-2599.

CHAPTER 18

Point-of-Care Ultrasound

Tyler Burke, Jennifer Frazee, and Jing Gao
Rocky Vista University, Montana College of Osteopathic Medicine, Billings, Montana, USA

Introduction

Point-of-care ultrasound (POCUS) was initially adopted by non-radiologists for the detection of intraperitoneal fluid in trauma patients through focused abdominal sonography exams [1, 2]. Due to its bedside accessibility and versatility, POCUS has evolved into an essential diagnostic tool with applications that extend well beyond the realms of both emergency medicine and critical care, including diagnostic assessment, surgical preparation, and interventional guidance [3, 4].

Ultrasound operators must complete formalized training and engage in regular practice to achieve proficiency in performing POCUS. Certification and training opportunities are provided via online webinars and in-person workshops presented by experienced physicians at local and national conferences. In addition, residency programs and medical schools have increasingly incorporated POCUS into their curriculum to reinforce anatomical principles and pathological findings during the early years of medical training. For fellowship-trained emergency physicians, the American Board of Emergency Medicine (ABEM) offers the Focused Practice Designation (FPD) in Advanced Emergency Medicine Ultrasonography (AEMUS) [5].

The use of POCUS is particularly advantageous for challenging patient anatomies who require further workup. Additional benefits of the use of POCUS include its noninvasive technique, lack of exposure to radiation (when compared to CT), and ability to expedite the diagnostic process. When performed by a certified operator, POCUS demonstrates diagnostic accuracy equivalent to that of radiologist-supervised ultrasound examinations; however, certification standards, whether established by radiology boards, ultrasound associations, or medical institutions, may drastically vary across regions [4–6]. Furthermore, compared with other imaging modalities, POCUS is highly cost-effective and can be life-changing in resource-limited areas.

While incorporation of POCUS has many potential benefits, its inter- and intra-operator variability should not be overlooked. The quality of images obtained by POCUS is heavily dependent on user training and experience. Ultrasound images are inherently subject to a handful of complicating factors, including artifact, patient body habitus, and inappropriate or inadequate patient positioning secondary to pain, patient cooperation, and various dressings and tubes in the scanning region [2].

There is no question that its incorporation can aid in quick diagnoses; however, POCUS is not as sensitive as either a CT or magnetic resonance imaging (MRI) in the assessment of bony structures, organs with air (lung parenchyma, intestine), and large fields of view with three-dimensional reconstruction. Keeping these potential benefits and limitations in mind, POCUS is capable of evaluating multiple organ systems, including cardiac, pulmonary, GI/GU, musculoskeletal, and neurovascular [3].

This chapter summarizes common uses of POCUS in clinical patient care. More detailed ultrasound examinations for each organ system are discussed in their associated chapters of this book.

Cardiac POCUS

Indications for cardiac POCUS scans include symptoms of chest pain, dizziness, hypotension, heart murmurs, abnormal EKG, or cardiac arrest. Patients with suspected pericardial effusions arrythmias, cardiac myopathies, heart failure, or shock may also benefit from a POCUS evaluation, particularly through Rapid Ultrasound for Shock and Hypotension (RUSH) examination [7–12]. Although the RUSH exam is a widely accepted POCUS assessment, its utility may be limited in patients with subcutaneous emphysema or thoracic dressings due to impaired image quality. [13]. In such cases, further workup with more advanced imaging, such as CT, is warranted. More details of cardiac ultrasound can be found in Chapter 4 of this book.

Cardiac 5 View Assessment

To perform a cardiac POCUS scan, five different views are obtained using a phased array transducer. The five views include long-axis (LAX) and short-axis (SAX) parasternal views, a subcostal (subxiphoid) four-chamber view, an IVC subcostal view, and an apical four-chamber view of the heart [14]. The multi-view assessment is completed to evaluate the anatomical structures, size, and function of the heart. Although cardiac POCUS is a quick and convenient scan, it is not meant to replace a comprehensive full-length echocardiogram [13, 14].

To obtain a parasternal LAX cardiac view, the ultrasound transducer is positioned between the second and third intercostal spaces along the left sternal border. The transducer indicator is directed toward the patient's right shoulder, and the image indicator should be displayed on the right side of the screen [14]. The parasternal LAX scan will show a cross section of the heart with the right ventricle (RV) in the near field and the left ventricle in the far field. This view allows the operator to identify mitral valvular function, atrial size, and visualize the aortic root, thickness of the interventricular septum (IVS), and left ventricle posterior wall. The RV, ascending aorta, and left atrium should have a roughly 1:1:1 ratio.

In a parasternal SAX view, the transducer is rotated clockwise toward the patient's left shoulder. This brings the interventricular septum and left ventricle into view in an axial, top-down view. To obtain a better view of the structures, the operator can adjust the transducer and sweep the sound beam from the base of the heart to its apex. Depending on the exact location of the ultrasound beams while in the parasternal SAX view, the operator can assess the aortic valve, pulmonary artery, interventricular septum, left ventricle, mitral valve, and papillary muscles for anatomical changes or functional abnormalities.

To perform a subcostal four-chamber view, the ultrasound machine should have the cardiac setting selected. The transducer should be placed below the xiphoid process with the indicator pointing to the left side of the patient's body. It is imperative to avoid gas in both the bowel and the stomach to obtain a high-quality image in this view. As such, the operator may use the left lobe of the liver as an acoustic window and fan the probe anteriorly from IVC to watch it enter the right atrium. The subxiphoid view allows the operator to compare the size of the atria and ventricles of the heart and pericardium. As the transducer is anatomically placed inferior to the heart, the right ventricle will appear in the near field, and the atria and left ventricle will be found in the far field [14].

In a subcostal IVC view, the transducer is placed in the same position as the subcostal four-chamber view, but the transducer indicator should be pointing toward the patient's head instead of the left side of the patient's body. The IVC will come into view in a longitudinal plane and will be seen entering the right atrium. Variations in IVC diameter measurements between inspiration and expiration will indirectly reflect volume status. This is best evaluated in the long axis of IVC [15].

The apical view of the heart is obtained by placing the transducer at the midclavicular line around the fifth intercostal space. The indicator on the transducer should be pointing toward the patient's left axilla [14]. Having the patient in the left lateral decubitus position can be useful in minimizing artifacts. An apical view can be used to assess pericardial effusions, to compare the size of all four chambers, and to observe the strength and symmetry of left ventricular segmental contraction [15].

Pulmonary POCUS

Bedside ultrasound of the lung can be extremely beneficial to those presenting with symptoms of acute shortness of breath, hypotension, labored breathing, or cough [16].

POCUS scans are commonly used to evaluate the lungs and expedite the diagnostic process of suspected pathologies, including, but not limited to, pneumothorax and pleural effusion [17]. Other lung pathologies, including pulmonary embolisms, asthma, COPD, and pneumonia, can be evaluated using POCUS; however, ultrasound is not the preferred method of diagnosis. The aforementioned pathologies should be evaluated by chest CT when available [18, 19].

POCUS of the lung is typically performed in three regions bilaterally (six total views) on the chest wall (anterior, lateral, and posterior). The anterior view assesses the right and left upper lobes. The lateral scan assesses the right middle lobe, while the posterior scan identifies the right and left lower lung lobes [20, 21]. A more detailed description of how lung ultrasound is performed and set up to assess both lung and pleural pathologies can be found in Chapter 3 of this book.

POCUS Anterior Lung

Pulmonary POCUS of the anterior chest wall is performed by placing the transducer (curvilinear or phased array) in the long axis orientation at the midclavicular line in the second intercostal space. Rib shadowing will characteristically have a "bat wing sign" appearance, as hyperechoic pleura will be visualized between posterior acoustic shadows from the ribs. Ideally, the pleura should move laterally on the screen, which indicates the visceral and parietal pleura sliding against each other [19]. Absent lung sliding heightens concern for a potential pneumothorax, pneumonia, or a pleural effusion, as fluid or air in the lung or pleural space can inhibit smooth movement of the pleural tissues. As a confirmatory measure, pleural sliding should be evaluated in M-mode. This setting will show a "barcode" or "stratosphere" sign with absent lung sliding, and a "seashore sign" in a healthy, normally functioning pleura evaluated using ultrasound [21].

POCUS Lateral Lung

To scan the middle right lobe of the lung, the transducer is placed in the long-axis orientation around the sixth or seventh intercostal space [20]. Manipulation of the transducer may be required by the operator to avoid significant rib shadowing. This can be accomplished by having the patient elevate their arm or engage in side bending. A-lines and B-lines are two pulmonary artifacts that are typically seen on lung ultrasound. A-lines are horizontal reverberations of the pleura interacting with the ultrasound waves, while B-lines are vertical, hyperechoic lines that represent comet tail artifacts. The change in B-lines is characteristically found in pathologies like bronchiolitis, pulmonary edema, or pneumonia, which reflects increase in lung interstitial fluid [21].

POCUS Posterior Lung

To scan the lower lobe of the lungs, the transducer is placed around the tenth to twelfth ribs at the posterior axillary line in long-axis orientation [20, 21]. In this position, the liver, spleen, diaphragm, and kidney will be seen with respiration. Pleural effusions may be visualized on this scan. If present, they will be located superior to both the diaphragm. Pleural effusion volumes can then be calculated via the Balik formula with ultrasound [21, 22]. The patients with large pleural effusions presenting with dyspnea, fever, or potential signs of septic shock will need further management, including other diagnostic tests and, potentially, therapeutic thoracentesis.

Bedside Lung Ultrasound Assessments

Once the operator becomes confident in scanning the lungs in these positions, point-of-care lung scanning may be applied to clinical algorithm assessments, including the Focused Assessment with Sonography in Trauma (FAST) exam, the Resuscitative Ultrasound for Shock and Hypotension (RUSH) exam, or the Bedside Lung Ultrasound in Emergency (BLUE) Protocol. More information on performing bedside ultrasound can be found in Chapters 12 and 14 of this book.

The FAST exam is a focused assessment with bedside sonography for trauma patients. This exam is used to quickly evaluate signs of internal bleeding that are indicative of organ damage in the abdomen, pelvis, or thoracic cavity post-blunt or penetrative trauma [23]. A meta-analysis with a sample of 24,000 patients found that the extended FAST (eFAST) exam detects pneumothorax and pericardial effusions with high specificity and sensitivity [24].

Similar to the FAST exam, the RUSH exam is performed at the bedside to evaluate patients in critical condition who may be suffering from pneumothorax. Additionally, the RUSH exam allows the sonographer to visualize vascular structures like the IVC and abdominal aorta for the sources of worsening patient conditions [4, 25]. It continues to be practiced in clinical settings secondary to its high sensitivity for screening patients with undifferentiated shock [25].

The Blue Protocol is another exam that utilizes ultrasound to distinguish among seven different lung pathologies: pulmonary edema, pulmonary embolism, pneumonia, COPD, asthma, pneumothorax, and pleural effusion [26]. It compares the presence of lung sliding and abnormal ultrasound artifacts to accomplish this feat. Due to its high clinical value for screening, clinicians consistently apply the Blue Protocol for the diagnosis of acute dyspneic conditions [26].

Abdominal and Pelvic Organs

The abdominal cavity is home to many organs, which makes identifying the cause of poorly localized abdominal pain challenging for clinicians. The incorporation of POCUS into clinical settings both improves diagnostic capabilities and allows for early identification of complicated pathologies.

The main indications for abdominal ultrasound include abdominal pain and trauma. While abdominal ultrasound has application for identifying bowel obstruction, appendicitis, intussusception, and diverticulitis, contrast-enhanced ultrasound (CEUS) is a novel application [27].

When conducting an abdominal ultrasound, it is imperative that the operator stands on the right side of the patient and has the ultrasound screen located directly in front of them. This allows the operator to scan with their right hand and operate the ultrasound machine with their left. A curvilinear probe is preferred for visualization of abdominal organs secondary to its optimized frequency, but a phased array probe is also acceptable. A linear probe may be necessary for pediatric patients and scans of the appendix. Regardless of which probe is used for these scans, an abdominal preset should be selected prior to scanning [27, 28]. Additional references for assessing abdominal pathologies can be found in Chapter 5 of this book.

Liver Ultrasound

Liver ultrasound is useful when a patient presents with complaints of right upper quadrant (RUQ) abdominal pain and/or has acute changes in liver function tests (LFTs).

When conducting a scan of the liver, the ultrasound probe should be placed on the patient's right mid-axillary line at the 10–11th intercostal space. The indicator should be oriented toward the patient's head. for imaging the long-axis view of the liver. The operator can ask the patient to put their arm above their head to widen the intercostal spaces and improve internal organ visualization. The diaphragm, liver, and right kidney should be visualized in the long-axis view [28]. Liver ultrasound is useful in detecting liver lacerations, hematomas, hepatosteatosis, hepatocellular carcinoma, or acute changes in the kidneys. It has applications in both acute and chronic patient presentations.

Gallbladder and Common Bile Duct Ultrasound

Unlike other organs, the gallbladder is not fixed to the abdominal wall. It can be found in various places in the RUQ of the abdomen and is commonly displaced during the third trimester of pregnancy. Operators should instruct patients to fast for about six hours prior to their scan and ensure that the gallbladder is dilated and contains bile [27, 28].

The patient can be positioned in either supine or left lateral decubitus to encourage the gallbladder migration toward the abdominal midline. Both intercostal and subcostal approaches are practical to image the gallbladder. The operator will know they have successfully identified the gallbladder when a hypoechoic sac is seen in the RUQ. Once located, the gallbladder can then be evaluated for wall thickness and presence of stones (hyperechoic foci with posterior shadowing). The ultrasound probe can then be rotated clockwise to obtain a short-axis view, which should help visualize the portal triad. Visualization of the portal triad is commonly referred to as the "Mickey Mouse Sign," where the common bile duct (CBD) and hepatic artery are the "ears," and the portal vein is Mickey's face or the "head" [28].

Splenic Ultrasound

To perform an ultrasound of the spleen, the operator should place the ultrasound probe on the patient's left side at the 7–8th intercostal space. The indicator should be directed toward the patient's head. A "knuckles to the bed" approach is often taught, as the spleen is positioned posteriorly in the abdominal cavity and will not be appropriately visualized if the ultrasound probe is too anterior on the patient's body. The spleen and adjacent left kidney will come into view in the long-axis plane. The Valsalva maneuver can be employed to expand the intercostal spaces and create a window for the ultrasound beams to travel through. This is accomplished by asking the patient to take a deep breath in and hold it. Ideally, the ultrasound beams will no longer be blocked by the ribs [28]. Once an appropriate view has been obtained, the spleen can be measured craniocaudally to assess splenomegaly. Additionally, the left kidney can be evaluated through this view.

Abdominal Free Fluid Ultrasound

In addition to examining individual organs, POCUS may be used to assess for free fluid in the abdominal cavity. Free fluid most typically occurs due to traumatic causes, but it can also be due to infectious or neoplastic causes and/or organ (heart, liver, kidney) failure. Free fluid tends to accumulate in the RUQ, LUQ, the rectovesical pouch (males), or the Pouch of Douglas (females), depending on the amount of free fluid.

Right Upper Quadrant View In the RUQ view, fluid can accumulate in the hepatorenal recess, colloquially referred to as "Morison's Pouch." Morison's Pouch is a potential space between the inferior surface of the right lobe of the liver and the upper pole of the right kidney [29]. Fluid can accumulate here because it is the most gravity-dependent space in the supramesocolic compartment [29].

Left Upper Quadrant View In the left upper quadrant view, the perisplenic recess can be visualized and evaluated. The spleen should be used as an acoustic window. With adequate positioning of the transducer, the operator should be able to evaluate the following organs: the spleen, perisplenic space, diaphragm, and the left kidney.

Rectovesical Pouch Free fluid may accumulate in the rectovesical pouch in biological males, as it is the most gravity-dependent portion of the peritoneal cavity. This space is formed by the anterior reflection of the peritoneum from the middle third of the rectum onto the superior aspect of the bladder [30].

Pouch of Douglas Free fluid may accumulate in the Pouch of Douglas (posterior cul-de-sac) in biological females, as it is the most gravity-dependent portion of the peritoneal cavity in biological females. The posterior cul-de-sac is positioned between the uterus and rectum. While it is normal to have a small amount of clear fluid in that area, which corresponds to the menstrual cycle. However, the presence of blood, pus, and/or excessive pain requires medical attention [31]. Abnormal fluid accumulation can be caused by various etiologies, including ectopic pregnancy, ruptured ovarian cyst, pelvic inflammatory disease, endometriosis, and retrograde menstruation [31].

Pneumoperitoneum Ultrasound

Similar to free fluid, free intraperitoneal air can also be detected using ultrasound. Perforation of a visceral organ is the most common cause of free air beneath the parietal peritoneum (pneumoperitoneum) and typically presents with acute abdominal pain and distention. When evaluating pneumoperitoneum using ultrasound, the most common finding is the Enhanced Peritoneal Stripe Sign (EPPS), which is an echogenic thin line caused by signal reflection beneath the parietal peritoneum [27, 32]. Pneumoperitoneum often presents other symptoms, including a rigid abdomen, fever, nausea, vomiting, and bowel changes, often necessitating surgical intervention.

Musculoskeletal and Neurovascular POCUS

In addition to its use to image various organ systems, POCUS is capable of visualizing more superficial structures, including nerves, muscles, and blood vessels. POCUS is not an effective option for visualization of structures like bone with very high density secondary to the limited ability of the ultrasound to penetrate those tissues. More detailed explanation of musculoskeletal (MSK) ultrasound can be found in Chapter 9 of this book.

Nerves

To optimize peripheral nerve visualization with POCUS, a high-frequency linear transducer should be used. While scanning in the short-axis orientation, nerves can be identified as round, speckled, hyperechoic tissues. They are often described as having a "honeycomb" appearance on B-mode ultrasound images. To distinguish nerves from surrounding structures, color flow imaging can aid in identification by emphasizing vasculature. Additionally, gentle transducer compression may help to further distinguish compressible venous structures from noncompressible neural tissue.

Clinicians can perform procedures on the identified nerves, including peripheral or central nerve blocks for pain management. Peripheral nerve blocks are superficial injections of an anesthetic that are designed to reduce pain by inhibiting neurotransmission to the spinal cord or brain. They play a key role in maintaining patient satisfaction, limiting perioperative pain, and reducing postoperative opioid use [33]. Common targets of peripheral nerve blocks include derivatives of the cervical, brachial, or lumbosacral plexus. An example of one such technique is targeting the supraclavicular nerve for analgesia during upper extremity surgical procedures or targeting the femoral nerve for lower extremity procedures [34].

In contrast, central nerve blocks interfere with neurotransmission of the central nervous system. Providers inject an anesthetic deep into the space surrounding the spinal cord. These are commonly performed in obstetric patients [33].

Vasculature

To identify vasculature on ultrasound, the operator must use a high-frequency transducer in either the long- or short-axis orientation. The normal lumen of vessels will appear anechoic on B-mode images. Color flow imaging and/or pulse wave Doppler can be applied to confirm blood flow in the vessels. Indications for vascular POCUS include symptoms of dizziness, hypotension, headaches, an acutely cold limb, and skin ulceration. Common vascular abnormalities seen on ultrasound include hemodynamically significant arterial stenosis in the common carotid artery and extremity arteries, defined as >75% of arterial lumen reduction or artery occlusion. Common causes of these arterial incidents include atherosclerotic plaque, arterial embolization, or aneurysmal formation, all of which are sequelae of chronic hypertension, smoking, or cardiac conditions (valvular diseases, ventricular septum defect, atrial fibrillation). Interventional procedures requiring the use of ultrasound guidance may include cannulation of vessels, which requires accurate placement, like that seen in central venous line catheters [35].

Ultrasound screening of major abdominal vascular structures like the abdominal aorta is primarily recommended by the US Preventive Services Task Force for male patients between 65 and 75 who have a history of smoking [36]. To perform this screen, the operator should place the probe just inferior to the xiphoid process. Visualization of the IVC and aorta should be obtained. The transducer indicator should be toward the patient's right while imaging a transverse plane of these vessels. The aorta will appear as a thick-walled, hypoechoic, pulsatile circle structure anterior to the vertebral body. The IVC will be next to the aorta and will demonstrate with respiratory variation (IVC diameter decreases in lumen diameter in the expiration and increases in a deep inspiration). Constant downward pressure can help displace bowel gas, if needed [36]. Aneurysms, a vascular pathology that can be identified with this ultrasound view, are considered severe and require surgical intervention if they are greater than 5.5 cm in diameter. Surgical interventions are recommended as large aneurysms may burst, leading to aortic dissection and accompanying hypotensive shock. More information about imaging carotid artery, extremity vasculature, aorta, and IVC can be found in other chapters of this book [36].

Muscle and Tendon

Indications for muscle POCUS include assessing muscle size, evaluating muscle fiber quality, and identifying tendon tears or ligamentous strains [37].

On ultrasound, muscle fascia, tendons, and ligaments appear hyperechoic due to the high density of fibrous tissue. Muscle fascia is often described as being "leaf-like," or "stringy." Muscle fibers are easier to identify in a dynamic state, as contraction causes them to slide laterally across the screen. Operators should keep in mind that tendons and muscles are anisotropic tissues. Anisotropy is an ultrasound artifact related to the decrease in tissue brightness when the angle between the direction of sound beam and orientation of the scanned tissue is off 90°. The operator should keep the ultrasound beam perpendicular to the longitudinal plane of the tissue (muscle, tendon, and nerve) to avoid this artifact, as well as potential misdiagnosis.

Medicine Specialties

Ultrasound has become a staple in modern clinical practice to meet the needs of all medical specialties. As previously mentioned, ultrasound is used to guide regional nerve blocks in anesthesiology. Ultrasound provides direct visualization of nerves, needle placement, and surrounding structures [38]. Similarly, ultrasound has become a staple for internists, as it enhances procedural skills, diagnostic capabilities, and patient management. The use of this modality empowers clinicians to provide bedside assessments, which saves time and cost for diagnosis, especially in rural regions, emergency medicine, and intensive care units. While the use of ultrasound in this and other settings can be incredibly beneficial, the main challenge in widespread implementation is the lack of trained ultrasound operators [39, 40].

While we have touched on ultrasound's application in two medical specialties, the possibilities of its incorporation into medical practice are endless, especially considering the ever-growing list of advances.

Recent Advancements of Point-of-Care Research

Trending areas of POCUS research include artificial intelligence, CEUS technology, and tele-ultrasound guidance.

Artificial Intelligence (AI)

Artificial intelligence is an advanced computer system that uses pattern recognition and algorithm-based learning to improve human tasks [41]. New versions of ultrasound software are beginning to incorporate AI-driven machine learning programs to improve scanning and diagnostic skills. AI can assist the operator in identifying pathology by highlighting target regions and automatically adjusting gain or depth options for optimal image acquisition [42]. Ultrasound operators may also use AI to receive suggestions on probe position and direction, allowing even novice operators the ability to achieve high-quality scans [40].

The incorporation of AI is not without limitations, as recent studies have found worse results with handheld POCUS devices than cart-based ultrasound machines [43]. While this study focuses on a select subset of ultrasound imaging, future studies should evaluate its use in more developed ultrasound machines to ensure the use of AI is advancing the field rather than setting it back. Additionally, further development with AI is warranted before its use can be incorporated into the standard of POCUS imaging devices.

Contrast-Enhanced Ultrasound

POCUS has traditionally been used to identify hydronephrosis and to assess the causes of both acute kidney injury (AKI) and chronic kidney disease (CKD) by using B-mode (anatomic structures) and Doppler (hemodynamic information) techniques. Unfortunately, its use in measuring the extent of disease without the support of serum creatinine, eGFR, and urine output levels is limited [44, 45]. Recent developments using CEUS may be the solution to this problem [45, 46]. CEUS uses micro gas bubbles, bound to a protein ligand in a nontoxic contrast solution, to increase signal intensity in the vasculature. This technique oscillates in blood vessels when exposed to acoustic ultrasound waves and allows for better flow visualization and better detection of small renal masses, cortical lesions, and hypo- or hyper-vascular tumors [46]. As the glomerulus and other vascular components of the kidney are significantly damaged in CKD or AKI, CEUS has the potential to significantly impact the future of ultrasound diagnostics in kidney health.

Tele-Ultrasound Guidance

Another recent addition to POCUS scanning is the introduction of tele-ultrasound guidance technology. This technology involves an online platform that allows the operator to talk to an ultrasound specialist in real time, who can guide them through both the scanning and diagnostic process [47]. Tele-ultrasound is designed to be especially useful for operators who would like a second opinion, given their limited exposure using a new ultrasound device, or for operators who are in resource-limited areas and require further expertise by a trained sonographer [48]. This real-time evaluation may change the conventional dynamic of ultrasound service, as radiologists or sonologists typically interpret ultrasound images after scanning.

Summary

The incorporation of POCUS into everyday medical practice has the potential to advance patient care. POCUS is a highly versatile imaging modality with a plethora of clinical applications. It entails using a portable ultrasound device at the bedside to aid in interventional or diagnostic procedures. As such, POCUS is a valuable tool in clinical settings, especially those that are resource-limited. Intensivists, emergency medical physicians, and surgical staff often use POCUS because of its ability to provide real-time information and quick results. POCUS is also helpful in the reinforcement of anatomical knowledge, and because of its noninvasive nature.

A primary limitation of POCUS, as with conventional ultrasound, is its operator dependence. Although POCUS is integrated into medical education in many medical schools, attending a formalized training to become a certified operator is recommended, especially for licensed providers. Certification and training are provided through online webinars, workshops, and medical school curricula. It is becoming increasingly common for residency programs to incorporate formal ultrasound training in their curriculum. This is especially true for emergency medicine, anesthesia, and internal medicine (i.e. cardiology and pulmonology) specialties.

In the cardiovascular system, POCUS can attain a multi-view assessment for quick identification of the size and function of the heart. Patients with symptoms of acute chest pain, EKG changes, dizziness, or hypotension may benefit from this expedited cardiac POCUS exam, as it can rule out pericardial effusions or cardiogenic shock.

Likewise, indications for POCUS in the respiratory system include symptoms of acute shortness of breath, hypotension, or labored breathing. Protocols such as the FAST exam, RUSH exam, and Blue Protocol now incorporate POCUS into their clinical assessments.

In the gastrointestinal system, POCUS can help to quickly identify intraperitoneal fluid, pneumoperitoneum, and assess for various abnormal organ pathologies, including hepatosteatosis, cirrhosis, cholecystitis, appendicitis, diverticulitis, splenomegaly, intussusception, and small bowel obstructions. Vascular irregularities such as abdominal aortic aneurysms or IVC collapse may also be visualized in these regions using ultrasound.

Selection of a higher frequency transducer will allow for visualization of superficial tissues like muscle, nerves, and peripheral vascular structures. MSK POCUS allows operators to assess for muscle tears, tendon ruptures, or ligamentous sprains. Nervous tissue will appear "honeycomb"-like, in contrast to densely fibrous tissues like tendons. Nerves will be noncompressible on ultrasound and can be targeted for guided pain management interventions like those necessary in surgical or obstetric care. Additionally, color flow imaging and pulse wave Doppler functions may help distinguish nervous tissue from vascular tissue. Vascular ultrasound is typically used to help with vessel cannulation, which requires extensive precision by the operator.

Although POCUS has many established applications, research advancements are underway. Trending areas of research include artificial intelligence, CEUS, and tele-ultrasound guidance. Further investigation into these fields of research is needed to evaluate and support POCUS's clinical significance.

Review Questions

1. A patient comes into the hospital with traumatic injuries to the epigastric region. The patient is initially stabilized with no free fluid seen on exam. However, hours later, the patient becomes more hypotensive and confused. Which bedside ultrasound procedure would be indicated to identify the source of worsening symptoms?

a. Blue Protocol exam

b. RUSH exam

c. FAST exam

d. Carotid ultrasound exam

e. Cardiac ultrasound

2. Upon auscultation of a routine examination, you hear a loud heart murmur in a 55-year-old patient. The patient is overweight, smokes, but denies shortness of breath or radiating chest pain. To evaluate the heart, you place the transducer indicator toward the right shoulder between the 2nd and 3rd ribs. Which view would you expect to see?
   - **a.** Parasternal long axis
   - **b.** Parasternal short axis
   - **c.** Apical four-chamber
   - **d.** Subcostal/subxiphoid
   - **e.** It is an incorrect transducer placement
3. A patient is in need of a bedside ultrasound procedure. Which of the following is a limitation of POCUS?
   - **a.** Exposure to low levels of radiation
   - **b.** Low diagnostic sensitivity to pneumothorax
   - **c.** Image quality
   - **d.** Cost-effectiveness
   - **e.** Visual artifacts secondary to abdominal gas, large body habitus, and/or inadequate patient positioning
4. True or False: Point-of-care ultrasound is a cost-effective modality capable of being implemented in resource-scarce settings.
5. While using a high-frequency transducer on the upper extremity, a speckled "honeycomb" like structure is visualized. What is this structure most likely to be?
   - **a.** Muscle tendon
   - **b.** Muscle belly
   - **c.** Ligament
   - **d.** Nerve
   - **e.** Vasculature/blood vessel
6. Contrast-enhanced ultrasound (CEUS) uses micro gas bubbles bound to a protein ligand in a nontoxic contrast solution to increase signal intensity in ______.
   - **a.** Vasculature allows for improved diagnosis of kidney failure
   - **b.** Dense tissues make it difficult to visualize potential neoplasms
   - **c.** Cysts are limited by the lack of signal intensity (anechoic)
   - **d.** Respiratory alveoli during gas exchange
   - **e.** Increase in the thickness of the renal cortex
7. A 46-year-old male presents to the emergency department with worsening abdominal pain after a bicycle accident. A physician decides to perform an abdominal ultrasound at the bedside using a curvilinear transducer. She positions herself on the patient's right side with the ultrasound screen directly in front of her and uses her right hand to visualize the appropriate acoustic window. Which of the following best describes the primary clinical indications for this type of ultrasound exam?
   - **a.** Screening for hepatic steatosis and evaluation of abnormal liver function tests
   - **b.** Assessment of blunt trauma for rapid identification of intraperitoneal bleed
   - **c.** Evaluation of suspected vascular abnormalities such as aneurysm or stenosis
   - **d.** Investigation of bowel obstruction
   - **e.** Assessment of gastric ulcer

8. Why is it important for patients to fast 6 hours prior to undergoing a gallbladder ultrasound?
   a. To prevent bowel gas interference
   b. To avoid gallbladder contraction
   c. To reduce peristalsis
   d. To enhance sound beam penetration
   e. To increase mechanical index on ultrasound scanner
9. A 24-year-old male is brought to the emergency department after a motor vehicle collision. He is hypotensive with a blood pressure of 88/56 mmHg and tachycardic at 120 bpm. Focused Assessment with Sonography for Trauma (FAST) exam is performed. On the RUQ view, you see an anechoic stripe between the inferior surface of the liver and the upper pole of the right kidney. Where is this fluid located, and why is this space clinically significant?
   a. Rectovesical pouch; it is the lowest point of the peritoneal cavity in males
   b. Pouch of Douglas; physiologic small fluid collection may be normal in females
   c. Morison's Pouch: it is the most gravity-dependent space in the supramesocolic compartment
   d. Perisplenic recess; it is commonly used as an acoustic window for LUQ fluid assessment
   e. This space is where the adrenal gland is located
10. A 54-year-old man with cirrhosis presents for evaluation of new ascites. The hepatology team considers using advanced point-of-care ultrasound (POCUS) techniques to improve diagnostic accuracy. They discuss recent research trends that include computer algorithms that optimize probe positioning, injectable microbubble solutions that enhance vascular signals, and remote guidance from an expert sonographer via a live video platform. Which of the following best summarizes these recent POCUS advancements?
    a. Artificial intelligence, contrast-enhanced ultrasound, and tele-ultrasound guidance
    b. Artificial intelligence, elastography, and fusion imaging
    c. Contrast-enhanced ultrasound, handheld portable devices, and tele-ultrasound guidance
    d. Artificial intelligence, contrast CT-ultrasound integration, and robotic probe navigation
    e. Combination of imaging modalities, including CT, MRI, and ultrasound

Correct answers: 1. b; 2. a; 3. e; 4. True; 5. d; 6. a; 7. b; 8. b; 9. c; 10. a.

References

1. Moore CL, Copel JA. Point-of-care ultrasonography. *N Engl J Med* 2011; 364: 749–757. https://doi.org/10.1056/NEJMra0909487.
2. Chelikam N, Vyas A, Desai R, et al. Past and present of point-of-care ultrasound (POCUS): a narrative review. *Cureus* 2023. https://doi.org/10.7759/cureus.50155.
3. Osterwalder J, Polyzogopoulou E, Hoffmann B. Point-of-care ultrasound—history, current and evolving clinical concepts in emergency medicine. *Medicina (Lithuania)* 2023; 59(12). https://doi.org/10.3390/medicina59122179.
4. Perera P, Mailhot T, Riley D, Mandavia D. The RUSH exam: rapid ultrasound in shock in the evaluation of the critically ill. *Emerg Med Clin North Am* 2010; 28(1): 29–56. http://10.1016/j.emc.2009.09.010.

5. Adhikari S, Leo M, Liu R, et al. The 2023 core content of advanced emergency medicine ultrasonography. *J Am Coll Emerg Physicians Open* 2023; 4: e13015. https://doi.org/10.1002/emp2.13015.
6. Sorensen B, Hunskaar S. Point-of-care ultrasound in primary care: a systematic review of generalist performed point-of-care ultrasound in unselected populations. *Ultrasound J* 2019; 11(1): 31. https://doi.org/10.1186/s13089-019-0145-4.
7. Hanson MG, Chan B. The role of point-of-care ultrasound in the diagnosis of pericardial effusion: a single academic center retrospective study. *Ultrasound J* 2021; 13(1): 2. https://doi.org/10.1186/s13089-021-00205-x.
8. Fox JC, Lahham S, Maldonado G, et al. Hypertrophic cardiomyopathy in youth athletes: successful screening with point-of-care ultrasound by medical students. *J Ultrasound Med* 2017; 36: 1109–1115. https://doi.org/10.7863/ultra.16.06044.
9. Popat A, Yadav S, Pethe G, et al. The role of POCUS in diagnosing acute heart failure in the emergency department: a meta-analysis. *J Cardiol* 2025. https://doi.org/10.1016/j.jjcc.2025.06.012.
10. Schmidt GA, Koenig S, Mayo PH. Shock. *Chest* 2012; 142: 1042–1048. https://doi.org/10.1378/chest.12-1297.
11. Volpicelli G, Lamorte A, Tullio M, et al. Point-of-care multiorgan ultrasonography for the evaluation of undifferentiated hypotension in the emergency department. *Intensive Care Med* 2013; 39: 1290–1298. https://doi.org/10.1007/s00134-013-2919-7.
12. Yoshida T, Yoshida T, Noma H, et al. Diagnostic accuracy of point-of-care ultrasound for shock: a systematic review and meta-analysis. *Crit Care* 2023; 27: 200. https://doi.org/10.1186/s13054-023-04495-6.
13. Kirkpatrick JN, Panebianco N, Díaz-Gómez JL, et al. Recommendations for cardiac point-of-care ultrasound nomenclature. *J Am Soc Echocardiogr* 2024; 37: 809–819. https://doi.org/10.1016/j.echo.2024.05.001.
14. Lee V, Ahn J, Deschamps J, et al. Cardiac ultrasound (echocardiography) made easy: step-by-step guide. POCUS 101. 2023 https://www.pocus101.com/cardiac-ultrasound-echocardiography-made-easy-step-by-step-guide.
15. Barr R. AIUM practice parameter for the performance of point-of-care ultrasound examinations. *J Ultrasound Med* 2019; 38: 833–849. https://doi.org/10.1002/jum.14972.
16. Ciumanghel I, Barbuta E, Ciumanghel AI, et al. Point-of-care lung ultrasound - a rapid and reliable diagnostic tool for emergency physicians treating patients with acute dyspnea in high-volume emergency departments. *Emerg Radiol* 2025; 32: 329–338. https://doi.org/10.1007/s10140-025-02343-4.
17. Zanobetti M, Scorpiniti M, Gigli C, et al. Point-of-care ultrasonography for evaluation of acute dyspnea in the ED. *Chest* 2017; 151: 1295–1301. https://doi.org/10.1016/j.chest.2017.02.003.
18. Okoli ML, Rao P, Kavuma S, et al. POCUS for thrombus: emphasizing the importance of initial point-of-care ultrasound in the management of pulmonary thromboembolism. *Cureus* 2024. https://doi.org/10.7759/cureus.58272.
19. Jia Y, Zhang Q. Research progress on diaphragm ultrasound in chronic obstructive pulmonary disease: a narrative review. *Ultrasound Med Biol* 2022; 48: 587–597. https://doi.org/10.1016/j.ultrasmedbio.2021.10.019.
20. Lichtenstein DA. Lung ultrasound in the critically ill. *Ann Intensive Care* 2014; 4(1): 1. https://doi.org/10.1186/2110-5820-4-1.
21. Marini TJ, Rubens DJ, Zhao YT, et al. Lung ultrasound: the essentials. *Radiol Cardiothorac Imaging* 2021; 3(2): e200564. https://doi.org/10.1148/ryct.2021200564.
22. Cruz-Rodríguez C, García-Cruz E, Gopar-Nieto R, et al. Utilidad de la fórmula de Balik para la cuantificación del derrame pleural por ultrasonido en el posoperatorio de cirugía cardiaca. *NCT Neumología y Cirugía de Tórax* 2023; 82: 72–78. https://doi.org/10.35366/115393.
23. Ritchie JD, Trujillo CN, Convissar DL, et al. Focused assessment with sonography for trauma (FAST) exam: image acquisition. *J Vis Exp* 2023; (199). https://doi.org/10.3791/65066.

24. Netherton S, Milenkovic V, Taylor M, Davis PJ. Diagnostic accuracy of eFAST in the trauma patient: a systematic review and meta-analysis. *CJEM* 2019; 21: 727–738. https://doi.org/10.1017/cem.2019.381.
25. Keikha M, Salehi-Marzijarani M, Soldoozi Nejat R, et al. Diagnostic accuracy of rapid ultrasound in shock (RUSH) exam; a systematic review and meta-analysis. *Bull Emerg Trauma* 2018; 6: 271–278. https://doi.org/10.29252/beat-060402.
26. Bekgoz B, Kilicaslan I, Bildik F, et al. BLUE protocol ultrasonography in emergency department patients presenting with acute dyspnea. *Am J Emerg Med* 2019; 37: 2020–2027. https://doi.org/10.1016/j.ajem.2019.02.028.
27. Li JJ, Boivin Z, Bhalodkar S, Liu R. Point of care abdominal ultrasound. *Semin Ultrasound CT MR* 2024; 45: 11–21. https://doi.org/10.1053/j.sult.2023.12.003.
28. Tooma D, Dinh V, Ahn J, et al. Abdominal ultrasound made easy: step-by-step guide. POCUS 101. 2023 https://www.pocus101.com/abdominal-ultrasound-made-easy-step-by-step-guide.
29. Kaur G, Kaur T, Das CJ. Morrison's pouch: anatomy and radiological appearance of pathological processes. *Indian J Radiol Imaging* 2023; 33: 80–88. https://doi.org/10.1055/s-0042-1758874.
30. Jahangiri A, Bell D, White R. Rectovesical pouch. In: Radiopaedia.Org. Radiopaedia.org, 2016. https://doi.org/10.53347/rID-48837.
31. Shwayder JM. Normal pelvic anatomy. *Obstet Gynecol Clin N Am* 2019; 46: 563–580. https://doi.org/10.1016/j.ogc.2019.06.001.
32. Hoffmann B, Nürnberg D, Westergaard MC. Focus on abnormal air. *Eur J Emerg Med* 2012; 19: 284–291. https://doi.org/10.1097/MEJ.0b013e3283543cd3.
33. Jogie J, Jogie JA. A comprehensive review on the efficacy of nerve blocks in reducing postoperative anesthetic and analgesic requirements. *Cureus* 2023. https://doi.org/10.7759/cureus.38552.
34. Chang A, Dua A. Peripheral nerve blocks. In: StatPearls [Internet]. Treasure Island, FL: StatPearls Publishing, 2025. https://www.ncbi.nlm.nih.gov/books/NBK459210.
35. Leibowitz A, Oren-Grinberg A, Matyal R. Ultrasound guidance for central venous access: current evidence and clinical recommendations. *J Intensive Care Med* 2020; 35: 303–321. https://doi.org/10.1177/0885066619868164.
36. Owens DK, Davidson KW, Krist AH, et al. Screening for abdominal aortic aneurysm: US preventive services task force recommendation statement. *JAMA* 2019; 322: 2211–2218. https://doi.org/10.1001/jama.2019.18928.
37. Nagae M, Umegaki H, Yoshiko A, Fujita K. Muscle ultrasound and its application to point-of-care ultrasonography: a narrative review. *Ann Med* 2023; 55: 190–197. https://doi.org/10.1080/07853890.2022.2157871.
38. Naji A, Chappidi M, Ahmed A, et al. Perioperative point-of-care ultrasound use by anesthesiologists. *Cureus* 2021. https://doi.org/10.7759/cureus.15217.
39. Lambrecht JE, Zhang K, Tierney DM, et al. Integration of point-of-care ultrasound education into the internal medicine core clerkship experience. *J Ultrasound Med* 2022; 41: 33–40. https://doi.org/10.1002/jum.15702.
40. Yazici MM, Yavaşi Ö. The development of point-of-care ultrasound. Worldwide contributions and publication trends. *J Clin Ultrasound* 2025; 53: 129–138. https://doi.org/10.1002/jcu.23846.
41. Bajwa J, Munir U, Nori A, Williams B. Artificial intelligence in healthcare: transforming the practice of medicine. *Future Healthc J* 2021; 8: e188–e194. https://doi.org/10.7861/fhj.2021-0095.
42. Yan L, Li Q, Fu K, et al. Progress in the application of artificial intelligence in ultrasound-assisted medical diagnosis. *Bioengineering* 2025; 12: 288. https://doi.org/10.3390/bioengineering12030288.
43. Blaivas M, Blaivas LN, Tsung JW. Deep learning pitfall: impact of novel ultrasound equipment introduction on algorithm performance and the realities of domain adaptation. *J Ultrasound Med* 2022; 41: 855–863. https://doi.org/10.1002/jum.15765.

44. Moses AA, Fernandez HE. Ultrasonography in acute kidney injury. *POCUS J* 2022; 7: 35–44. https://doi.org/10.24908/pocus.v7iKidney.14989.
45. Hull TD, Agarwal A, Hoyt K. New ultrasound techniques promise further advances in AKI and CKD. *J Am Soc Nephrol* 2017; 28: 3452–3460. https://doi.org/10.1681/ASN.2017060647.
46. Kazmierski B, Deurdulian C, Tchelepi H, Grant EG. Applications of contrast-enhanced ultrasound in the kidney. *Abdom Radiol (NY)* 2018; 43: 880–898. https://doi.org/10.1007/s00261-017-1307-0.
47. Nix K, Liu EL, Oh L, et al. A distance-learning approach to point-of-care ultrasound training (ADAPT): a multi-institutional educational response during the COVID-19 pandemic. *Acad Med* 2021; 96: 1711–1716. https://doi.org/10.1097/ACM.0000000000004399.
48. Britton N, Miller MA, Safadi S, et al. Tele-ultrasound in resource-limited settings: a systematic review. *Front Public Health* 2019; 7. https://doi.org/10.3389/fpubh.2019.00244.

Index

D

E

H

Q

R

V

W

Y

Z